S0-BQM-283

Progress in
Cancer Research and Therapy
Volume 30

GENE TRANSFER AND CANCER

Progress in Cancer Research and Therapy

Vol. 30: Gene Transfer and Cancer
Mark L. Pearson and Nat L. Sternberg, editors, 1984

Vol. 29: Markers of Colonic Cell Differentiation
Sandra R. Wolman and Anthony J. Mastromarino, editors, 1984

Vol. 28: The Development of Target-Oriented Anticancer Drugs
Yung-Chi Cheng, Barry Goz, and Mimi Minkoff, editors, 1983

Vol. 27: Environmental Influences in the Pathogenesis of Leukemias and Lymphomas
Ian T. Magrath, Gregory T. O'Conor, and Bracha Ramot, editors, 1984

Vol. 26: Radiation Carcinogenesis: Epidemiology and Biological Significance
John D. Boice, Jr. and Joseph F. Fraumeni, editors, 1983

Vol. 25: Steroids and Endometrial Cancer
Valerio Maria Jasonno, Italo Nenci, and Carlo Flamigni, editors, 1983

Vol. 24: Recent Clinical Developments in Gynecologic Oncology
*C. Paul Morrow, John Bonnar, Timothy J. O'Brien, and
William E. Gibbons, editors, 1983*

Vol. 23: Maturation Factors and Cancer
Malcolm A. S. Moore, editor, 1982

Vol. 22: The Potential Role of T Cells in Cancer Therapy
Alexander Fefer and Allen L. Goldstein, editors, 1982

Vol. 21: Hybridomas in Cancer Diagnosis and Treatment
Malcolm S. Mitchell and Herbert F. Oettgen, editors, 1982

Vol. 20: Lymphokines and Thymic Hormones: Their Potential Utilization in Cancer
Therapeutics
Allen L. Goldstein and Michael A. Chirigos, editors, 1982

Vol. 19: Mediation of Cellular Immunity in Cancer by Immune Modifiers
Michael A. Chirigos, Malcolm S. Mitchell, and Michael J. Mastrangelo, editors, 1982

Vol. 18: Carninoma of the Bladder
John G. Connolly, editor, 1981

Vol. 17: Nutrition and Cancer: Etiology and Treatment
Guy R. Newell and Neil M. Ellison, editors, 1981

Vol. 16: Augmenting Agents in Cancer Therapy
E. M. Hersch, M. A. Chirigos, and M. J. Mastrangelo, editors, 1981

Vol. 15: Role of Medroxyprogesterone in Endocrine-Related Tumors
Stefano Iacobelli and Aurelio Di Marco, editors, 1980

Vol. 14: Hormones and Cancer
Stefano Iacobelli, R. J. B. King, Hans R. Lindner, and Marc E. Lippman, editors, 1980

Vol. 13: Colorectal Cancer: Prevention, Epidemiology, and Screening
Sidney J. Winawer, David Schottenfield, and Paul Sherlock, editors, 1980

Vol. 12: Advances in Neuroblastoma Research
Audrey E. Evans, editor, 1980

Vol. 11: Treatment of Lung Cancer
Marcel Rozencweig and Franco Muggia, editors, 1978

Vol. 10: Hormones, Receptors, and Breast Cancer
William L. McGuire, editor, 1978

Vol. 9: Endocrine Control in Neoplasia
R. K. Sharma and W. E. Criss, editors, 1978

Vol. 8: Polyamines as Biochemical Markers of Normal and Malignant Growth
D. H. Russell and B. G. M. Durie, editors, 1978

Vol. 7: Immune Modulation and Control of Neoplasia by Adjuvant Therapy
Michael A. Chirigos, editor, 1978

Vol. 6: Immunotherapy of Cancer: Present Status of Trials in Man
William D. Terry and Dorothy Windhorst, editors, 1978

Vol. 5: Cancer Invasion and Metastasis: Biologic Mechanisms and Therapy
*Stacey B. Day, W. P. Laird Myers, Philip Stansly, Silvio Garattini, and
   Martin G. Lewis, editors, 1977*

Vol. 4: Progesterone Receptors in Neoplastic Tissues
William L. McGuire, Jean-Pierre Raynaud, and Etienne-Emile Baulieu, editors, 1977

Vol. 3: Genetics of Human Cancer
*John J. Mulvihill, Robert W. Miller, and Joseph F. Fraumeni, Jr.,
   editors, 1977*

Vol. 2: Control of Neoplasia by Modulation of the Immune System
Michael A. Chirigos, editor, 1977

Vol. 1: Control Mechanisms in Cancer
Wayne E. Criss, Tetsuo Ono, and John R. Sabine, editors, 1976

Progress in
Cancer Research and Therapy
Volume 30

Gene Transfer and Cancer

Editors

Mark L. Pearson, Ph.D.

and

Nat L. Sternberg, Ph.D.

NCI-Frederick Cancer Research Facility
Frederick, Maryland

RC 267
A1
P97
v. 30
1984

Raven Press ■ New York

Raven Press, 1140 Avenue of the Americas, New York, New York 10036

© 1984 by Raven Press Books, Ltd. All rights reserved. This book is protected by copyright. No part of it may be reproduced, stored in a retrieval system, or transmitted, in any form or by any means, electronic, mechanical, photocopying, recording, or otherwise, without the prior written permission of the publisher.

Made in the United States of America

Library of Congress Cataloging in Publication Data
Main entry under title:

Gene transfer and cancer.

Papers derived from the Fourth Litton Technology
Transfer Workshop, held in Apr. 1982 at the Frederick
Cancer Research Facility and sponsored by Litton Bionetics,
Inc.
    Includes bibliographical references and index.
    1. Cancer—Genetic aspects—Congresses. 2. Genetic
transformation—Congresses. 3. Oncogenes—Congresses.
4. Gene expression—Congresses. I. Pearson, Mark L.
II. Sternberg, Nat L. III. Litton-Bionetics, Inc.
IV. Litton Technology Transfer Workshop (4th : 1982 :
Frederick Cancer Research Facility) [DNLM: 1. Transfor-
mation, Genetic—Congresses. 2. Oncogenes—Congresses.
3. Cell transformation, Neoplastic—Congresses. 4. DNA,
Recombinant—Congresses. QZ 202 G3265 1982]
RC268.4.G42   1984   616.99′4071   84-3266
ISBN 0-89004-899-1

Papers or parts thereof have been used as camera-ready copy as submitted by the authors whenever possible; when retyped, they have been edited by the editorial staff only to the extent considered necessary for the assistance of an international readership. The views expressed and the general style adopted remain, however, the responsibility of the named authors. Great care has been taken to maintain the accuracy of the information contained in the volume. However, neither Raven Press nor the editors can be held responsible for errors or for any consequences arising from the use of information contained herein.

The use in this book of particular designations of countries or territories does not imply any judgment by the publisher or editors as to the legal status of such countries or territories, of their authorities or institutions or of the delimitation of their boundaries.

Some of the names of products referred to in this book may be registered trademarks or proprietary names, although specific reference to this fact may not be made: however, the use of a name with designation is not to be construed as a representation by the publisher or editors that it is in the public domain. In addition, the mention of specific companies or of their products or proprietary names does not imply any endorsement or recommendation on the part of the publisher or editors.

Authors were themselves responsible for obtaining the necessary permission to reproduce copyright material from other sources. With respect to the publisher's copyright, material appearing in this book prepared by individuals as part of their official duties as government employees is only covered by this copyright to the extent permitted by the appropriate national regulations.

Preface

In the late 1970s, the twin technologies of DNA gene splicing and DNA-mediated gene transfer had advanced to a point where it was feasible to think that any gene could be placed in an appropriate expression vector and be expressed in a variety of mammalian cell types. The significance of these results was reinforced by the appearance in 1981 of the first reports of the successful transfer of cellular oncogenes from carcinogen-treated rodent cell lines to NIH-3T3 mouse fibroblasts. Soon thereafter, whole new sets of transforming genes were discovered in birds and various mammalian species, and the nucleotide sequence of the human bladder and lung carcinoma genes was found to be similar to those of the Harvey and Kirsten rat sarcoma viruses, respectively. In a very short time, these experiments shifted the focus of much of the national effort in cancer research to the study of the structure and function of cellular oncogenes using gene splicing and DNA transfer techniques.

These developments provided the impetus for this volume, which addresses the following questions that relate to the development of gene transfer techniques and the analysis of the transformed cell phenotype: How best might DNA be delivered to mammalian cells? How might one avoid the complications of DNA rearrangements associated with the DNA transfer process? What might be the best vector systems? How might one maximize stable gene expression after the DNA transfer step? How are oncogenes activated to result in the appearance of the transformed phenotype? Is there a differential expression of these genes during development? How many different oncogenes might there be? Can analysis of these genes ultimately lead to improved diagnosis and treatment of human malignancy?

Collectively, this book provides an overview of the advances in genetic approaches to cancer research. In addition, the chapters serve to illustrate that discoveries in one area of research can be the key to unlocking answers to old questions in a seemingly unrelated area. This volume summarizes important work in specific areas of research, and we believe this aspect of the book will prove useful to researchers in the laboratory.

Mark L. Pearson
Nat L. Sternberg

Acknowledgments

We wish to express our gratitude to Michael G. Hanna, Jr., the Director of the NCI-FCRF, and to James Nance, the President of Litton Bionetics, Inc., for their encouragement and generous financial support of the Fourth Litton Technology Transfer Workshop, on which this volume was based.

This workshop would not have been possible without the dedicated assistance of many people on the NCI-FCRF staff. In particular, we would like to thank Linda Davis for making the local arrangements and Bridget Traynor and Betty Cramer who assisted in the scheduling of the meeting.

NCI-FCRF staff members also provided invaluable help in the preparation of this book. We are grateful to Hilda Marusiodis for collecting and organizing the manuscripts in this volume and for managing the authors and editors alike patiently and cheerfully. We owe a special debt to Kelly Bivens and Vickie Koogle, our editors at NCI-FCRF, for their efforts in supervising the preparation and production of the camera-ready manuscripts, and to Hilda Marusiodis, Jan Jenkins, and Bobbie Jones, who carefully and diligently retyped all the manuscripts.

Finally, we would like to thank the scientists who contributed their expertise and enthusiasm to make the workshop a success and the authors who contributed the manuscripts to make the book possible.

Contents

Bacterial Transformation

1 Sequence-Specific and Non-Sequence-Specific Components of DNA
Recognition in *Haemophilus* Transformation
D. B. Danner and H. O. Smith

9 Sequence-Specific DNA-Binding Vesicles Are Released from *Haemophilus Influenzae* Cells During Loss of Competence for Transformation
R. A. Deich

15 Gene Transfer Between Plasmid and Chromosome in *Haemophilus Influenzae*
J. K. Setlow, D. McCarthy, and N. L. Clayton

Gene Transfer and Rescue

21 Transfer of Single Specific Chromosomes by Microcell Fusion and Gene
Mapping in Mammalian Cells
R. S. Athwal and V. Dhar

31 Gene Transfer in CHO Cells
I. Abraham and M. M. Gottesman

37 DNA-Mediated Transfer of Genes into Mammalian Cells: Evidence for
Homologous Recombination Between Transfected DNAs
*B. Pomerantz, M. Naujokas, W. Muller, A.-M. Mes, M. Featherstone,
P. Moreau, and J. A. Hassell*

47 Homologous Recombination Between Segments of the Herpes Simplex
Virus Thymidine Kinase Gene in Mouse L Cells
F.-L. Lin and N. Sternberg

53 DNA-Mediated Transfer of Multidrug Resistance and Expression of P-
Glycoprotein
*V. Ling, N. Kartner, P. Debenham, A. Chase, L. Siminovitch, and
J. R. Riordan*

59 Development of a Cloning System for the Gene for Asparagine Synthetase
P. N. Ray, I. L. Andrulis, and L. Siminovitch

67 DNA-Mediated Transfer of an RNA Polymerase II Gene
C. J. Ingles, J. K-C. Wong, and M. Shales

73 Gene Transfer of an RNA Polymerase II Mutation that Affects Muscle
Differentiation
C. W. Shearman, P. Benfield, R. Zivin, D. Graf, and M. L. Pearson

Vectors

81 Bovine Papillomavirus/pML2 Hybrid Vector: A Dual Host Replicon
N. Sarver, S. Mitrani-Rosenbaum, M.-F. Law, J. C. Byrne, and P. M. Howley

89 Development of Friend Spleen Focus-Forming Virus as a Mammalian Gene Transfer Vector
A. L. Joyner and A. Bernstein

97 Construction of a Small Retrovirus Cloning Vector and Splicing of Genomic Mouse α-Globin DNA Inserted in this Vector
S. Watanabe, K. Shimotohno, and H. M. Temin

105 Defective Virus Vectors (Amplicons) Derived from Herpes Simplex Viruses
N. Frenkel, L. P. Deiss, A. D. Kwong, and R. R. Spaete

DNA Transforming Viruses

115 Structure of the Polyoma Virus Early Promoter: Sequences Required for Expression and Tumor Antigen Binding
C. Mueller, A.-M. Mes, B. Pomerantz, M. Featherstone, M. Naujokas, and J. A. Hassell

125 Human Papilloma Virus Type 1 RNA Transcription and Processing in COS-1 Cells
L. T. Chow and T. R. Broker

135 Identification of an Adenovirus Function Required for Initiation of Cell Transformation Possibly at the Level of DNA Integration
D. T. Rowe, M. Ruben, S. Bacchetti, and F. L. Graham

RNA Transforming Viruses

143 Comparison of the Sequences of the Murine and Gibbon Ape Retrovirus LTR: Analysis of Elements Involved in Transcriptional Control and Provirus Integration
S. P. Clark and T. W. Mak

157 DNA Transfection Studies of Endogenous Ecotropic MuLV
R. Risser, J. McCubrey, P. Green, J. Horowitz, and C. Sinaiko

163 Origins of the Structural and Transforming (*rel*) Genes of Reticuloendotheliosis Virus
R. V. Gilden, N. R. Rice, R. M. Stephens, R. R. Hiebsch, and S. Oroszlan

169 Isolation of New Mammalian Type C Transforming Viruses
U. R. Rapp, F. H. Reynolds, Jr., and J. R. Stephenson

179 Isolation of v-*fes*/v-*fps* Homologous Sequences from a Human Lung Carcinoma Cosmid Library
J. Groffen, N. Heisterkamp, and J. R. Stephenson

Transforming Genes

189   Characterization of Four Members of the P21 Gene Family Isolated from
      Normal Human Genomic DNA and Demonstration of Their Oncogenic
      Potential
      *E. H. Chang, M. A. Gonda, M. E. Furth, J. L. Goodwin, S. S. Yu,
      R. W. Ellis, E. M. Scolnick, and D. R. Lowy*

197   Chromosomal Mapping of Tumor Virus Transforming Gene Analogs in
      Human Cells
      O. W. McBride, D. C. Swan, K. C. Robbins, K. Prakash, and S. A. Aaronson

207   Cellular Oncogenes: Enhancement of Their Expression in Animal and
      Human Tumors
      U. G. Rovigatti and S. M. Astrin

219   Cellular Transforming Genes in Cancer
      M.-A. Lane, A. Sainten, D. Neary, D. Becker, and G. M. Cooper

227   Genetic Analysis of the Transformed Phenotype in Mouse Cells
      *M. B. Small, E. Simmons, K. K. Jha, H. L. Ozer, L. A. Feldman, J. Pyati,
      S. Hann, and D. Dina*

Methylation

237   DNA Methylation and Gene Activity
      W. Doerfler, L. Vardimon, I. Kruczek, D. Eick, B. Kron, and I. Kuhlmann

249   Concerted Hypermethylation and Stable Shutdown of a Cluster of
      Thymidine Kinase Genes
      S. C. Hardies, D. E. Axelrod, M. H. Edgell, and C. A. Hutchison III

259   DNA Methylation Controls Expression of Transferred Genes in a Mouse L
      Cell Derivative
      B. Christy and G. Scangos

265   Gene Inactivation and Reactivation at the *emt* Locus in Chinese Hamster
      Cells
      R. G. Worton, S. G. Grant, and C. Duff

273   Inhibition of DNA Methylation by 5-Azacytidine and Chemical
      Carcinogens
      P. A. Jones, S. M. Taylor, and V. L. Wilson

281   DNA Methylase-Dependent Transcription of the Phage Mu *mom* Gene
      S. Hattman

Gene Expression

289   High Frequency Alterations of Transfected Thymidine Kinase Gene
      Expression Are Mediated by Changes in Chromatin Structure
      R. L. Davies, S. Fuhrer-Krusi, and R. Kucherlapati

297   Structural and Functional Analysis of the Glucocorticoid-Regulated MMTV Transcriptional Promoter
M. C. Ostrowski and G. L. Hager

303   Are Glucocorticoid Receptor Binding Domains Regulatable "Enhancer" Elements?
V. L. Chandler, B. A. Maler, and K. R. Yamamoto

311   Study of DNA Modification and X Inactivation in the Mouse Using DNA-Mediated Gene Transfer
R. M. Liskay, V. M. Chapman, P. G. Kratzer, and L. D. Siracusa

315   Alternative View of Mammalian Repetitive DNA Sequence Organization
R. K. Moyzis, J. Bonnet, B. D. Crawford, M. Dani, P. J. Jackson, J.-R. Wu, and P. O. P. Ts'o

325   Host Specificity of Enhancement of Gene Expression by Activator Elements
L. Laimins, G. Khoury, C. Gorman, B. Howard, and P. Gruss

331   Use of Gene Transfer to Study the Properties of Long Terminal Repeats of Retroviral DNA
S.-M. Cheng and N. Sternberg

337   Molecular Cloning and Expression of a Gene that Encodes a Novel Transplantation-Related Antigen
M. Kress, D. Cosman, E. Jay, G. Khoury, and G. Jay

345   DNA Sequences that are Required for the Alcohol Dehydrogenase Gene Expression in *Drosophila*
C. Benyajati

351   Amplification and Regulated Expression of a Modular Dihydrofolate Reductase cDNA Gene
R. J. Kaufman and P. A. Sharp

361   Mouse *dhfr* Minigenes: Transfer, Expression, and Amplification
G. F. Crouse, R. N. McEwan, and M. L. Pearson

369   *Subject Index*

Contributors

S. A. Aaronson
Laboratory of Cellular and Molecular Biology
National Cancer Institute
National Institutes of Health
Bethesda, Maryland 20205

Irene Abraham
Laboratory of Molecular Biology
Molecular Cell Genetics Section
National Cancer Institute
National Institutes of Health
Bethesda, Maryland 20205

*French Anderson
National Cancer Institute
National Institutes of Health
Bethesda, Maryland 20205

Irene L. Andrulis
Department of Genetics
The Hospital for Sick Children
555 University Avenue
Toronto, Ontario, M5G 1X8 Canada

S. M. Astrin
The Institute for Cancer Research
The Fox Chase Cancer Center
Philadelphia, Pennsylvania 19111

Raghbir S. Athwal
Department of Microbiology
New Jersey College of Medicine
Newark, New Jersey 07006

David E. Axelrod
Waksman Institute of Microbiology
Busch Campus
Rutgers University
Piscataway, New Jersey 08854

S. Bacchetti
Department of Pathology
McMaster University
Hamilton, Ontario, L8S 4J9 Canada

*Mariano Barbacid
Laboratory of Molecular and Cellular Biology
National Cancer Institute
National Institutes of Health
Bethesda, Maryland 20205

Dorothea Becker
Laboratory of Molecular Carcinogenesis
Department of Pathology
Harvard Medical School
Sidney Farber Cancer Institute
44 Binney Street
Boston, Massachusetts 02115

Pamela Benfield
Cancer Biology Program
National Cancer Institute-
Frederick Cancer Research Facility
Frederick, Maryland 21701

Cheeptip Benyajati
National Cancer Institute-
Frederick Cancer Research Facility
P.O. Box B
Frederick, Maryland 21701

Alan Bernstein
Department of Medical Biophysics
The Ontario Cancer Institute
University of Toronto
500 Sherbourne Street
Toronto, Ontario, M4X 1K9 Canada

*Donald Blair
Laboratory of Molecular Oncology
National Cancer Institute
Frederick Cancer Research Facility
P.O. Box B
Frederick, Maryland 21701

Jacques Bonnet
Division of Biophysics
School of Hygiene and Public Health
The Johns Hopkins University
Baltimore, Maryland 21205

Thomas R. Broker
Cold Spring Harbor Laboratory
P.O. Box 100
Cold Spring Harbor, New York 11724

Janet C. Byrne
Laboratory of Pathology
National Cancer Institute
National Institutes of Health
Bethesda, Maryland 20205

*Conference participants.

Vicki L. Chandler
Department of Biochemistry and Biophysics
University of California
San Francisco, California 94143

Esther H. Chang
Dermatology Branch
National Cancer Institute
National Institutes of Health
Bethesda, Maryland 20205

Verne M. Chapman
Department of Molecular Biology
Roswell Park Memorial Institute
Buffalo, New York 14263

Sheau-Mei Cheng
National Cancer Institute-
Frederick Cancer Research Facility
P.O. Box B
Frederick, Maryland 21701

A. Chase
The Ontario Cancer Institute
University of Toronto
Toronto, Ontario, M4X 1K9 Canada

Louise T. Chow
Cold Spring Harbor Laboratory
P.O. Box 100
Cold Spring Harbor, New York 11724

Barbara Christy
Department of Biology
The Johns Hopkins University
Charles and 34th Streets
Baltimore, Maryland 21218

Stephen P. Clark
Department of Medical Biophysics
University of Toronto
Toronto, Ontario, M4X 1K9 Canada

Nancy-Lee Clayton
Department of Biology
Brookhaven National Laboratory
Upton, New York 11973

Geoffrey M. Cooper
Laboratory of Molecular Carcinogenesis
Department of Pathology
Harvard Medical School
Sidney Farber Cancer Institute
44 Binney Street
Boston, Massachusetts 02115

David Cosman
Laboratory of Molecular Virology
National Cancer Institute
National Institutes of Health
Bethesda, Maryland 20205

Brian D. Crawford
Genetics Group
Los Alamos Scientific Laboratory
Los Alamos, New Mexico 87545

Gray F. Crouse
National Cancer Institute-
Frederick Cancer Research Facility
P.O. Box B
Frederick, Maryland 21701

Maria Dani
Division of Biophysics
School of Hygiene and Public Health
The Johns Hopkins University
Baltimore, Maryland 21205

David B. Danner
Department of Molecular Biology and Genetics
The Johns Hopkins University
School of Medicine
725 North Wolfe Street
Baltimore, Maryland 21205

Robin L. Davies
Department of Biochemical Sciences
Princeton University
Princeton, New Jersey 08544

P. Debenham
The Hospital for Sick Children
University of Toronto
Toronto, Ontario, M4X 1K9 Canada

Robert A. Deich
National Cancer Institute-
Frederick Cancer Research Facility
P.O. Box B
Frederick, Maryland 21701

Louis P. Deiss
Department of Biology
The University of Chicago
920 East 58th Street
Chicago, Illinois 60637

Veena Dhar
Department of Microbiology
New Jersey School of Medicine
Newark, New Jersey 07006

Dino Dina
Department of Genetics
Albert Einstein College of Medicine
Bronx, New York 10461

Walter Doerfler
Institute of Genetics
University of Cologne
5000 Cologne 41, Federal Republic of Germany

Catherine Duff
Genetics Department and Research Institute
Hospital for Sick Children and Department of
    Medical Genetics
University of Toronto
Toronto, Ontario, M5G 1X8 Canada

Marshall H. Edgell
Department of Microbiology and Immunology
University of North Carolina
Chapel Hill, North Carolina 27514

Dirk Eick
Institute of Genetics
University of Cologne
5000 Cologne 41, Federal Republic of Germany

Ronald W. Ellis
Laboratory of Tumor Virus Genetics
National Cancer Institute
National Institutes of Health
Bethesda, Maryland 20205

*Ron Evans
Tumor Virology Laboratory
The Salk Institute
San Diego, California 92138

Mark Featherstone
Department of Microbiology and Immunology
McGill University
3775 University Street
Montreal, Quebec, H3A 2B4 Canada

Lawrence A. Feldman
Department of Microbiology
University of Medicine and Dentistry
Newark, New Jersey 01703

Niza Frenkel
Department of Biology
University of Chicago
920 East 58th Street
Chicago, Illinois 60637

Stelia Fuhrer-Krusi
Department of Biochemical Sciences
Princeton University
Princeton, New Jersey 08544

Mark E. Furth
Laboratory of Tumor Virus Genetics
National Cancer Institute
National Institutes of Health
Bethesda, Maryland 20205

*Raymond Gesteland
Howard Hughes Medical Institute
University of Utah
Department of Biology
205 Life Sciences Building
Salt Lake City, Utah 94112

Raymond V. Gilden
Biological Carcinogenesis Program
National Cancer Institute-
Frederick Cancer Research Facility
P.O. Box B
Frederick, Maryland 21701

*Yakov Gluzman
Cold Spring Harbor Laboratory
P.O. Box 100
Cold Spring Harbor, New York 11724

*Mitchell Goldfarb
Cold Spring Harbor Laboratory
P.O. Box 100
Cold Spring Harbor, New York 11724

Mathew A. Gonda
National Cancer Institute-
Frederick Cancer Research Facility
Frederick, Maryland 21701

Jerome L. Goodwin
Department of Pathology
Uniformed Services University of the Health
    Sciences
Bethesda, Maryland 20014

Cornelia Gorman
Laboratory of Molecular Biology
National Cancer Institute
National Institutes of Health
Bethesda, Maryland 20205

Michael M. Gottesman
Laboratory of Molecular Biology
Molecular Cell Genetics Section
National Cancer Institute
National Institutes of Health
Bethesda, Maryland 20205

David Graf
Cancer Biology Program
National Cancer Institute-
Frederick Cancer Research Facility
Frederick, Maryland 21701

Frank L. Graham
Departments of Pathology and Biology
McMaster University
Hamilton, Ontario, L83 4J9 Canada

Stephen G. Grant
Genetics Department and Research Institute
Hospital for Sick Children and
*   Department of Medical Genetics*
University of Toronto
Toronto, Ontario, M5G 1X8 Canada

P. Green
McArdle Laboratory for Cancer Research
University of Wisconsin
Madison, Wisconsin 53706

*Terri Grodzicker
Cold Spring Harbor Laboratory
P.O. Box 100
Cold Spring Harbor, New York 11724

John Groffen
Laboratory of Viral Carcinogenesis
National Cancer Institute
Frederick Cancer Research Facility
Frederick, Maryland 21701

Peter Gruss
Laboratory of Molecular Virology
National Cancer Institute
National Institutes of Health
Bethesda, Maryland 20205

Gordon L. Hager
Laboratory of Tumor Virus Genetics
National Cancer Institute
National Institutes of Health
Bethesda, Maryland 20205

Stephen Hann
Department of Genetics
Albert Einstein College of Medicine
Bronx, New York 10461

Stephen C. Hardies
Department of Bacteriology and Immunology
University of North Carolina
Chapel Hill, North Carolina 27514

John A. Hassell
Department of Microbiology and Immunology
McGill University
3775 University Street
Montreal, Quebec, H3A 2B4 Canada

Stanley Hattman
Department of Biology
University of Rochester
Rochester, New York 14627

Nora Heisterkamp
Laboratory of Viral Carcinogenesis
National Cancer Institute
Frederick Cancer Research Facility
Frederick, Maryland 21701

Ronald R. Hiebsch
Biological Carcinogenesis Program
National Cancer Institute-
Frederick Cancer Research Facility
P.O. Box B
Frederick, Maryland 21701

J. Horowitz
McArdle Laboratory for Cancer Research
University of Wisconsin
Madison, Wisconsin 53706

Bruce Howard
Laboratory of Molecular Biology
National Cancer Institute
National Institutes of Health
Bethesda, Maryland 20205

Peter M. Howley
Laboratory of Pathology
National Cancer Institute
National Institutes of Health
Bethesda, Maryland 20205

*Stephen Hughes
Cold Spring Harbor Laboratory
P.O. Box 100
Cold Spring Harbor, New York 11724

Clyde A. Hutchison III
Department of Microbiology and Immunology
University of North Carolina
Chapel Hill, North Carolina 27514

C. James Ingles
Banting and Best Department of Medical Research
University of Toronto
112 College Street
Toronto, Ontario, M5G 1L6 Canada

Paul J. Jackson
Genetics Group
Los Alamos Scientific Laboratory
Los Alamos, New Mexico 87545

Ernest Jay
Laboratory of Molecular Virology
National Cancer Institute
National Institutes of Health
Bethesda, Maryland 20205

Gilbert Jay
Laboratory of Molecular Virology
National Cancer Institute
National Institutes of Health
Bethesda, Maryland 20205

Krishna K. Jha
Department of Biological Sciences
Hunter College
New York, New York 10021

Peter A. Jones
Division of Hematology-Oncology
Childrens Hospital of Los Angeles
4650 Sunset Boulevard
Los Angeles, California 90027

Alexandra L. Joyner
Department of Medical Biophysics
The Ontario Cancer Institute
University of Toronto
Toronto, Ontario, M4X 1K9 Canada

N. Kartner
The Ontario Cancer Institute
University of Toronto
Toronto, Ontario, M4X 1K9 Canada

Randal J. Kaufman
Genetics Institute
Boston, Massachusetts 02115

George Khoury
Laboratory of Molecular Virology
National Cancer Institute
National Institutes of Health
Bethesda, Maryland 20205

Paul G. Kratzer
Department of Molecular Biology
Roswell Park Memorial Institute
Buffalo, New York 14263

Michel Kress
Laboratory of Molecular Virology
National Cancer Institute
National Institutes of Health
Bethesda, Maryland 20205

Birgitt Kron
Institute of Genetics
University of Cologne
5000 Cologne 41, Federal Republic of Germany

Inge Kruczek
Institute of Biochemistry
University of Munich
Munich, Federal Republic of Germany

Raju Kucherlapati
Center for Genetics
University of Illinois
808 South Wood Street
Chicago, Illinois 60612

Ingrid Kuhlmann
Institute of Virology
University of Cologne
5000 Cologne 41, Federal Republic of Germany

Ann D. Kwong
Department of Biology
The University of Chicago
920 East 58th Street
Chicago, Illinois 60637

Laimonis Laimins
Laboratory of Molecular Virology
National Cancer Institute
National Institutes of Health
Bethesda, Maryland 20205

Mary-Ann Lane
Laboratory of Immunobiology
Department of Pathology
Harvard Medical School
Sidney Farber Cancer Institute
44 Binney Street
Boston, Massachusetts 02115

Ming-Fan Law
Laboratory of Pathology
National Cancer Institute
National Institutes of Health
Bethesda, Maryland 20205

Fwu-Lai Lin
National Cancer Institute-
Frederick Cancer Research Facility
P.O. Box B
Frederick, Maryland 21701

Victor Ling
The Ontario Cancer Institute
University of Toronto
Toronto, Ontario, M4X 1K9 Canada

R. Michael Liskay
Departments of Therapeutic Radiology and Human
  Genetics
Yale School of Medicine
333 Cedar Street
New Haven, Connecticut 06510

Douglas R. Lowy
Dermatology Branch
National Cancer Institute
National Institutes of Health
Bethesda, Maryland 20205

Tak W. Mak
Department of Medical Biophysics
The Ontario Cancer Institute
University of Toronto
500 Sherbourne Street
Toronto, Ontario M4X 1K9 Canada

Bonnie A. Maler
Department of Biochemistry and Biophysics
University of California, San Francisco
San Francisco, California 94143

O. Wesley McBride
Laboratory of Biochemistry
National Cancer Institute
National Institutes of Health
Bethesda, Maryland 20205

David McCarthy
Department of Biology
Brookhaven National Laboratory
Upton, New York 11973

J. McCubrey
McArdle Laboratory for Cancer Research
University of Wisconsin
Madison, Wisconsin 53706

Robert N. McEwan
Cancer Biology Program
National Cancer Institute-
Frederick Cancer Research Facility
Frederick, Maryland 21701

Anne-Marie Mes
Department of Microbiology and Immunology
McGill University
3775 University Street
Montreal, Quebec, H3A 2B4 Canada

Stella Mitrani-Rosenbaum
Laboratory of Pathology
National Cancer Institute
National Institutes of Health
Bethesda, Maryland 20205

P. Moreau
Department of Microbiology and Immunology
McGill University
3775 University Street
Montreal, Quebec, H3A 2B4 Canada

Robert K. Moyzis
Division of Biophysics
School of Hygiene and Public Health
The Johns Hopkins University
Baltimore, Maryland 21205

Christopher Mueller
Department of Microbiology and Immunology
McGill University
3775 University Street
Montreal, Quebec, H3A 2B4 Canada

W. Muller
Department of Microbiology and Immunology
McGill University
3775 University Street
Montreal, Quebec, H3A 2B4 Canada

*Daniel Nathans
Department of Microbiology
The Johns Hopkins University
The School of Medicine
725 North Wolfe Street
Baltimore, Maryland 21205

Monica Naujokas
Department of Microbiology and Immunology
McGill University
3775 University Street
Montreal, Quebec, H3A 2B4 Canada

Dorothy Neary
Laboratory of Immunobiology
Department of Pathology
Harvard Medical School
Sidney Farber Cancer Institute
44 Binney Street
Boston, Massachusetts 02115

Stephen Oroszlan
Biological Carcinogenesis Program
National Cancer Institute-
Frederick Cancer Research Facility
P.O. Box B
Frederick, Maryland 21701

Michael C. Ostrowski
Laboratory of Tumor Virus Genetics
National Cancer Institute
Bethesda, Maryland 20205

Harvey L. Ozer
Department of Biological Sciences
Hunter College
New York, New York 10021

Mark L. Pearson
Cancer Biology Program
National Cancer Institute
Frederick Cancer Research Facility
Frederick, Maryland 21701

*Sonia Pearson-White
Department of Microbiology
The Johns Hopkins University
School of Medicine
725 North Wolfe Street
Balitmore, Maryland 21205

Betsy Pomerantz
Department of Microbiology and Immunology
McGill University
3775 University Street
Montreal, Quebec, H3A 2B4 Canada

K. Prakash
Laboratory of Cellular and Molecular Biology
National Cancer Institute
National Institutes of Health
Bethesda, Maryland 20205

Jayashree Pyati
Department of Genetics
Albert Einstein College of Medicine
Bronx, New York 10461

Ulf R. Rapp
Laboratory of Viral Carcinogenesis
National Cancer Institute
Frederick Cancer Research Facility
Frederick, Maryland 21701

Peter N. Ray
Department of Genetics
The Hospital for Sick Children
555 University Avenue
Toronto, Ontario, M5G 1X8 Canada

Fred H. Reynolds, Jr.
Carcinogenesis Intramural Research Program
National Cancer Institute
Frederick Cancer Research Facility
Frederick, Maryland 21701

Nancy R. Rice
Biological Carcinogenesis Program
National Cancer Institute-
Frederick Cancer Research Facility
P.O. Box B
Frederick, Maryland 21701

*Arthur Riggs
City of Hope Research Institute
Duarte, California 91010

J. R. Riordan
The Hospital for Sick Children
University of Toronto
Toronto, Ontario, M4X 1K9 Canada

Rex Risser
McArdle Laboratory for Cancer Research
University of Wisconsin
Madison, Wisconsin 53706

K. C. Robbins
Laboratory of Cellular and Molecular Biology
National Cancer Institute
National Institutes of Health
Bethesda, Maryland 20205

U. G. Rovigatti
Laboratory of Molecular Oncology
National Cancer Institute-
Frederick Cancer Research Facility
Frederick, Maryland 21701

D. T. Rowe
Department of Biology
McMaster University
Hamilton, Ontario, L8S 4J9 Canada

M. Ruben
Department of Pathology
McMaster University
Hamilton, Ontario, L8S 4J9 Canada

*Ruth Sager
Sidney Farber Cancer Institute
Harvard Medical School
44 Binney Street
Boston, Massachusetts 02115

Adrienne Sainten
Laboratory of Immunobiology
Department of Pathology
Harvard Medical School
Sidney Farber Cancer Institute
44 Binney Street
Boston, Massachusetts 02115

Nava Sarver
Laboratory of Pathology
National Cancer Institute
National Institutes of Health
Bethesda, Maryland 20205

George Scangos
Department of Biology
The Johns Hopkins University
Charles and 34th Streets
Baltimore, Maryland 21218

Edward M. Scolnick
Laboratory of Tumor Virus Genetics
National Cancer Institute
National Institutes of Health
Bethesda, Maryland 20205

Jane K. Setlow
Department of Biology
Brookhaven National Laboratory
Upton, New York 11973

Michael Shales
Banting and Best Department of Medical Research
University of Toronto
Toronto, Ontario, M5G 1L6 Canada

*Larry Shapiro
Department of Pediatrics
Division of Medical Genetics
Harbor/UCLA Medical Center
100 West Carson Street
Torrance, California 90509

Phillip A. Sharp
Center for Cancer Research
Department of Biology
Massachusetts Institute of Technology
Cambridge, Massachusetts 02139

Clyde W. Shearman
NCI-Frederick Cancer Research Facility
P.O. Box B
Frederick, Maryland 21701

Kunitada Shimotohno
National Cancer Center Research Institute
Tokyo, Japan

L. Siminovitch
The Hospital for Sick Children
University of Toronto
Toronto, Ontario, M4X 1K9 Canada

Esau Simmons
Department of Biological Sciences
Hunter College
New York, New York 10021

C. Sinaiko
McArdle Laboratory for Cancer Research
University of Wisconsin
Madison, Wisconsin 53706

Linda D. Siracusa
Department of Molecular Biology
Roswell Park Memorial Institute
Buffalo, New York 14263

Michael B. Small
Department of Biological Sciences
Hunter College
New York, New York 10021

Hamilton O. Smith
Department of Molecular Biology and Genetics
The Johns Hopkins University
School of Medicine
725 North Wolfe Street
Baltimore, Maryland 21205

*Tom Sneider
Department of Biochemistry
Colorado State University
Fort Collins, Colorado 80526

Richard R. Spaete
Department of Medical Microbiology
Stanford University School of Medicine
Palo Alto, California 94305

*Clifford Stanners
Department of Medical Biophysics
Ontario Cancer Institute
500 Sherbourne Street
Toronto, Ontario, M4X 1K9 Canada

Robert M. Stephens
Biological Carcinogenesis Program
National Cancer Institute-
Frederick Cancer Research Facility
P.O. Box B
Frederick, Maryland 21701

John R. Stephenson
Laboratory of Viral Carcinogenesis
National Cancer Institute
Frederick Cancer Research Institute
Frederick, Maryland 21701

Nat L. Sternberg
Cancer Biology Program
National Cancer Institute-
Frederick Cancer Research Facility
P.O. Box B
Frederick, Maryland 21701

*William Summers
Department of Therapeutic Radiology
Yale University Medical School
333 Cedar Street
New Haven, Connecticut 06510

D. C. Swan
Laboratory of Cellular and Molecular Biology
National Cancer Institute
National Institutes of Health
Bethesda, Maryland 20205

Shirley M. Taylor
Division of Hematology-Oncology
Childrens Hospital of Los Angeles
Los Angeles, California 90027

Howard M. Temin
McArdle Laboratory for Cancer Research
University of Wisconsin
450 North Randall Street
Madison, Wisconsin 53706

*Gary Temple
Bethesda Research Labs
P.O. Box 6009
Gaithersburg, Maryland 20877

Paul O. P. Ts'o
Division of Biophysics
School of Hygiene and Public Health
The Johns Hopkins University
Baltimore, Maryland 21205

*George Vande Woude
Laboratory of Molecular Virology
National Cancer Institute
National Institutes of Health
Bethesda, Maryland 20205

Lily Vardimon
Massachusetts Institute of Technology
Boston, Massachusetts 02139

Shinichi Watanabe
National Cancer Institute
National Institutes of Health
Bethesda, Maryland 20205

Vincent L. Wilson
Division of Hematology-Oncology
Childrens Hospital of Los Angeles
Los Angeles, California 90027

Jerry K-C. Wong
Banting and Best Department of Medical Research
University of Toronto
Toronto, Ontario, M5G 1L6 Canada

Ronald G. Worton
Genetics Department and Research Institute
Hospital for Sick Children and Department of
*   Medical Genetics*
University of Toronto
555 University Avenue
Toronto, Ontario, M5G 1X8 Canada

Jung-Rung Wu
Division of Biophysics
School of Hygiene and Public Health
The Johns Hopkins University
Baltimore, Maryland 21205

Keith R. Yamamoto
Department of Biochemistry and Biophysics
University of California, San Francisco
San Francisco, California 94143

Shirley S. Yu
Meloy Laboratory
Springfield, Virginia 22151

*Robert Yuan
National Cancer Institute-
Frederick Cancer Research Facility
P.O. Box B
Frederick, Maryland 21701

Robert Zivin
Cancer Biology Program
National Cancer Institute-
Frederick Cancer Research Facility
Frederick, Maryland 21701

Gene Transfer and Cancer, edited by M. L. Pearson and N. L. Sternberg. Raven Press, New York © 1984.

Sequence-Specific and Non-Sequence-Specific Components of DNA Recognition in *Haemophilus* Transformation

David B. Danner and Hamilton O. Smith

Department of Molecular Biology and Genetics, Johns Hopkins University School of Medicine, Baltimore, Maryland 21205

ABSTRACT. Cells of the bacterial genus Haemophilus have evolved a highly efficient system for genetic transformation. In the appropriate culture medium, nearly 100% of H. influenzae cells can become competent to take up exogenous DNA and incorporate it into the cell chromosome. Transformable gram-positive bacteria such as Bacillus subtilis show no selectivity in terms of what DNAs may be taken up, but gram-negative Haemophilus cells show a 25- to 100-fold preferential uptake of Haemophilus DNA. Fragments of Haemophilus DNA cloned in Escherichia coli retain the ability to direct preferential uptake, ruling out the possibility that Haemophilus DNA is recognized on the basis of its methylation pattern. Four cloned Haemophilus DNA fragments ranging from 92 bp to 256 bp in size which can direct preferential uptake have been sequenced and found to contain a common 11-bp sequence, 5'-AAGTGCGGTCA-3'. This sequence has been chemically synthesized and cloned at various locations in the plasmid pBR322. Those restriction fragments to which the 11-mer has been added are found to be preferentially taken up; however, the extent of fragment uptake may vary as much as 48-fold depending on the surrounding DNA context. Uptake activity correlates with the A+T richness of the flanking DNA. Southern hybridization with the radioactively labeled synthetic 11-bp sequence indicates that Haemophilus genomic DNA is highly enriched for this sequence compared to E. coli DNA. The Haemophilus cell appears to have modeled its DNA uptake system and its genome around the recognition of a specific 11-bp sequence embedded in A+T-rich DNA.

INTRODUCTION

During the process of genetic transformation, cells take up naked DNA from the surrounding environment and incorporate it into their own chromosome to acquire an altered genotype which can then be passed on to daughter cells (13). Many types of cells can be genetically transformed by artificial means such as calcium or enzymatic treatment, but few cell types - only certain bacteria and perhaps yeasts - have evolved machinery for carrying out this process in nature. Those bacteria which have developed such natural systems rely on them for the distribution of valuable new mutations throughout the gene pool, and for these organisms, transformation is as useful for this task as are the analogous processes

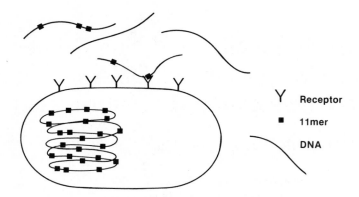

FIGURE 1. A model for the uptake of DNA by a competent Haemophilus cell.
Each cell has a small number of receptors which bind to exogenous DNA,
recognizing and preferentially taking up fragments containing an 11-bp
sequence. This sequence is present in many copies in the Haemophilus
genome.

of conjugation and transduction. Transformation was first described in
the pneumococcus by Griffith in 1928 (5) and was used by Avery in 1944
to show that DNA carries genetic information (1). Much work has been
done since this time on the mechanisms of transformation, especially in
species of Bacillus, Streptococcus, Haemophilus and Neisseria. It has
become evident that gram-positive and gram-negative bacteria, which have
quite different cell envelope structures, also have quite different methods of transporting DNA through that envelope. Of particular interest in
our laboratory has been the observation, first made by Scocca concerning
Haemophilus cells (10), that unlike the gram-positive bacteria, gram-
negative bacteria preferentially take up DNA from the same genus and ex-
clude other DNAs (Fig. 1). The experimental finding that Haemophilus
DNA cloned in E. coli retains the ability to direct preferential uptake
ruled out the idea that the Haemophilus modification methylase pattern
might be the basis of DNA recognition and made it likely that recognition was based on a specific sequence characteristic of Haemophilus DNA
(12). Our approach to defining this sequence was to assemble several
cloned DNA fragments which could direct preferential uptake, to examine
them for a common sequence and then to insert a chemically synthesized
version of this sequence into non-Haemophilus DNA to see if the addition
of this sequence to a DNA fragment would be both necessary and sufficient
to direct preferential uptake.

Identifying an Uptake Sequence by Comparison of Haemophilus DNA Fragments

   Two recombinant plasmids were constructed by cloning BamHI-cut fragments of H. parainfluenzae DNA into the BamHI site of the plasmid pBR322
(12). Plasmid pKS17 was found to contain an 8.1-kb insert of Haemophilus
DNA and plasmid pKS11 a 5.5-kb insert. As previously mentioned, DNA from
these plasmids retained the ability to be preferentially taken up by
competent cells (12). In addition, when these plasmids were cut into
several fragments with a restriction enzyme, ^{32}P end-labeled, and exposed
to competent Haemophilus cells, certain fragments could be preferentially
recovered from cell lysates. For each plasmid, those fragments preferentially taken up were found to be a subset of the fragments derived from

the Haemophilus DNA insert, indicating that each insert contained more than one recognition sequence. Using this assay, it was possible to narrow down the location of these sequences to progressively smaller fragments, until four such fragments could be isolated, two from pKS17 and two from pKS11, which were as small as could be produced with commercially available restriction enzymes. These fragments were then sequenced by the method of Maxam and Gilbert (6), and found to contain a common 11-bp sequence, 5'-AAGTGCGGTCA-3' (3). (This sequence and some of the flanking DNA for each fragment is shown in Figure 3). It is evident that the sequence is nondegenerate in these fragments (unlike, for example, bacterial promoters), and that the flanking DNA is A+T rich.

Proving That the 11-mer Is the Recognition Sequence by Cloning It in pBR322

Finding the same 11-bp sequence on all four Haemophilus DNA fragments strongly indicated that this was the DNA recognition sequence, but did not provide a clear proof of this idea. For example, recognition might have involved a degenerate (and therefore less recognizable) sequence, with which the 11-mer was associated for some unknown reason. Our approach to obtaining this proof was to show that the addition of a chemically synthesized version of the 11-bp sequence to a DNA fragment was both necessary and sufficient to direct the preferential uptake of that fragment (4). We decided to use the plasmid pBR322 as a source of these DNA fragments because it was known from sequence data that pBR322 had no 11-bp sequence and from our own uptake experiments that pBR322 had no functional DNA uptake site. To avoid the possibility that some sequence flanking the 11-mer might be fortuitously recreated during the construction, the chemically synthesized 11-bp sequence was inserted in several different contexts in pBR322.

An A+T-rich context was obtained by adding 3' poly-dT extensions to the synthetic 11-mer (7), mixing with PstI-cut pBR322 to which 3' poly-dA extensions had been added, transfecting E. coli cells and screening for ampicillin-sensitive, tetracycline-resistant colonies.

A somewhat less A+T-rich environment was obtained using two synthetic 15-mers which, when mixed together, gave the synthetic 11-mer duplex and 5' four-base overhangs complementary to EcoRI-produced ends. EcoRI sites are not regenerated when such molecules are ligated to EcoRI-produced ends. Therefore, this synthetic molecule was ligated to EcoRI-cut pBR322 in the presence of EcoRI so that self-annealed pBR322 molecules would be re-cleaved and the reaction driven toward the formation of the recombinant plasmid.

An essentially random DNA environment for the 11-mer was obtained by ligating it into the RsaI site at base 164 of pBR322 DNA (in the tetra-cycline-resistance gene). Since pBR322 has three RsaI sites, a partial digest of the plasmid was used, and the recombinant plasmid was selected on the basis of loss of tetracycline-resistance (2).

A G+C-rich environment for the 11-mer was obtained by ligating the synthetic 11-mer with an excess of BamHI and cloning these molecules into the BamHI site of pBR322. The recombinant plasmids were all sequenced in the region of the 11-mer to verify their structure (see Figure 3 for context of each 11-bp sequence).

To examine the uptake activity of each synthetic recognition site, we digested each pBR322 derivative with HindIII and AvaI, ^{32}P end-labeled the resulting two fragments and exposed them to competent cells to measure uptake. To obtain a quantitative comparison with the naturally occurring sites, EcoRI fragments of pKS17 were end labeled and mixed

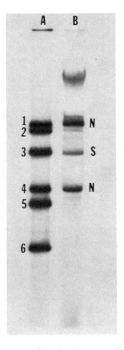

FIGURE 2. A typical uptake experiment comparing the ability of synthetic and naturally occurring recognition sites to direct the preferential uptake of DNA fragments. Seen is an autoradiogram of ^{32}P end-labeled DNA fragments separated on a 1% agarose gel. Lane A shows a mix of six DNA fragments. Fragments 1, 2, 4 and 6 are EcoRI fragments of the plasmid pKS17; fragments 3 and 5 are produced by HindIII-AvaI digestion of the plasmid pEUP1 (see Figure 3). Fragments 1 and 4 bear naturally occurring uptake sites; fragment 3 bears a synthetic site. Lane B shows the radioactive material obtained when the fragments in lane A are treated as follows. They are exposed to competent Haemophilus cells, the cells are treated with DNase I and washed with high salt to remove unabsorbed material, and the cells are then lysed and the lysate is extracted with phenol and run out on an agarose gel. The relative enrichment of bands 3 and 4 as measured by densitometer tracing is used to quantitate uptake activity (see Figure 3).

with the two pBR322-derived fragments prior to uptake. Thus fragments bearing natural sites were mixed before uptake at a certain ratio with fragments bearing synthetic sites; after uptake, fragments were recovered and this ratio was found to be changed. Densitometer tracings of the appropriate autoradiograms were used to quantitate this change in relative abundance and derive an "uptake activity" relative to one of the natural site-bearing fragments. These experiments were done under saturating DNA conditions (>1 µg/ml) to ensure maximum competition between synthetic and natural recognition sequences. Figure 2 shows an autoradiogram obtained by this approach; Figure 3 documents the results obtained for each fragment examined. It is evident that the addition of the 11-mer to a DNA fragment is necessary and sufficient for prefer-

PLASMID	SEQUENCE	ACTIVITY
pPUP3	AAAAAAAAAAAAAAA AAGTGCGGTCA TTTTTTTTTTTTTTT	191%
pKS17	AAAATTAAAATTTAA AAGTGCGGTCA TTTTGACCGAGATTT	117%
pKS17	GGTTGTGCATTGTTG AAGTGCGGTCA AAAAATCGGAAATTT	100%
pKS11	GTTCGCCCCAAAGGA AAGTGCGGTCA TTTTATAGGTTGGAT	ND
pKS11	TTACTTATAAAATAA AAGTGCGGTCA ATTTCAAAACAGTTT	ND
pKS11	GTAATCCTAAACAGA AAGTGCGGTCA ATTTTAAAACTGTTT	ND
pEUP1	TCGTCTTCAAGAATT AAGTGCGGTCA AATTCTCATGTTTGA	40%
pRSUP1	CTTGGTTATGCCGGT AAGTGCGGTCA ACTGCCGGGCCTCTT	27%
pBUP2	GCGTAGAGGATCCGG AAGTGCGGTCA CCGGATCCACAGGAC	4%
pBR322	NO 11 bp-SEQUENCE	<1%

FIGURE 3. Five naturally occurring and four synthetic DNA recognition sites are compared for 15 nucleotides to either side of the 11-bp sequence. Uptake activity as determined by the assay shown in Figure 2 is listed in the right-hand column (ND = not done).

ential uptake of that fragment. However, it is also clear that sites may vary at least 48-fold in uptake activity, and that this variation correlates with the A+T richness of the flanking DNA.

DISCUSSION

These data provide reasonable proof that the 11-bp sequence is the DNA recognition site for Haemophilus transformation. Additional data, obtained during the course of these experiments, support this idea. A 2.2-kb fragment of H. haemolyticus DNA, sequenced by Brigitte Schoner in this laboratory (personal communication), has no 11-bp sequence and exhibits no preferential uptake. Robert A. Deich has shown that chemically adding ethyl groups to DNA will interfere with DNA uptake, but only if the ethyl groups are added in the region of the 11-bp sequence (3). Presumably these groups sterically hinder the interaction between the recognition site and the cellular receptor. One idea that has not been ruled out by these experiments is that degenerate versions of the uptake sequence may exist which we have not yet observed, but which do have uptake activity.

Although 5'-AAGTGCGGTCA-3' appears to specify preferential uptake, it seems evident that the effectiveness of this sequence depends to a large extent on the DNA context in which it is embedded. We have not proven that the effect of flanking DNA depends on A+T richness, however, the correlation between A+T richness and uptake is strong, and the other alternative i.e., base-pair degeneracies (11) such as those recognized by restriction enzymes, does not seem to fit the observed data. Three physical properties distinguish A+T-rich DNA from G+C-rich DNA: A-T base pairs lack a 2-amino group in the minor grove (11), A+T-rich DNA melts at a lower temperature than G+C-rich DNA, and even short runs of A or T result in a different helical twist than other DNA sequences (8,9). Any of these differences could play a role in recognition.

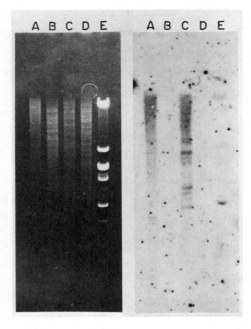

FIGURE 4. Southern hybridization analysis showing that Haemophilus
genomic DNA is highly enriched for the 11-bp sequence compared to
E. coli DNA. On the left, an ethidium bromide-stained agarose gel;
on the right, an autoradiogram obtained when DNA is transferred from
the gel to nitrocellulose and hybridized with ^{32}P end-labeled synthetic
11-mer DNA at 14°C. Lanes A and B, PstI-cut H. influenzae and E. coli
DNA, respectively; lanes C and D, EcoRI-cut H. influenzae and E. coli
DNA, respectively. Lane E, a set of molecular-weight standards.

Competition experiments between Haemophilus genomic DNA and cloned
DNA bearing two recognition sites indicate that Haemophilus cells have
about 600 sites per genome or one every 4 kb (12). Southern hybridization of Haemophilus and E. coli genomic fragments with ^{32}P-labeled synthetic 11-mer demonstrates the presence of hundreds of copies of this
sequence in the Haemophilus genome and essentially none in E. coli DNA
(Figure 4). Since one can calculate that this sequence should occur
at random every 4^{11} bases or 0.5×4^{11} bp (1 per 2×10^6 bp, one or two
copies per genome), it is evident that Haemophilus DNA is highly en-
riched for this sequence. Random genetic drift should act to reduce the
number of copies of this sequence in the cell; therefore it is clear
that some selection pressure must exist to maintain the high copy number.
Probably the transformation system itself provides this pressure, since
new sites created by mutation will spread throughout the gene pool,
whereas defective sites created by mutation will not be taken up and
will eventually be corrected by the spread of the corresponding non-
mutated sites. In theory, these recognition sites may continue to
spread throughout the genome until their number begins to compromise
cell survival.

ACKNOWLEDGEMENTS

We wish to thank Mildred Kahler and JoAnn Olsen for excellent preparation of the manuscript. This work was funded by NIH grant PO1-CA16519 to H.O.S. D.B.D. was supported by NIH predoctoral training grant 5-T32-GM07445 and more recently received predoctoral fellowship support from the Monsanto Company. H.O.S. is an American Cancer Society Distinguished Research Professor.

REFERENCES

1. Avery OT, MacLeod C, McCarty M (1944): J Exp Med 79:137
2. Bochner BR, Huang H, Schieven GL, Ames BN (1980): J Bacteriol 143:926
3. Danner DB, Deich RA, Sisco KL, Smith HO (1980): Gene 11:311
4. Danner DB, Smith HO, Narang SA (1982): Proc Natl Acad Sci USA 79:2392
5. Griffith F (1928): J Hyg 27:113
6. Maxam AM, Gilbert W (1980): Methods Enzymol (Grossman L, Moldave K, (eds) New York: Academic Press, 65:499
7. Nelson T, Brutlag D (1970) Methods Enzymol (Wu R, ed), New York: Academic Press, 68:41
8. Peck LJ, Wang JC (1981) Nature 292:375
9. Rhodes D, Klug A (1981) Nature 292:378
10. Scocca JJ, Poland RL, Zoon KD (1974) J Bacteriol 118:369
11. Seaman NC, Rosenberg JM, Rich A (1976) Proc Natl Acad Sci USA 73:804
12. Sisco KL, Smith HO (1979) Proc Natl Acad Sci USA 76:972
13. Smith HO, Danner DB, Deich RA (1981) Annu Rev Biochem 50:41

Gene Transfer and Cancer, edited by M. L. Pearson and N. L. Sternberg. Raven Press, New York © 1984.

Sequence-Specific DNA-Binding Vesicles Are Released from *Haemophilus Influenzae* Cells During Loss of Competence for Transformation

Robert A. Deich

Cancer Biology Program, National Cancer Institute, Frederick Cancer Research Facility, Frederick, Maryland 21701

ABSTRACT. Competence for genetic transformation in Haemophilus influenzae is inducible; over 99% of a cell population can be made competent by maintaining the cells in appropriate nongrowth conditions. When induced H. influenzae cells are returned to normal growth conditions, competence is rapidly lost. Electron microscopy studies of H. influenzae cells showed that membranous extensions (blebs) are generated on the cell surface during induction of competence and that these structures are shed as free vesicles during loss of competence. Free vesicles have been isolated and shown to retain the ability to bind DNA in a nuclease-resistant, salt-stable form. The vesicle binding is specific for DNAs containing the 11-bp H. influenzae DNA uptake sequence and has similar pH, temperature, and cofactor requirements to those of DNA binding to whole competent cells. Vesicles contain the major H. influenzae outer membrane proteins and are enriched for several minor proteins.

INTRODUCTION

Many bacterial species undergo genetic transformation by interacting with DNA molecules in solution and stably incorporating the information in these molecules into their genome. To accomplish this, bacterial cells have developed genetically defined systems for specifically binding, absorbing, and processing free DNA molecules (for recent review, see 12).

The gram-negative bacterium H. influenzae has proven to be an excellent model system for studying these processes for several reasons. First, high levels of competence can be attained in H. influenzae; over 99% of a cell population can be made transformable (6). Second, competent Haemophilus cells have the ability to specifically recognize and bind their own DNA (10). This recognition has been shown to be based on the presence of an 11-base sequence, 5'-AAGTGCGGTCA-3', which occurs in multiple copies in the Haemophilus genome (1,2,10,11). This specificity of DNA uptake makes Haemophilus transformation an excellent system for studying site-specific DNA membrane interactions and for looking at the processes of DNA binding and uptake.

Finally, competence for transformation in H. influenzae is a reversibly inducible phenomenon. Under normal conditions of exponential growth in rich medium, competence frequencies of less than 10^{-4} are observed. High levels of competence in H. influenzae are induced by transferring growing cells into an appropriate medium that allows continued protein synthesis but does not permit cell division (6). Once attained, the competent state is stable for several hours under growth-limiting conditions. However, when induced cells are returned to rich growth medium, competence is rapidly lost (9). After 1 hr in rich broth, the level of competence drops to the background level.

We have examined morphological changes on the surface of cells by means of scanning electron microscopy and observed that membranous extensions or blebs are generated during competence induction. These structures are shed as free vesicles and found that they contain a Haemophilus-specific DNA-binding activity similar to that of whole competent cells. Our results suggest that the blebs are the initial site of DNA binding to cells and may be involved in subsequent uptake and processing of DNA for genetic transformation.

RESULTS

Morphological Changes During Competence Induction

Scanning electron microscopy studies revealed distinct morphological changes on the cell surface during competence induction in H. influenzae (4). Cells became rough and wrinkled in appearance, and blebs formed on the cells. About a dozen blebs formed per cell and were distributed apparently randomly on the cell surface. Blebs were roughly spherical extensions of 80 to 100 µm diameter as determined by scanning electron microscopy and 60 to 80 µm diameter as determined by thin-section transmission electron microscopy. When competent cells were returned to rich growth medium, the blebs were spontaneously shed from the cell surface with approximately the same kinetics as the loss of cellular competence.

This temporal correspondence of the appearance and loss of blebs with the ability of H. influenzae cells to bind and absorb DNA molecules (Figure 1) suggested that these structures might be directly involved in cell-DNA interactions. We therefore purified these vesicles to see whether they retained any of the lost cellular DNA-binding activity.

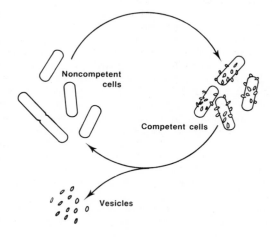

FIGURE 1. Model of the generation and loss of blebs by H. influenzae cells during the competence induction cycle.

Purification and Properties of Vesicles

Vesicles were purified by differential centrifugation. Cells were pelleted by a slow-speed spin (8000 rpm x 10 min), and vesicles were pelleted by a high-speed spin (20,000 rpm x 3 hr). Final purification of this crude vesicle pellet was done by chromatography on heparin-agarose (vesicle fractions eluted at 0.4 to 0.5 M NaCl). An essentially pure population of vesicles was obtained as determined by electron microscopy (4).

Purified vesicles retained the ability to bind double-stranded DNA molecules in a nuclease-resistant complex that could be retained on nitrocellulose. The vesicle binding resembled whole-cell DNA binding in that it showed a strong requirement for the presence of the Haemophilus uptake sequence on the bound DNA duplex. DNA of plasmid pPUP3, a derivative of pBR322 containing a single, chemically synthesized uptake site (10), bound about 50-fold more efficiently to vesicles than pBR322 DNA. DNA binding to vesicles also showed identical requirements for salt, temperature, and pH as DNA binding to whole competent cells (Table 1). We can therefore infer that loss of cellular competence for transformation is attributable to the physical removal of the DNA-binding apparatus from the cell surface via shed vesicles.

Vesicles have been shown to contain the six major outer membrane proteins of H. influenzae Rd and to be enriched for several minor polypeptides between 40 and 60 kd. In particular, two polypeptides of 51 and 56 kd are very strongly enriched in vesicle preparations.

DISCUSSION

We have shown that induction of competence for transformation in H. influenzae is accompanied by the generation of membranous extensions of the outer membrane (blebs) and loss of competence by the shedding of these structures as free vesicles which retain a DNA binding activity essentially identical to that of whole cells. These results strongly

TABLE 1. Conditions for DNA Binding to Competent H. influenzae
Cells and to Purified Vesicles

	Purified vesicles	Cells
Haemophilus uptake sequence	Required	Required
Optimal binding conditions:		
Temperature	37°	36°
pH	7	7
Na^+	100 mM	100–150 mM
Mg^{2+}/Ca^{2+}	1 mM	0.5 mM
Inhibitors:		
EDTA	1 mM	1 mM
Na^+	0.5 M	0.4 M
Heparin	50 µg/ml	50 µg/ml
Cold	<25°C	<20°C

suggest that the blebs are involved in the binding of DNA to competent cells for transformation. This conclusion is further supported by the observation that the number of blebs per cell as determined by scanning electron microscopy is in agreement with the estimated number of DNA receptors per cell determined biochemically (5). In addition, certain nontransformable mutants of Haemophilus that cannot bind DNA are known to shed DNA binding vesicles when placed in competence-inducing conditions (7).

An important question that arises from the study of DNA binding to free vesicles is the nature of the nuclease-resistant complex formed. Vesicles are capable of protecting large DNA molecules from nuclease digestion. Lambda Charon 4 recombinant DNA molecules carrying Hameophilus DNA inserts (about 45 kb in length) were protected from DNAse I digestion by vesicles (R.A. Deich, unpublished observations). The simplest explanation is that bound DNA is internalized into the vesicles. Vesicles should be able to bind large amounts of DNA internally, being about the same dimension as T4 phage heads, which contain about 200 kb of duplex DNA. Such internalization into the vesicles would require a mechanism for folding and compacting DNA analogous to phage head packaging with the 11-bp uptake sequence acting as an initiating site. On the other hand, we cannot rule out the possibility that DNA is somehow "collapsed" on the surface of the vesicles in a nuclease-resistent complex analogous to that reported during mammalian cell transformation by Loyter et al. (8). However, it is difficult to see how a surface collapse mechanism of DNA binding could continue to show such a high degree of specificity for Haemophilus DNA.

In addition vesicles clearly must contain the specific receptor for the Haemophilus uptake sequence. To date, all attempts to identify this protein biochemically have failed; dissociation of the vesicle membrane has always led to rapid inactivation of all specific binding activity. Probably more genetic data on the mechanism of transformation will be required to positively identify the receptor protein(s).

The role of the blebs in DNA uptake into competent cells remains unclear. One possibility is that DNA is initially bound into the vesicles and the entire DNA-vesicle complex is transported into the cytoplasm for processing. This model is attractive for two reasons. First, it is consistent with our presumption that DNA is internalized into free vesicles. Second, it explains the relative stability of transforming DNA molecules within cells after uptake: bound DNA is not attacked by cellular exonucleases or restriction endonucleases, although it is sensitive to both in vitro. On the other hand, the model raises the question of how such a large, complex structure could be transported through the outer and inner cell membranes without disrupting them. Obviously, other models for the role of blebs in DNA uptake by competent cells are possible. Indeed, we cannot rule out the possibility that blebs are not directly involved in DNA uptake by whole cells at all but are merely a mechanism for shedding the DNA-binding apparatus during competence loss. Clearly more work in this area is needed.

In any event, use of purified vesicles should provide a simplified system for studying the initial, site-specific interaction between transforming DNA and the Haemophilus cell surface. It may also provide a useful system for studying the initial steps in DNA transport into cells and processing of DNA for genetic transformation.

ACKNOWLEDGEMENT

Research sponsored by the National Cancer Institute, DHHS, under Contract No. NO1-CO-75380 with Litton Bionetics, Inc. The contents of this publication do not necessarily reflect the views or policies of the Department of Health and Human Services, nor does mention of trade names, commercial products, or organizations imply endorsement by the U.S. Government.

REFERENCES

1. Chung GC, Goodgal SH (1979): Biochem Biophys Res Commun 88:208
2. Danner DB, Deich RA, Sisco KS, Smith HO (1980): Gene 11:311
3. Danner DB, Smith HO, Narang SA (1982): Proc Natl Acad Sci USA 79:2392
4. Deich RA, Hoyer LC (1982): J Bacteriol, in press
5. Deich RA, Smith HO (1980): Mol Gen Genet 177:369
6. Herriott RM, Meyer EM, Vogt M (1970): J Bacteriol 101:517
7. Kahn M, Concino M, Gromkova R, Goodgal SH (1979): Biochem Biophys Res Commun 87:764
8. Loyter A, Scangos GA, Ruddle FH (1982): Proc Natl Acad Sci USA 79:422
9. Scocca JJ, Haberstat M (1978): J Bacteriol 135:961
10. Scocca JJ, Poland RL, Zoon KC (1974): J Bacteriol 118:369
11. Sisco KL, Smith HO (1979): Proc Natl Acad Sci USA 76:972
12. Smith HO, Danner DB, Deich RA (1981): Annu Rev Biochem 50:41

Gene Transfer and Cancer, edited by M. L. Pearson
and N. L. Sternberg. Raven Press, New York © 1984.

Gene Transfer Between Plasmid and Chromosome in *Haemophilus Influenzae*

Jane K. Setlow, David McCarthy, and Nancy-Lee Clayton

Department of Biology, Brookhaven National Laboratory, Upton, New York 11973

ABSTRACT. Recombination can readily occur between a large cloned
piece of chromosomal DNA in an otherwise nonhomologous plasmid and the
recipient chromosome upon transformation of Haemophilus influenzae by
the plasmid. As a result of this recombination, the plasmid can acquire
homologous DNA from the chromosome and the chromosome can also acquire a
homologous marker from the plasmid, but not in the same event. Both
processes require wild-type rec1 and rec2 genes. Another smaller cloned
piece of chromosomal DNA in another vector only very rarely recombines
with the chromosome. The piece of cloned DNA contains an antibiotic-
resistance marker that is recessive to antibiotic sensitivity. This
marker on the plasmid is only expressed when there is Rec-dependent recombination with the chromosome, so that the marker is both on the plasmid and on the chromosome.

INTRODUCTION

H. influenzae is a microorganism particularly suitable for studies of
recombination because under optimal conditions an entire population of
cells can be made to recombine at the same time. The study of recombination between plasmid and chromosome in this bacterium is interesting
because such recombination can play a role in the establishment of plasmids (10). These phenomena may be of practical importance, since in the
last decade the spread of antibiotic resistance, presumably mediated
through plasmids, has severely compromised antibiotic treatment of serious H. influenzae infections (3).

In the present work two questions are addressed: a) What are the
conditions governing gene transfer between plasmid and chromosome? b)
What are the factors governing expression of antibiotic resistance coded
for by a plasmid where the corresponding genetic information for sensitivity to that antibiotic is on the chromosome?

RESULTS AND DISCUSSION

We constructed the plasmids used for this work by cloning fragments of
chromosomal DNA from H. influenzae cells resistant to eight different
antibiotics. Two plasmid vectors were used. The first (RSF0885) confers
ampicillin resistance on the host cell (7) and contains a single PvuII
site used for cloning (10). The other plasmid vector was constructed by
combining RSF0885 with a portion of the 34-megadalton plasmid p2265 (1,

2). The resulting hybrid pDM2 carries the ampicillin-resistance marker of RSF0885 and the chloramphenicol-resistance marker of p2265.

Cloning with pDM2 was done by insertion of chromosomal fragments into the PstI site in the ampicillin-resistance gene. Plasmid transformants were obtained by selection for chloramphenicol resistance. Neither of the cloning vectors contains an active transposon, and we have obtained evidence that the ampicillin- and chloramphenicol-resistance genes of these vectors do not recombine into the chromosome. Thus whenever the resistance to these antibiotics was lost from the cell, the plasmid was also lost, as judged by the disappearance of the plasmid band from agarose gels of crude lysates (9).

Neither of the two cloning vectors has appreciable homology with the H. influenzae chromosome, but with the insertion of chromosomal DNA, both plasmids become partially homologous and are likely to acquire a particular 11-bp sequence necessary for efficient uptake into H. influenzae (4,5). Thus the recombinant plasmid will be taken up by a competent cell about two orders of magnitude better than the parent plasmid vector. In addition, we found that the presence of homologous DNA on part of the plasmid increases the probability by about three orders of magnitude that the plasmid once inside the cell can become established. This increase in efficiency of plasmid establishment is strictly dependent on wild-type rec1 and rec2 genes (10).

Some of the properties of two recombinant plasmids are shown in Table 1. Both these plasmids contain a cloned novobiocin-resistance marker. The high-level marker of pNov1 consists of a complex of two closely linked markers individually conferring resistance to at least 1 and 2.5 µg/ml novobiocin (6), whereas pNov2 contains only one of the lower-level markers. Table 1 shows the results of transformation of competent wild-type H. influenzae by purified preparations of the two plasmids. Whereas the 2.5 µg/ml novobiocin marker when it is on the chromosome is about twice as efficiently transformed as the high-level marker (11), the 2.5 µg/ml novobiocin marker of pDM2 is transformed two orders of magnitude less well than the 25 µg/ml novobiocin marker of pNov1. This may reflect the fact that the sizes of the chromosomal inserts differ by about a factor of 10. Establishment of the plasmid, as indicated by transformation of the plasmid marker (ampicillin or chloramphenicol resistance) is also considerably less efficient for pNov2, probably because its small size hinders the ability of the insert to stabilize the plasmid so that it can replicate.

TABLE 1. Transformation of H. influenzae with plasmids pNov1 and pNov2

Plasmid	Level of novobiocin resistance (µg/ml)	Mol. wt.	Mol. wt. of chromosomal insert	% Transformation	
				Plasmid marker	Chromosomal marker
pNov1 (in vector RSF0885)	25	9.6×10^6	5.9×10^6	1	10
pNov2 (in vector pDM2)	2.5	6.9×10^6	5.3×10^5	10^{-3}	10^{-1}

In the case of both plasmids, the novobiocin marker is transformed much more efficiently than the plasmid marker. In most of the novobiocin transformation events, the plasmid donates a homologous part of its DNA to the chromosome and then the remainder of the plasmid disintegrates (10). When the pNov1 plasmid becomes established after entering the competent cell, three-quarters of the time the novobiocin-resistance marker is not present in the cell, but the established plasmid has the same size and restriction pattern as the original pNov1. The difference between the plasmids of such transformants, called pNov1s, and pNov1 is that the former have acquired DNA specifying novobiocin sensitivity from the chromosome by a rec1- and rec2-dependent recombination. Purified preparations of pNov1s can readily transform novobiocin-resistant cells to sensitivity. The recombination event that generates pNov1s is not reciprocal, i.e., the chromosome does not at the same time acquire the novobiocin-resistance gene.

Establishment of plasmid pNov2 in the wild-type cell does not cause a subculture of the transformant to be phenotypically novobiocin-resistant. However, the novobiocin-resistance marker is not lost as it is in most pNov1 plasmid-containing transformants, as shown by the fact that lysates of pNov2 chloramphenicol transformants can transform novobiocin-sensitive cells to resistance. Thus the novobiocin-resistance marker in these transformants is present, but not expressed. However, when a culture of such a transformant is grown for a long time in 2.5 µg/ml novobiocin, it becomes resistant to the antibiotic, with a probability considerably higher than that indicated by the known frequency of spontaneous mutation to that level of novobiocin resistance (8). Furthermore, a culture of a pNov2 transformant that has not been exposed to novobiocin contains a very small fraction of cells that are novobiocin-resistant, but this fraction is four orders of magnitude higher than the fraction of novobiocin-resistant cells that are lacking the plasmid (Table 2). However, the fact that the corresponding Rec$^-$ cells only show the spontaneous mutation level of novobiocin resistance suggests that a recombination event causes the Rec$^+$ cultures to become phenotypically novobiocin-resistant. When the rare, resistant cells in the Rec$^+$ (pNov2) population were isolated and plasmid-free variants obtained, these were also found to be novobiocin-resistant. On the other hand, unselected transformants cured of their plasmids were novobiocin-sensitive. Thus a cell containing the pNov2 plasmid only becomes novobiocin-resistant when the novobiocin-re-

TABLE 2. The effect of host Rec function on expression of novobiocin resistance with plasmid pNov2

Bacterial strains	Fraction of cells resistant to 2.5 µg/ml novobiocin
Rec$^+$ (no plasmid)	3×10^{-8}
Rec$^+$ (pNov2)	2×10^{-4}
Rec$^-$ (no plasmid)	3×10^{-8}
Rec$^-$ (pNov2)	3×10^{-8}

sistance marker has been donated to the chromosome by a Rec[+]-dependent process. However, a novobiocin-resistance marker in a cell containing pNov1 renders the cell novobiocin-resistant, whether or not the marker is on both the chromosome and the plasmid (10).

The difference between these two situations could result from cloning in different sites in the vectors RSF0885 and pDM2 and/or the difference between the 2.5 µg/ml novobiocin-resistance marker pNov2 and the 25 µg/ml novobiocin-resistance marker of pNov1. It is possible that the marker in pNov2 cannot be expressed when it is exclusively on the plasmid because of the lack of an adequate promoter or because only part of the gene product is made following transcription from the plasmid. We have obtained the following evidence that there is a difference in dominance of novobiocin sensitivity over the two markers. A rec1 mutant carrying either the 2.5 µg/ml novobiocin or the 25 µg/ml novobiocin-resistance markers was transformed with the pNov1s plasmid carrying novobiocin sensitivity. The mutation precludes recombination between the plasmid and the chromosome. The question was then asked, what is the phenotypic character of the transformants with respect to novobiocin sensitivity?

The 2.5 µg/ml novobiocin transformants all appeared sensitive to 2.5 µg/ml novobiocin, indicating that sensitivity was clearly dominant over resistance. The 25 µg/ml novobiocin transformants behaved for several hours like sensitive cells in 25 µg/ml novobiocin, and then the growth rate steadily increased to that of resistant cells. During this period the plasmid copy number as measured in ethidium bromide-cesium chloride gradients decreased from about 30 to less than 10. Thus resistance to 25 µg/ml novobiocin is dominant over sensitivity, provided that the ratio of sensitivity to resistance genes is not too overwhelming.

CONCLUSIONS

a) Gene transfer between plasmid and chromosome in the absence of transposons is profoundly affected by the size of the region in the plasmid that is homologous to some part of the chromosome.

b) Gene transfer from a plasmid to a chromosome, the most frequently observed result of plasmid-chromosome interaction after a plasmid has entered the competent cell, is a nonreciprocal event and is therefore not usually accompanied by establishment of a plasmid.

c) Gene transfer from chromosome to plasmid is also nonreciprocal and thus can result in the loss of the homologous plasmid marker from a cell transformed by a plasmid originally bearing a homologous resistance marker.

d) Expression of some antibiotic-resistance markers initially on a plasmid does not occur unless there is recombination between plasmid and chromosome, causing the chromosome to acquire the marker.

e) All the types of plasmid-chromosomal interaction described, including that which increases the probability of plasmid establishment after it enters the cell, are Rec[+]-dependent processes.

ACKNOWLEDGEMENTS

This work was carried out at the Brookhaven National Laboratory under the auspices of the U.S. Department of Energy.

REFERENCES

1. Albritton WL, Bendler JW, Setlow JK (1981): J Bacteriol 145:1099

2. Albritton WL, Slaney L (1980): In: Plasmids and Transposons: Environmental Effects and Maintenance Mechanisms (Studdard C, Rozee KR, eds), New York: Academic Press, pp 107–116

3. Broda P (1979): Plasmids, San Francisco: Freeman WH

4. Danner DB, Smith HO (1983): This volume

5. Danner DB, Smith HO, Narang SA (1982): Proc Natl Acad Sci USA 79: 2393

6. Day RS III, Rupert CS (1971): Mutat Res 11:293

7. deGraaf J, Elwell L, Falkow S (1976): J Bacteriol 126:439

8. Kimball RF, Setlow JK, Liu M (1971): Mutat Res 12:21

9. Notani NK, Setlow JK, McCarthy D, Clayton N-L (1981): J Bacteriol 148:812

10. Setlow JK, Notani NK, McCarthy D, Clayton N-L (1981): J Bacteriol 148:804

11. Voll MJ, Goodgal SH (1965): J Bacteriol 90:873

Gene Transfer and Cancer, edited by M. L. Pearson and N. L. Sternberg. Raven Press, New York © 1984.

Transfer of Single Specific Chromosomes by Microcell Fusion and Gene Mapping in Mammalian Cells

Raghbir S. Athwal and Veena Dhar

*Department of Microbiology, New Jersey School of Medicine,
Newark, New Jersey 07006*

ABSTRACT. We have used a combination of chromosome-mediated gene transfer (CMGT) and microcell fusion techniques to transfer two Chinese hamster chromosomes (1 and 2) individually to mouse cells. Clonal cell lines of Chinese hamster cells (transgenotes) expressing human hypoxanthine guanine phosphoribosyl transferase (hprt) were produced following CMGT. Microcells prepared from the subclones of two independent transgenotes (GT1 and GT8) were size fractionated and fused with mouse cells. The resultant hybrids were isolated by selection in HAT medium. Cytogenetic analysis of microcell hybrids revealed that clones originating from independent transgenotes contained single intact hamster chromosomes 1 and 2, respectively. The transferred chromosomes carry an integrated selectable marker and thus can be retained in cells by selection. Microcell hybrids were subcloned to isolate single-cell subclones for the retention or loss of hprt by selection in HAT or 6-thioguanine medium. Parent hybrids and selected subclones were analyzed for the expression of 32 isozymes. These data were used to map seven markers (Est-D, PEP-B, PEP-S, PGM-1, GSR, NP, and ADK) to hamster chromosome 1 and four markers (AK-2, Eno-1, PGM-2, and 6-PGD) to chromosome 2. We were able to determine the gene order of four markers assigned to chromosome 2 from the sequential loss of these markers which occurred in the back selected clones.

INTRODUCTION

The application of parasexual methods for the genetic analysis of cultured cells has provided a highly productive approach to the mapping of genes and the study of the regulation of gene expression in eucaryotic organisms (for reviews, see Refs 18 and 25). These experimental systems depend upon the analysis of clonal cell populations, each carrying a different subset of another species genome. Such cell lines are normally generated by cell/cell hybridization and random segregation of chromosomes of one of the parent species (18,20,25). Although considerable progress in mapping of genes has been made by cell hybridization, the technique has limitations for high-resolution gene mapping of the type achieved in procaryotes. The lengthy interval required for chromosome segregation is technically undesirable, and it is very difficult if not impossible to achieve a perfectly stable karyotype in the segregating hybrids (25). At the same time it is difficult to construct clones from hybrid cells in which only a single chromosome of one of the parent types persists even when the selective pressure can be maintained for the retention of this chromosome alone.

A more direct approach to the production of cell lines possessing a limited amount of genetic material of another species would be to introduce only a single donor chromosome into the recipient cells. It is possible to achieve such a result by the microcell hybridization technique (2,4,8,16). Mammalian cells when treated with mitotic inhibitors for an extended period of time (30 to 40 hr) form multiple small nuclei (micronuclei) in the cells, and each micronucleus contains only a subset of the cell genome (4). Experimentally isolated micronuclei surrounded with a thin layer of cytoplasm and plasma membrane are called microcells (4,25). Microcells can be fused with cultured cells by conventional methods, and hybrids can be isolated by selection for the transfer of a selectable marker and corresponding chromosome(s) contained in the microcell (2,4-8,16,19,32). The size of the micronuclei has been found to correlate with the amount of the genetic material (29) or conversely with the number of chromosomes they contain (2). Thus, the fusion of size-fractionated microcells allows us to construct hybrids containing only a single donor cell chromosome (2,8).

Like any other genome transfer method, chromosome transfer by microcell fusion requires a selection system. The limitations of this technique, therefore, relate to the fact that most chromosomes in the mammalian cells do not carry loci for phenotypic markers that are subject to selection. However, the selectable markers transferred by CMGT (for review, see 11,15, 17) or by DNA-mediated gene transfer (24,26,31) could become integrated at random into multiple integration sites in the recipient cell genome. This property of random integration of transferred genes into nonhomologous sites can be utilized to produce clonal cell lines, each carrying the selectable marker integrated into a different chromosome (2,7,16). The chromosome carrying the selectable marker can then be transferred to a recipient cell by microcell hybridization technique (2,7,16). We have used this combination approach of gene transfer and microcell fusion to transfer Chinese hamster chromosomes 1 and 2 individually to the mouse cells (2,16 and V. Dhar and R.S. Athwal, unpublished results). The mouse cell lines harboring hamster chromosomes 1 and 2 individually have been used to map genes on these chromosomes.

RESULTS AND DISCUSSION

Preparation of Donor Cell Lines

The human gene for hprt was first transferred to Chinese hamster hprt⁻ cells by CMGT and independent gene transfer clones GT1 and GT8 (transgenote) were isolated (1) by selection in HAT (13) medium. In order to promote the integration of the transferred gene (transgenome) into the recipient cell chromosomes, transgenotes GT1 and GT8 were cultured continuously in selective medium for 30 to 40 cell generations (11,17). The results of several studies on CMGT indicate that a transgenome probably becomes integrated only into a single site in one cell rather than several transgenomes being integrated into different sites (for reviews, see 11,17). A stable transgenote thus may be composed of different cells each with a transgenome integrated into a different chromosome. In our experiments following the stable expression of human hprt, we isolated single-cell subclones GT1-1, GT1-2, and GT8-2 from GT1 and GT8, respec-

tively. The progeny of a single-cell subclone produced in this manner
would constitute a homogeneous cell population carrying the selectable
marker integrated into the same chromosome. These clonal cell lines
(GT1-1, GT1-2 and GT8-2) were then used as microcell donor in our experiments.

Microcell Preparation

   The preparation of microcells involve two distinct processes, i.e.,
induction of micronuclei formation (micronucleation) and isolation of the
individual micronuclei thus formed. The micronucleation is induced by
prolonged exposure (30 to 50 hr) of cultured cells to mitotic inhibitors
(colchicine, colcemid, nocodozole and vinblastin) (4,25). The mitotic
poisons inhibit the assembly of microtubules and thus interfere with the
spindle formation. Lack of a functional spindle leads to an aberrant
movement of chromosomes at anaphase, and the nuclear membrane reassembles
around an individual chromosome or a group of chromosomes scattered in
the cell, without the occurrence of cytokinesis (4,25). In our experiments, microcell donor cell lines GT1-1, GT1-2, and GT8-2 cultured at 50%
confluency level in 100-mm plates were treated with colchicine (1 µg/ml)
for 30 to 40 hr to induce micronucleation. The frequency of micronucleated cells under these conditions varied from 30 to 60% in different experiments. Treatment of Chinese hamster cells (V79 and Don) with colchicine (1 µg/ml) for 18 hr with subsequent cultivation in drug-free
medium increased the number of micronucleated cells to 80 to 90%. At the
same time, the micronuclei were formed with relatively shorter periods of
mitotic arrest (V. Dhar and R.S. Athwal, unpublished results). A regimen
of sequential treatment with colcemid (0.02 µg/ml) and cytochalasin B
(1 µg/ml) has also been found to increased the frequency of micronucleation in human and mouse cells (5). Additionally micronucleation required a much shorter exposure time to the mitotic inhibitors (5). The
duration of mitotic arrest is an important variable in the microcell
fusion experiments. The recovery of viable microcell hybrids has been
found to correlate inversely with the length of the mitotic arrest (5).
   Treatment of cells with dimethylsulfoxide (DMSO) has also been found
to induce micronuclei formation in several cell lines of human and hamster origin. Chinese hamster cells (V79) cultured in the medium containing DMSO (5% final concentration) formed micronuclei in 16 to 24 hr
(Figure 1). The frequency of micronucleated cells observed following
DMSO treatment varied from 60 to 80% (V. Dhar and R.S. Athwal, unpublished results). The mechanism of micronuclei formation by DMSO is not
yet clear. However, formation of multiple nuclei in the absence of
spindle microtubes and cytokinesis has been shown to occur in cells of
Dictyostelium that are treated with DMSO (9).
   Micronuclei formed in the cells can be isolated with cytochalasin B
treatment (10 µg/ml) followed by centrifugation of micronucleated
cells either attached to the solid surface (4,5,19) or in suspension by
zonal sedimentation in Ficoll gradients (2,16). In our experiments we
used the zonal sedimentation method for the isolation of Chinese hamster
microcells. This procedure provides the advantage of working with large
populations of cells (1 x 10^8 to 2 x 10^8) for each fusion experiment. A
microcell preparation constitutes a heterogeneous population of various
sizes. In order to produce hybrids containing only a single donor chromosome, microcells are size fractionated by sedimentation at unit gravity
using bovine serum albumin or Ficoll gradients (14). Different size

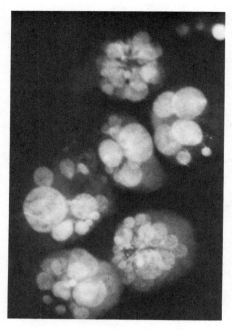

FIGURE 1. Chinese hamster micronucleated cells. Micronucleation induced by DMSO treatment.

classes can also be separated by filtration through nucleopore filters with pore diameter of 1 to 5 µg (19).

Microcells prepared from GT-1, GT1-2, and GT8-2 were size fraction- ated and fused with mouse hprt⁻ cells in a series of experiments. Microcell fusion was performed by the described procedures using poly- ethylene glycol (4) or inactivated Sendai virus (23), and microcell hybrids were isolated by selection in HAT medium (13). In one set of experiments, when the smallest size class of microcells from GT1-1 and GT1-2 were fused with mouse TG8 (hprt⁻) cells, we recovered two hybrid clones. These hybrids originated with a frequency of 10^{-6}.

In a second series of experiments, microcells prepared from GT8-2 cells were fused with mouse RAG (hprt⁻) cells. In these experiments, eight different size classes of fractionated microcells were fused sepa- rately with the recipient cells, and we recovered a total of 22 hybrids. The frequency of hybrids recovered (10^{-5}) in these experiments was an order of magnitude higher than in previous ones. The increase in the frequency of hybrid formation in the second series of experiments is attributed to shorter mitotic arrest used for the induction of micronu- cleation (data not shown).

Analysis of Microcell Hybrids

All microcell hybrids were analyzed cytologically by a sequential staining procedure involving Giemsa banding followed by Hoechst 33258 fluorescent staining (12). Mouse chromosomes display a characteristic

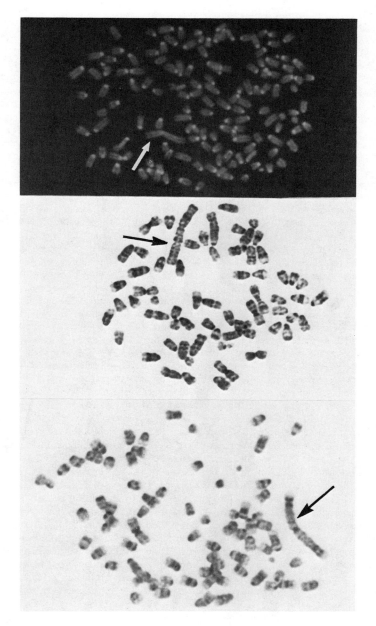

FIGURE 2. Top. Metaphase spread of microcell hybrid MCH1 stained with
Hoechst 33258. A single Chinese hamster chromosome present in a mouse
cell is identified by characteristic staining. Middle. Giemsa-banded
metaphase spread of microcell hybrid CR1. The Chinese hamster chromosome
present was identified as chromosome 1. Bottom. Giemsa-banded metaphase
spread of microcell hybrid MCH-1 Chinese hamster chromosome present in
this hybrid was identified as chromosome 2.

intense fluorescence of the centromeric region when stained with Hoechst 33258, whereas hamster chromosomes show uniform staining throughout the length of the chromosome (Figure 2, top). Thus, hamster chromosomes present in mouse cells can be readily detected (Figure 2, top). Giemsa banding was used to assign the hamster chromosome to the standard karyo-type. The number of Chinese hamster chromosomes present in different microcell hybrids varied from 1 to 12. Of a total of 24 hybrids ana-lyzed, four clones (MCH-1, MCH-2, CR-1, and CR-2) were found to contain only a single Chinese hamster chromosome (Figure 2). The chromosome present in hybrids MCH-1 and MCH-2 was identified to be hamster chromo-some 2 (Figure 2, bottom), whereas hybrids CR1 and CR2 contained hamster chromosome 1 (Figure 2, middle).

The monochromosomal hybrids, MCH-1, MCH-2, CR-1, and CR-2 were ana-lyzed further for the expression of 32 isozymes (Table 1) which could be separated between these two species. Crude extracts prepared as a high-speed supernate of cell lysate (10^8 cells/ml) in Tris-HCl buffer (pH 7.4) were electrophoresed in starch gels and stained histochemically with appropriate reaction mix to determine the presence of mouse and hamster isozymes in the hybrids (10,22). A summary of the isozyme data for all the microcell hybrids is presented in Table 1. The isozyme data shows (Table 1) the expression of only four hamster-specific enzymes (Eno-1; AK-2, PGM-2, and 6-PGD) in monochromosomal hybrids MCH-1 and MCH-2. Since these clones contained only hamster chromosome 2, the loci for these four markers therefore are assigned to this chromosome. Isozyme data (Table 1) on microcell hybrids CR1 and CR2 shows the expression of seven hamster specific enzymes (EST-D, PEP-B, PEP-S, GSR, NP, PGM-1, and ADK) associated with the presence of hamster chromosome 1. There-fore, loci for these seven markers can be assigned to this chromosome. The assignment of these loci to chromosomes 1 and 2 has also been re-ported previously from cell/cell hybridization studies (27,30).

Four single-cell subclones were isolated from each of MCH-1 and MCH-2 by selection in HAT medium. From each HAT-selected subclone, we further isolated one subclone by selection in 6-thioguanine for the loss of human hprt and consequently the Chinese hamster chromosome. All the HAT-selec-ted subclones and their back selections were analyzed again for the ex-pression of four Chinese hamster markers (Eno-1, AK-2, PGM-2, and 6-PGD) assigned to Chinese hamster chromosome 2. In the HAT-selected subclones, all four hamster-specific enzymes were expressed. However, cytogenetic analysis revealed the presence of only the long arm (9) of chromosome 2 in some clones while others contained the complete chromosome 2. These observations allow us to assign these four markers to the long arm of this chromosome. In the clones selected for the loss of hprt, a differ-ent combination of Chinese hamster markers was lost in addition to the human hprt gene: hprt was lost alone in two clones; with AK-2 in two clones; with Ak-2 and Eno-1 in two clones; with Ak-2, Eno-1, and PGM-2 in one clone; and with all four markers in one clone. Since the microcell hybrid contained only a single hamster chromosome (no 2), these results are consistent with the model that independent back-selected isolates lost different-sized fragments of the donor chromosome with the loss of hprt. The sequential loss of different markers along with the loss of hprt provides a system to determine the gene order for these markers. A tentative gene order for these markers is proposed to be 6-PGD, PGM-2, Eno-1, Ak-2 (R.S. Athwal and O.W. McBride, unpublished results). De-tailed cytogenetic analysis of back-selected clones would allow a precise assignment of each marker to the defined regions of the chromosome.

TABLE 1. Chinese hamster isozymes associated with specific chromosomes in different microcell hybrids

Microcell donor	Microcell hybrid	Hamster chromosome	Hamster-specific enzymes[a] expressed
GT8-2	CR-1	1	EST-D; PEP-S; PEP-B; GSR; NP; PGM-1; ADK
GT8-2	CR-2	1	EST-D; PEP-S; PEP-B; GSR; NP; PGM-1; ADK
GT1-2	MCH-1	2	AK-2; Eno-1; PGM-2; 6-PGD
GT1-2	MCH-2	2	AK-2; Eno-1; PGM-2; 6-PGD

[a] The following isozymes were analyzed: acid phosphatases 1 and 2 (ACP; EC 3.1.3.2); adenine phosphoribosyltransferase (APRT; EC 2.4.2.7); adenosine kinase (ADK; EC 2.7.1.20); adenylate kinases 1 and 2 (AK-1 and -2; EC 2.7.4.3); enolase 1 (ENO-1; EC 4.2.1.11), esterase D (EsTD; EC 3.1.1.1); galactokinase (Galk; EC 2.7.1.6); glutamate-oxaloacetate transaminase (GOT; EC 2.6.1.1); glucose phosphate isomerase (GP1; EC 5.3.1.9); glutathione reductase (GSR; EC 1.6.4.2); glyoxalase (GLO; EC 4.4.1.5); isocitrate dehydrogenase (IDH; EC 1.1.1.27); malic enzyme (ME; EC 1.1.1.40); mannose phosphate isomerase (MPI; EC 5.3.1.8); nucleoside phosphorylase (NP; EC 2.4.2.1); 6-phosphogluconate dehydrogenase (6-PGD; EC 1.1.1.44); phosphoglucomutases 1,2, and 3 (PGM-1, -2, and -3; EC 2.7.5.1), pyruvate kinase (PK-3; EC 2.7.1.40); peptidases A, B, C, and S (PEP-A, -B, -C, and -S; EC3.4.11), and (PEP-D; EC 3.4.13.9); superoxide dismutase (SOD-1; EC 1.15.1.1) triosephosphate isomerase (TPI; EC 5.3.1.1); hypoxanthine phosphoribosyl transferase (HPRT; EC 2.4.2.8); hexokinase (HK; EC 2.7.1.1); creatine kinase (CK; EC 2.7.3.2).

An alternate approach to the production of hybrid colonies retaining only a segment of the donor chromosome would be to induce the chromosome breaks and then select clones for the retention or loss of the selectable marker. Associated loss of the known markers then would allow determination of the gene order. Cells from monochromosomal hybrid CR-1 were X-irradiated at doses of 50 to 150 rads to induce random breaks in Chinese hamster chromosome. Following the irradiation, we isolated 32 independent single-cell clones, 15 being selected in medium containing HAT and 17 selected in 6-thioguanine. All these clones were then analyzed for the expression of Chinese hamster markers previously assigned to chromosome 1 (Table 1). Of 15 HAT-selected clones, 13 retained the expression of all seven hamster markers, and cytogenetic analysis of two of these 13 clones revealed the presence of an intact hamster chromosome 1. Of the other two clones, one showed the expression of six enzymes (Est-D, PEP-S, PEP-B, GSR, NP, and PGM-1), whereas the second retained only four markers (PEP-B, PGM-2, EST-D and ADK). Seven of 17 clones selected in 6-thioguanine for the loss of hprt lost all seven markers. Each of the other ten lost a different combination of markers along with human hprt (data not presented). These data will allow us to determine the gene order for the markers assigned to chromosome 1. Correlation of biochemical markers with chromosomal segment present in these clones will permit regional localization of these genes. Preliminary cytogenetic analysis reveals a correlation between the number of enzymes expressed in 6-thioguanine-selected clones and the size of chromosomal segment being retained.

CONCLUSIONS

Data presented in this report show the feasibility of the combination of gene transfer and microcell fusion strategy to transfer single specific chromosomes between cells. In two independent gene transfer clones, a transgenome was integrated into two different chromosomes. By randomly selecting donor clones, we were able to transfer Chinese hamster chromosomes 1 and 2 to the mouse cells. A very elegant approach, employing naturally existing Robertsonian (Rb) translocations in which one of the partner chromosome carries a selectable marker, has been utilized by Fournier and Frelinger (8) to transfer individual mouse chromosomes to the Chinese hamster cells. This selection scheme provides the advantage of identification of the donor chromosome prior to the microcell fusion experiments. An alternative approach is to design a selection scheme using dominant cloned selectable markers for integration into chromosomes of microcell donor cells. A radiolabeled probe that is specific for the transferred gene can then be used for in situ hybridization to identify the chromosome of integration. Dominant cloned procaryotic markers such as Escherichia coli xanthine guanine phosphoribosyl transferae (xgprt) are now available and can be transferred to the mammalian cells even in the presence of an analogous cellular gene (21). This technique eliminates the requirement for a mutant cell line as the recipient in these experiments.

Cell lines harboring a single chromosome of another species have obvious implications in the genetic and molecular studies. They will simplify the process of gene mapping with enhanced efficiency and resolution (28) and it will be possible to determine the gene order by deletion mapping strategy (8,28). In our experiment, the sequential loss of various markers in the subclones of a monochromosomal hybrid selected for the loss of the selectable marker allowed us to determine the gene order for four markers assigned to the long arm of Chinese hamster chromosome 2. In addition, the transfer and continuous maintenance of a single chromosome under selective pressure will be particularly helpful in studying the expression or suppression of malignant transformation. It will be possible to study the effect of a single donor chromosome on the phenotype of the recipient cells.

Chromosomes of different species often differ in size or in the amount of DNA. The monochromosomal hybrids thus can be used to purify a large population of transferred chromosomes by fractionation procedures. Thus, a DNA probe specific for a chromosome or segment of a chromosome can be prepared for cloning experiments. This will facilitate the construction of subgenomic clone libraries for eucaryotic organisms and, therefore, the process for the isolation of specific genes will be simplified.

ACKNOWLEDGEMENTS

This work was supported in part by grant CD124 from the American Cancer Society and March of Dimes Birth Defects Foundation grant no. 5-267. We greatly appreciate the help provided by Helen Beale-Holcombe and Michelle Vitale in the preparation of this manuscript.

REFERENCES

1. Athwal RS, McBride OW (1977): Proc Natl Acad Sci USA 74:2943
2. Athwal RS, McBride OW (1980): In: Emergent Techniques (Rubenstein I, Genenback B, Phillips, R, Green E, eds), Minneapolis: University of Minnesota Press, p 153
3. Davidson RL, O'Malley KA, Wheller TB (1976): Somatic Cell Genet 2: 271
4. Ege T, Ringertz NR (1974): Exp Cell Res 87:378
5. Fournier REK (1981): Proc Natl Acad Sci USA 78:6349
6. Fournier REK, Ruddle FH (1977): Proc Natl Acad Sci USA 74:319
7. Fournier REK, Ruddle FH (1977): Proc Natl Acad Sci USA 74:3937
8. Fournier REK, Frelinger JA (1982): Mol Cell Biol 2:526
9. Fukui Y (1980): J Cell Biol 86:181
10. Harris H, Hopkins DA (1976): Handbook of Enzyme Electrophoresis in in Human Genetics, New York: Elsevier
11. Klobutcher LA, Ruddle FH (1981): Annu Rev Biochem 50:533
12. Kozak CA, Lawrence JB, Ruddle FH (1977): Exp Cell Res 105:109
13. Littlefield JW (1964): Science 145:709
14. McBride OW, Peterson EA (1970): J Cell Biol 47:132
15. McBride OW, Athwal RS (1977): Proc Brookhaven Symp Biol 29:116
16. McBride OW, Athwal RS (1979): In: Concepts of the Structure and Function of DNA, Chromatin and Chromosomes (Dion AS, ed), Miami, Florida: Symposia Specialists, p 229
17. McBride OW, Peterson JL (1980): Annu Rev Genet 14:321
18. McKusick VA, Ruddle FH (1977): Science 196:390
19. McNeill CA, Brown RL (1980): Proc Natl Acad Sci USA 77:5394
20. Minna JD, Coon HG (1974): Nature 252:401
21. Mulligan RC, Berg P (1981): Proc Natl Acad Sci USA 78:2027
22. Nichols EA, Ruddle FH (1973): J Histochem Cytochem 21:1066
23. Okada Y, Tadokero, J (1963): Exp Cell Res 32:417
24. Perucho M, Hanahan D, Wigler M (1980): Cell 22:309
25. Ringertz NR, Savage RE (1976): Cell Hybrids, New York: Academic Press
26. Robbins DM, Ripley S, Henderson A, Axel R (1981): Cell 23:29
27. Roberts M, Ruddle FH (1980): Exp Cell Res 127:47
28. Ruddle FH (1981): Nature 294:115
29. Sekiguchi T, Shelton K, Ringertz NR (1978): Exp Cell Res 113:247
30. Stalling RL, Siciliano (1981): Somatic Cell Genet 7:683
31. Wigler M, Sweet R, Sim GK, Wold B, Pellicer A, Lacy E, Maniatis T, Silverstein S, Axel R (1979): Cell 16:777
32. Worton R, Duff C, Flintoff W (1980): Mol Cell Biol 1:330

Gene Transfer and Cancer, edited by M. L. Pearson
and N. L. Sternberg. Raven Press, New York © 1984.

Gene Transfer in CHO Cells

Irene Abraham and Michael M. Gottesman

Laboratory of Molecular Biology and Molecular Cell Genetics Section, National Cancer Institute, National Institutes of Health, Bethesda, Maryland 20205

ABSTRACT. The introduction of foreign genes into animal cells is a powerful tool for studying gene function and regulation. Using Chinese hamster ovary (CHO) cells as host cells because of the wide array of available mutants and because of their stable karyotype we have begun studying gene transfer by the DNA–CaPO$_4$ method. Thymidine kinase (Tk) negative CHO cells can be transformed with whole genomic CHO Tk$^+$ DNA (frequency 10^{-7}) or with the herpes simplex virus (HSV)-tk gene cloned in pBR322 (pX1-tk) (frequency 10^{-5}). CHO HSV-Tk$^+$ transformants were very stable, and in several clones HSV-tk gene copies were found integrated in high-molecular-weight DNA, as were unselected cotransforming DNA sequences. The transformation frequency can be increased by digesting pX1-tk with BamHI. The transformation frequency can be further increased to 5 x 10^{-3} by transforming the cells with a pBR322 vector containing both tk and a portion of SV40. Wild-type CHO cells can be transformed at a similar frequency by the recombinant pSV2-gpt plasmid, which carries the bacterial gene gpt (xanthine–guanine phosphoribosyl transferase) and SV40 sequences. Of the cells transformed with the HSV-tk gene and the Eco-gpt gene, 80% of the clones selected for growth on HAT could also subsequently be grown on MXHAT, indicating cotransformation of the unselected gpt sequences with tk. These results suggest that the pSV2-vector system might be useful for enhancing transformation of single-copy genomic sequences in CHO cells.

INTRODUCTION

CHO cells have been extensively used for genetic studies probing the structure and organization of the mammalian genome. In our laboratory we are studying mutants conferring resistance to cAMP and mutants affecting tubulin and microtubule structure in these cells. We would like to transfer unpurified mutant and wild-type genes between different lines of CHO cells by transfer of whole genomic DNA. This transfer will allow study of the regulation of these genes in various CHO backgrounds and also facilitate cloning of these genes through gene rescue.

As a model system for gene transfer in CHO cells, we have initially studied the transfer of the tk gene from HSV into CHO cells using the CaPO$_4$ method (2,12), and selecting for transformants in HAT media (11). The characteristics of this system have been reported in detail (1).

In the studies reported here, we used a plasmid derived from pBR322 that carries the HSV-tk gene (pX1-tk) [kindly given to us by L. Enquist (5)]. All transformations were done with calf thymus DNA or CHO DNA as carrier DNA. After transformation with pX1-tk plasmid DNA, several independent HAT^R colonies were selected and studied for the presence of the tk gene and the stability of the expressed HAT^R phenotype. Cotransformation of unselected DNA sequences was also studied. As described below, stable transformation and cotransformation of CHO cells was observed, albeit at a frequency somewhat less than that seen with mouse L cells. With the goal of improving transformation frequency, we also studied the effect of the presence of sequences from SV40 in the plasmid containing the tk gene.

RESULTS AND DISCUSSION

Our initial results indicated that Tk^- CHO cells (sent to us by L. Siminovitch) can be readily transformed with the tk-gene-containing plasmid, pX1-tk. The DNA-$CaPO_4$ precipitate was left on the cells for 16 to 24 hr (4), and the medium was then replaced with selective HAT media. Treatment of cells with dimethysulfoxide, DEAE-dextran, or high serum concentration, methods that have been recommended by other laboratories, did not improve transformation frequency in the CHO system. Transformation of 5×10^5 cells per 10-cm dish with 0.5 µg purified pX1-tk plasmid and 20 µg calf thymus DNA resulted in a transformation frequency of up to 2×10^{-4} Tk^+ transformants per cell. Comparison with mouse L Tk^- cells (given to us by R. Axel) demonstrated that CHO cells have a 50-fold lower frequency of transformation to HAT^R than L cells.

We have found that simply digesting the pX1-tk plasmid with BamHI restriction enzyme before transformation results in an over 100-fold increase in the transformation frequency of CHO cells, when compared with the uncut pX1-tk plasmid (Table 1). The basis of this effect is not clear, but we are currently investigating whether the effect is specific to this particular plasmid or whether it might be more general.

Many transformants of mouse L cells, transformed with DNA for different genes such as aprt (13), tk (9) and methotrexate resistance (6), have been characterized as generally unstable in that they lose their ability to grow in selective medium after being grown for a period of

TABLE 1. Transformation of CHO Tk^- cells with pX1-tk, with or without digestion with BamHI[a]

Transforming DNA	HAT^R colonies/µg/cell	Total cells
pX1-tk, undigested	4×10^{-6}	2.3×10^6
pX1-tk, digested with BamHI	5×10^{-4}	2.5×10^6

[a] 2.5×10^5 CHO Tk^- cells per 10-cm plate were transformed with 0.5 µg uncut pX1-tk or pBR322/SV-0/tk DNA and 20 µg calf thymus carrier DNA in the form of a $CaPO_4$ precipitate. DNA was removed after 18 hr and replaced with HAT medium. Cells were stained and colonies were counted after 2 weeks (1). These results are the average of two separate experiments.

time in nonselective medium. Because this seemed a frequent attribute of transformed cells, we examined the stability of some of our HAT[R] colonies. CHO Tk[-] cells were transformed with pX1-tk DNA cut with the restriction enzyme BamHI (which cuts the 3.5-kb tk gene fragment free from the pBR322 plasmid); calf thymus DNA was used as carrier. HAT[R] colonies were picked and grown on HAT medium for 40 (four colonies) or 75 days (one colony). These independently derived clones were then grown on nonselective HT media (media identical to HAT but lacking aminopterin; both Tk[+] and Tk[-] cells can survive on this media) and tested for retention of the HAT[R] phenotype at various times after this switch to nonselective media. Cells were plated on HAT and HT media and stained for colonies after 10 days. HAT[R] colonies would grow on both media; revertants that had lost the HAT[R] phenotype would grow only on HT media. The results indicated that of the five independent colonies tested, all were stable during a period of 30 days. In preliminary tests, another HAT[R] transformant clone was found to be relatively unstable. Therefore, our evidence to date indicates that five of six independently derived colonies showed a high level of stability of their HAT[R] phenotype. While these studies were not done in parallel with mouse L cells, they suggest that CHO cells transformed with DNA may be relatively more stable for their selected phenotype.

These five independently selected HAT[R] colonies, transformed with the 3.5-kb Tk BamHI fragment were also studied for the molecular presence of the tk gene by Southern analysis (10). DNA was isolated from these five colonies and cut with the restriction enzyme HindIII. This enzyme does not cut within the 3.5-kb fragment. The DNA was electrophoresed on an agarose gel, denatured, transferred to a nitrocellulose filter, and hybridized with the nick-translated, ^{32}P-labeled 3.5-kb tk gene fragment. Hybridization occurred to the DNAs of all the HAT[R] colonies, but not to HindIII-digested DNA from the parent Tk[-] cell line. All the hybridization to DNA from the HAT[R] lines was of a molecular weight higher than 3.5 kb, indicating that the tk gene or genes present in these cells no longer exists as the free 3.5-kb fragment. These results are consistent with the tk gene having been incorporated into higher molecular weight DNA: either carrier or CHO chromosomal DNA or both. Four of the HAT[R] transformed colonies showed multiple bands that hybridized to the tk probe, suggesting the presence of multiple tk genes per cell.

In another experiment CHO Tk[-] cells were transformed with HSV tk gene DNA as well as calf thymus carrier DNA and DNA from the plasmid pSR1 (14). After selection on HAT, Southern analysis of two of these colonies showed the presence of both the pBR322 and the pSR1 sequences, indicating that CHO cells can be cotransformed for unselected DNA sequences along with the sequences for which the colonies are selected.

We performed another cotransformation experiment to determine whether cotransformed sequences would be functional in CHO cells. For this purpose we used the pSV2-gpt plasmid (7). This plasmid carries the bacterial gene Eco-gpt (xanthine-guanine phosphoribosyltransferase) in a background of SV40 and pBR322 sequences. The SV40 sequences present include the origin and the 72-bp repeats as well as sites for the small t intervening sequence and sites for polyadenylation of mRNA and termination. The plasmid is constructed so that the Eco-gpt gene can be expressed in mammalian cells. The presence of this enzyme allows the mammalian cells to survive de novo purine synthesis inhibition by aminopterin and mycophenolic acid in the presence of exogenously added xanthine. We have previously shown that CHO cells can be transformed with pSV2-gpt alone $(3.6 \times 10^{-4}$ colonies/µg/cell) (1).

Tk$^-$ CHO cells were transformed simultaneously with pX1-tk and pSV2-gpt. Transformants were selected in HAT medium. HAT^R clones were transferred to either HAT or MXHAT (mycophenolic acid, 25 μg/ml; xanthine, 1.6×10^{-3} M; hypoxanthine, 10^{-4} M; aminopterin, 4.5×10^{-6} M; thymidine, 4×10^{-5} M) and studied for continued growth. In this cotransformation experiment, more than 80% of the colonies grew on both HAT and MXHAT, indicating the functional cotransformation of the Eco-gpt gene. In no cases did cells transformed with pX1-tk alone survive on MXHAT medium. This shows that CHO cells selected for one transferred marker can simultaneously take up other DNA and can subsequently be selected for this other marker with a high percentage of success.

The stability of CHO gene transferants suggested that the introduced genes were present in a stable form, as would be expected if they were integrated in the host chromosomes. We have begun a preliminary study of alterations in the CHO karyotype after gene transfer that might occur if integration caused chromosome breaks or occurred at sites of chromosome breakage. The CHO karyotype in a particular subline is relatively stable, and in the Tk$^-$ line used here, the modal chromosome number is stable at 23 chromosomes. In three HAT^R colonies studied, one showed the normal modal chromosome number of 23, one showed a modal number of 24, indicating an extra chromosome, and one showed a modal number of 22, indicating a loss of a chromosome. Robins and coworkers (8) have shown that after gene transfer in Buffalo rat liver cells the new DNA is sometimes found integrated at the site of a chromosome rearrangement. This phenomenon of chromosome rearrangement and DNA integration may also be occurring in CHO cells, but much more extensive karyotypic analysis would be needed to confirm these observations.

We next studied CHO Tk$^-$ cells for their ability to be transformed by whole genomic Tk$^+$ DNA. For this study, high-molecular-weight DNA was isolated from Tk$^-$ and Tk$^+$ CHO cells. CHO Tk$^-$ cells were transformed with these DNAs, and HAT^R colonies were selected at a frequency of 10^{-7}. No colonies were HAT^R after transfer of Tk$^-$ DNA (frequency less than 2×10^{-8}). In a parallel experiment using Tk$^+$ DNA, mouse L cells were transformed at a frequency of 10^{-6}.

Transformation of CHO cells with whole genomic DNA is therefore possible, but the frequency (10^{-7}) is quite low. This frequency is similar to or less than the rate of spontaneous mutation for many of the dominant mutations that we would like to transfer. In order to be able to distinguish transformants from spontaneous mutations, it would be helpful to be able to transform at a higher frequency. One way to attempt this is to utilize sequences shown to increase transformation in other systems.

We have evidence that the frequency of transformation of CHO Tk$^-$ cells with pX1-tk plasmid DNA can be increased in the presence of sequences from the virus SV40. Cappechi (3) showed that microinjection of the chimeric plasmid pBR322/SV-0/tk, which contains the HSV-tk gene, pBR322 sequences, and SV40 origin sequences, including the 72-bp repeats, gave increased frequencies of transformation of mouse Tk$^-$ L cells as compared to microinjection with the HSV-tk gene simply cloned into pBR322 (a clone equivalent to the plasmid pX1-tk). Utilizing these two uncut plasmids in the CaPO$_4$-DNA mediated transformation of Tk$^-$ CHO cells, we have demonstrated a 200-fold increase in the frequency of transformation of these cells by pBR322/SV-0/tk as compared to pX1-tk (Table 2). We are currently identifying the sequences responsible for this effect and determining whether these sequences can be used to enhance transformation with other genes.

TABLE 2. Transformation of CHO-Tk⁻ cells[a]

Transforming DNA	HAT^R colonies/µg/cell	Total cells
pX1-tk	2.4×10^{-5}	1.5×10^6
pBR322/SV-0/tk	4.8×10^{-3}	2.0×10^6

[a] The procedure was as described in Table 1, except cells were initially plated at 5×10^5.

CONCLUSION

We have shown that CHO cells can be transformed with both cloned and whole genomic DNAs. The transformant cells from DNA-mediated gene transfer using cloned DNA are relatively stable, and their frequency is about 50-fold lower than for comparable transfer into mouse L Tk⁻ cells. Southern analysis shows that the transformed DNA is incorporated into higher molecular weight DNA and appears to undergo some rearrangement after transformation. Unselected DNA can be cotransformed with selected DNA, and in some cases, unselected cotransformed DNA is present in a functional state (Eco-gpt gene of pSV2-gpt).

The frequency of transformation in CHO cells with the cloned HSV-tk gene, appears to be influenced by the presence of other DNA sequences. A striking increase in the frequency of transformation is associated with the presence of tk on a plasmid pBR322/SV-0/tk containing sequences near the origin of SV40. The exact DNA sequences responsible for this effect have not been identified. We have also shown that using pX1-tk plasmids digested with the restriction enzyme BamHI increases the frequency of transformation in these cells. The basis of these effects is unknown, but they may be useful in our attempts to increase the DNA transformation frequency with whole genomic DNA in CHO cells.

REFERENCES

1. Abraham I, Tyagi JS, Gottesman MM (1982): Somatic Cell Genet 8:23
2. Bacchetti S, Graham FL (1977): Proc Natl Acad Sci USA 74:1590
3. Capecchi MR (1980): Cell 22:479
4. Corsaro C, Pearson M (1981): Somatic Cell Genet 7:603
5. Enquist LW, Vande Woude GF, Wagner M, Smiley JR, Summers WC (1979): Gene (Amst.) 7:335
6. Lewis WH, Srinivasan PR, Stokoe N, Siminovitch L (1980): Somatic Cell Genet 6:333
7. Mulligan RC, Berg P (1981): Proc. Natl. Acad. Sci. USA 78:2072
8. Robins DM, Ripley S, Henderson AS, Axel R (1981): Cell 23:29
9. Scangos GA, Huttner KM, Juricek DK, Ruddle FH (1981): Mol Cell Biol 1:111
10. Southern EM (1975): J Mol Biol 98:503
11. Szybalska EH, Szybalski W (1962): Proc Natl Acad Sci USA 48:2026
12. Wigler M, Silverstein S, Lee, L-S, Pellicer A, Cheng Y, Axel R (1977): Cell 11:223
13. Wigler M, Pellicer A, Silverstein S, Axel R, Urlaub G, Chasin L (1979): Proc Natl Acad Sci USA 76:1373
14. Yamamoto T, Jay G, Pastan I (1980): Proc Natl Acad Sci USA 77:176

Gene Transfer and Cancer, edited by M. L. Pearson and N. L. Sternberg. Raven Press, New York © 1984.

DNA-Mediated Transfer of Genes into Mammalian Cells: Evidence for Homologous Recombination Between Transfected DNAs

B. Pomerantz, M. Naujokas, W. Muller, A.-M. Mes, M. Featherstone, P. Moreau, and J. A. Hassell

Department of Microbiology and Immunology, McGill University, Montreal, Quebec, H3A 2B4 Canada

ABSTRACT. We have performed an extensive analysis of the fate and final structure of recombinant plasmid molecules introduced into rat cells by DNA-mediated transfection. We found that the plasmid DNA invariably becomes integrated within the genome of the transformed cell and often is arranged as a head-to-tail tandem. Examination of the factors that might promote the formation of such integrated structures revealed that, while plasmids capable of replicating in the transfected host transformed them at higher frequency, the capacity to replicate did not insure integration of the plasmid as a tandem. Rather, the use of relatively high concentration of transforming DNA (100 to 1000 ng of recombinant plasmid DNA per 5×10^5 cells) facilitated the frequent isolation of transformed cell lines with tandemly arranged, integrated plasmid sequences. Because the fraction of dimers or multimers of the recombinant plasmid DNA present in the population of molecules used to transform the cells was far lower than the frequency of isolation of transformed cell lines bearing tandem insertions of plasmid sequences, we hypothesize that tandems arise by homologous recombination between plasmid molecules either prior or subsequent to integration within cellular DNA. To determine whether homologous recombination can occur after transfection with DNA, we made use of pairs of recombinant plasmids that bear physically separated mutations within their transforming sequences. Transfection with pairs of such mutant genomes resulted in transformation of the recipient cells at high frequency. By contrast, each mutant alone was incapable of causing transformation. Moreover, examination of the plasmid sequences within several independent transformants revealed the presence of "recombinant" DNA fragments that could only have been generated by homologous recombination.

INTRODUCTION

Polyoma virus is a member of the papovavirus group that includes among its members simian virus 40 and the papilloma viruses. It was isolated from C3H mice by Ludwig Gross and is commonly found as an apparently harmless passenger in both wild and laboratory-reared mice. Polyoma virus lytically infects mouse cell strains and lines in culture and transforms a wide variety of rodent cells. The virus is also tumor-igenic in rodents, inducing both carcinomas and sarcomas. The oncogenic potential of the virus resides in its DNA, and the maintenance of cellular transformation is mediated by proteins encoded therein. Only part of the viral genome, the transforming region, is required for oncogenicity in vivo or transformation in vitro. This region encodes two complete proteins, small T-antigen and middle T-antigen, and the amino-terminal half of large T-antigen. The entire large T-antigen molecule is required to initiate viral DNA replication, and this protein also acts as a repressor of early gene transcription. Middle T-antigen is the transforming protein of the virus, while the role of small T-antigen in either lytic or transforming infections remains mysterious.

Infection of nonpermissive cells at high multiplicity (100 to 1000 plaque-forming units per cell) with polyoma virus leads to the stable transformation of from 0.1 to 1.0% of the cell population (7). Such transformed cells harbor integrated viral genomes, and in more than 50% of the lines examined, the viral sequences are arranged in a head-to-tail tandem array (1). When these transformed cells are fused by cell hybridization techniques to permissive mouse cells, the viral genome is excised and virus progeny produced (8). We are interested in utilizing these features of the virus-cell system to implant and later retrieve foreign genes from transformed cells. This capacity could facilitate studies of mutagenesis and recombination in mammalian cells. Because the manipulations leading to the establishment of transformed cells as well as the recovery of excised viral sequences are more readily performed with recombinant plasmid DNAs, we investigated whether the outcome of transformation with polyoma virus (viz., the frequent integration of the viral genome as a head-to-tail tandem structure) could be duplicated by transfection with plasmid-cloned, viral DNA.

RESULTS

Transformation With Polyoma Virus Plasmid DNAs

The formation of tandemly arranged viral genomes in transformed cells is thought to result from the integration of long tandem arrays of viral sequences, and the latter are believed to arise from a rolling-circle type replicational mechanism (2). This model suggests that replication of the viral genome is a prerequisite to the formation of tandem insertions. Indeed, Della-Valle and his colleagues (3) have provided evidence that only viral DNA capable of replication will give rise to transformed cells harboring tandemly arranged viral genomes. Moreover, they observed that viral DNA capable of replicating in mouse cells transformed rat cells at a 20-fold higher frequency than viral DNA defective in its capacity to replicate. Their results apparently contradict observations made previously by us that showed no relationship between the transforming potential of cloned viral DNAs and their capacity to encode large T-antigen of polyoma virus (4). The latter protein is required to initiate viral DNA replication but is not essential for the maintenance of transformation (8). We therefore examined in greater detail the relationship between the specific transforming activity of a recombinant plasmid and its capacity to replicate in the cell line acting as recipient. We utilized a clone of F2408 rat cells, named Rat-1, for these experiments (4). Polyoma virus DNA replicates poorly within Rat-1 cells by comparison to permissive mouse cells (W. Muller and J. Hassell, unpublished data). To rigorously test the relationship between the replicational capacity of a recombinant plasmid and its transforming potential, we constructed a variety of recombinant DNAs whose compositions are presented in Table 1. Two different plasmids,

TABLE 1. The composition of polyoma virus-plasmid recombinants

Recombinant plasmid	Composition
pdPB1A	Polyoma virus DNA cloned at its BamHI site in PML2
pdPR1A	Polyoma virus DNA cloned at its EcoRI site in PML2
pdPtsA	Polyoma virus mutant DNA (tsA) cloned at its BamHI site in PML2
pPB1A	Polyoma virus DNA cloned at its BamHI site in pBR322
pPR1A	Polyoma virus DNA cloned at its EcoRI site in pBR322
pPtsA	Polyoma virus mutant DNA (tsA) cloned at its BamHI site in pBR322
pPBR2	The small transforming BamHI to EcoRI fragment of polyoma virus DNA cloned in pBR322
pPdlBgK	A derivative of pPBR2 from which sequences between the BglI and KpnI sites of polyoma virus DNA have been deleted. The deleted sequences include those required for viral DNA replication
ptk1	The thymidine kinase gene of herpes simplex virus cloned in pBR322
pPH1-8	The HindIII-1 fragment of polyoma virus DNA cloned in pBR322
pPdl15	A derivative of pPBR2 which has a 10-bp deletion at the SstI site in polyoma virus DNA at nucleotide number 1373
pPdl3	A derivative of pPBR2 which has a 15-bp deletion at the PstI site in polyoma virus DNA at nucleotide number 484
pPdl1-8	A derivative of pPH1-8 which has a 20-bp deletion at the PvuII site in polyoma virus DNA at nucleotide number 1144
pPin2	A derivative of pPH1-8 which has a 4-bp insertion at the AvaI site at nucleotide number 657 in polyoma virus DNA
pPin67	A derivative of pPH1-8 which has a 4-bp insertion at the AvaI site at nucleotide number 1016 in polyoma virus DNA

pBR322 and PML2, were employed as vectors, and both wild-type and tsA mutant polyoma virus DNA were cloned within each of these. PML2 is a deletion derivative of pBR322. When replication-competent viral DNA is cloned in PML2, it will replicate in mammalian cells 10- to 20-fold more efficiently than that same DNA cloned in pBR322 (5; W. Muller and J. Hassell, unpublished data). The transforming activity and replicational capacity of each DNA species shown in Table 1 was measured and the results are displayed in Table 2.

Comparison of the specific transforming activity of polyoma virus-pBR322 recombinant DNAs capable of synthesizing functional large T-antigen (pPB1A and pPtsA at 32°C) with that of pBR322 recombinants incapable

TABLE 2. The transforming activity of various polyoma virus-plasmid DNAs[a]

Plasmid	Temperature (°C)	Capacity to replicate in Rat-1 cells	Capacity to produce functional T-antigen	Specific transforming activity (foci/µg)
Experiment 1				
pdPB1A	37	–	+	3,444
pPR1A	37	–	–	2,893
Experiment 2				
pPtsA	32	–	+	8,019
pPtsA	38.5	–	–	5,540
Experiment 3				
pdPB1A	37	+	+	15,000
pdPR1A	37	–	–	2,350
pdPtsA	32	+	+	15,000
pdPtsA	38.5	–	–	2,500

[a]Rat-1 cells were transfected in triplicate with recombinant plasmid DNAs at three different DNA concentrations (from 1 to 50 ng/5 x 10^5 cells). The medium was changed every 3 days, and foci were scored 2 to 3 wk post transfection. To measure the replicational capacity of each DNA species in Rat-1 cells, 1 µg of recombinant plasmid DNA was used to inoculate 10^5 cells in duplicate. At 48 hr post transfection, low-molecular-weight DNA was isolated and digested with DpnI and BclI. DpnI cleaves only methylated DNA, or the input plasmid DNA, whereas BclI cleaves only unmethylated DNA, which arises by replication. Because the plasmids used carry only one BclI site, replication can be assayed as the appearance of linear plasmid DNA.

of producing functional large T-antigen (pPR1A and pPtsA at 38.5°C) revealed no significant difference. None of the aforementioned plasmids
are capable of replicating in Rat-1 cells (our limit of detection is 0.1
molecules of replicated DNA per cell). By contrast, all the polyoma
virus-PML2 recombinant DNAs capable of replicating in Rat-1 cells (pdPB1A
and pdPtsA at 32°C) transformed these cells at a much higher frequency
(approximately 6-fold) by comparison to their replication-incompetent
counterparts (pdPR1A and pdPtsA at 38.5°C). Two conclusions can be drawn
from these observations. First, large T-antigen facilitates transformation indirectly by promoting replication of the transfecting DNA. Recombinant plasmids that encode large T-antigen but which fail to replicate
because they carry pBR322 sequences (viz., pPB1A) also fail to transform
Rat-1 cells at enhanced frequencies (Table 2). Second, the capacity of a
recombinant plasmid to replicate in the transfected host is directly correlated with its transforming potential. Replication-competent plasmids
may transform cells at elevated frequencies by providing altered substrates for integration (i.e., replicative intermediates) or by effectively increasing through replication the number of copies of plasmid DNA
per cell.

The Occurrence of Tandem Insertions in Cell Lines Transformed with Various Recombinant Plasmid DNAs

To determine whether there is a relationship between the replicative
capacity of a recombinant plasmid and its propensity to become arranged
as a tandem within transformed cell DNA, we transfected Rat-1 cells with
either replication-competent or replication-incompetent DNA. The arrangement of the plasmid sequences within the DNA of many of the resulting transformed cell lines was then assessed. Briefly, the cellular DNA
was digested with restriction endonucleases that have only one cleavage
site in the transforming plasmid DNA (so called one-cut enzymes). The
resulting fragments were fractionated through agarose gels and then
transferred to nitrocellulose sheets (Southern blotting). Hybridization
with radiolabeled plasmid sequences then allowed detection by autoradiography of those fragments homologous to the probe. The release of DNA
fragments from cellular DNA that comigrate with unit-length, linear forms
of the transforming plasmid DNA indicates that the restriction endonuclease cleavage site is tandemly repeated in a head-to-tail fashion within
the integrated plasmid sequences. The release of unit-length plasmid DNA
from the cell's genome after cleavage with several different one-cut restriction endonucleases provides confidence that the plasmid DNA is arranged as at least a partial head-to-tail tandem repeat within cellular
DNA.

The data from such an analysis of 58 independent transformed cell
lines is shown in Table 3. They reveal no correspondence between the
replicative potential of a recombinant plasmid and the likelihood that
cell lines transformed with its DNA will contain tandem insertions of
the plasmid sequences. For example, among eight independent transformed
cell lines derived by transfection with pPR1A DNA (a plasmid incapable
of replicating in Rat-1 cells), four carried tandemly repeated pPR1A
genomes integrated within their DNA. By comparison, pdB1A DNA, a replication-competent plasmid, yielded no transformed cell lines with tandems
among seven lines examined. Upon careful inspection of our results we
noted that the occurrence of tandems in the various transformed cell
lines was correlated with the amount of transforming DNA used to inoculate the cultures. High concentrations of transforming DNA (500 to 1000

TABLE 3. The occurrence of head-to-tail, tandemly integrated
recombinant plasmid genomes in transformed cells[a]

Transforming DNA	Nanograms DNA per 5 x 10⁵ cells	Capacity of transforming DNA to		Frequency with which tandems occur
		Replicate	Encode large T-antigen	
pPBR2	1000	−	−	0.57 (4/7)
pPdlBgK	1000	−	−	0.43 (3/7)
pPR1A	1000	−	−	0.50 (4/8)
pPB1A	1000	−	+	0.43 (3/7)
pdPB1A	2	+	+	0.00 (0/7)
pdPR1A	3	−	−	0.00 (0/8)
ptk1	25	−	−	0.00 (0/8)
pPBR2*	500	−	−	0.66 (4/6)
ptk1*	5	−	−	0.17 (1/6)

[a] Rat-1 cells were transfected with recombinant plasmids at the concentrations indicated. In one case, denoted by asterisks, the two DNAs were
co-transfected. DNA from the various transformed cell lines was digested
with at least two one-cut restriction enzymes and analyzed by Southern
blot hybridization for the presence of tandemly integrated plasmid genomes. The numbers in parentheses refer to the fraction of cell lines
with tandems (number of cell lines with tandems/number of cell lines
examined).

ng/5 x 10⁵ cells) yielded transformed cell lines which frequently carried
tandemly arranged copies of the transforming species (40 to 60% of cell
lines examined), regardless of the replicational capacity of the transforming DNA. To test this directly we transfected a thymidine kinase
negative (Tk⁻) derivative of the Rat-1 cell line, named Rat-2, with two
DNA species simultaneously, one at high concentrations (pPBR2; 500 ng/
5 x 10⁵ cells), and the other at low concentrations (ptk1; 5 ng/5 x 10⁵
cells). We selected for the Tk⁺ phenotype and then independently
assessed the status of the integrated ptk1 and pPBR2 DNA in six of the
resulting cotransformants with probes unique to each plasmid DNA. The
results presented at the bottom of Table 3 show that the DNA species
present in highest concentration during transfection becomes integrated
within cellular DNA as a tandem in 66% of the cell lines examined. By
contrast, only one among these same six lines carried tandemly arranged
copies of ptk1 DNA (the DNA whose expression was selected for and which

was present in the lowest concentration during transfection). All of
the recombinant DNAs utilized for these experiments were isolated from
the recA⁻ E. coli strain HB101. The fraction of dimers or multimers of
plasmid DNA present in the various DNA preparations in no case exceeded
5% of the total DNA population. Moreover, supercoiled DNA (90% supercoiled and 10% circular in the worst preparations) was used to establish
the various transformed cell lines reported here. Therefore, it is very
unlikely that the preferential integration of multimer supercoiled or
circular species of the recombinant plasmids gave rise to the different
cell lines carrying tandems. Instead the relationship between the concentration of transforming DNA and the occurrence of tandems in transformed cell lines suggests that tandems arise by homologous recombination between plasmid molecules either prior or subsequent to their integration within cellular DNA.

Homologous Recombinations Between Transfected DNAs

To determine whether homologous recombination can occur after transfection of mammalian cells with DNA, we made use of pairs of polyoma
virus-plasmid recombinant DNAs that bear physically separated mutations
within their transforming sequences (6). The transforming region of
polyoma virus DNA encodes two complete proteins, small T-antigen and
middle T-antigen, and a portion (the amino-terminal half) of large T-
antigen. Only middle T-antigen is required to convert normal cell lines
in culture to the transformed phenotype (4,9). We have constructed a
variety of mutations within the polyoma virus sequences of recombinant
plasmids and derived mutants from such manipulations that bear lesions
(insertions or deletions) in middle T-antigen coding sequences (6).
Many of these mutant DNAs are incapable of transforming Rat-1 cells in
culture. We reasoned that if homologous recombination could occur between the mutations borne by different nontransforming mutant DNAs during DNA-mediated transfection, then wild-type genomes could result. The
latter when integrated and expressed should yield wild-type middle T-antigen and result in the malignant transformation of the cell. Moreover,
we expected that the greater the distance between the mutations carried
by the mutant pairs, the greater would be the frequency of occurrence of
foci of transformed cells. The outcome of an experiment of this sort is
illustrated in Table 4. Transfection of Rat-1 cells with each mutant
DNA alone (1000 ng of mutant DNA per 5 x 10⁵ cells) yielded no foci. By
contrast, transfection with mixtures of two mutant DNAs (1000 ng of each
species per 5 x 10⁵ cells) yielded a large number of foci, and the greater
the distance between the mutations borne by the mutant DNA pairs, the
higher was the frequency of occurrence of foci (Table 4). As a control,
two wild-type recombinant plasmid DNAs were also tested for transforming
potential. The use of 1000 ng of each of these DNAs yielded approximately 500 foci. By comparison, from 20 to 100 foci resulted from
transfection with pairs of mutant DNAs. We have isolated a total of six
transformed cell lines that resulted from transfection with two pairs of
mutant DNAs (three lines from the cross pPd13 x pPdl1-8 and three lines
from the cross pPin2 x pPin67) and examined their DNA for "recombinant"
fragments. In all six lines, recombinant restriction endonuclease fragments were found that could only have been generated by homologous recombination between the transfected mutant DNAs. Moreover, immunoprecipitation of the polyoma virus T-antigens resident in these six lines
revealed the presence of the wild-type middle and small T-antigens.

TABLE 4. Transformation with mixtures of mutant DNAs

Recombinant Plasmid	Distance between mutations (bp)	Average no. foci/dish
pPdl15	-	0
pPdl3	-	0
pPdl1-8	-	0
pPin2	-	0
pPin67	-	0
pPin2 + pPin67	359	21
pPdl3 + pPdl1-8	660	28
pPdl15 + pPdl3	889	98
pPH1-8	-	500
pPBR2	-	500

Therefore, it is very unlikely that the phenotype of these lines can be accounted for by complementation. These results show that homologous recombination does occur during DNA-mediated transfection and that it occurs at relatively high frequency.

CONCLUSION

We have sought to determine the mechanism of formation of head-to-tail, tandemly arranged plasmid sequences in the DNA of transformed cells. We found that the occurrence of tandems correlated with the concentration of transforming DNA used during transfection and not with the replicative capacity of this DNA. Therefore, it is unlikely that tandem arrays generated by replication are a precursor to integrated plasmid DNA. Instead we propose that tandems arise by homologous recombination between plasmid DNA molecules either prior or, less likely, subsequent to integration within cellular DNA. Our data suggest that the recombination frequency is high and can account for the high frequency of tandemly arranged plasmid insertions found in transformed cells.

ACKNOWLEDGEMENTS

This research was supported by funds from the National Cancer Institute and the Medical Research Council of Canada. J.A.H. is a research scholar of the National Cancer Institute, A.M.M. and M.F. are research students of the National Cancer Institute, and W.M. is a research student of the Medical Research Council.

REFERENCES

1. Birg F, Dulbecco R, Fried M, Kamen R (1979): J Virol 29:633
2. Chia W, Rigby PWJ (1981): Proc Natl Acad Sci USA 78:6638
3. Della Valle G, Fenton RG, Basilico C (1981): Cell 23:347
4. Hassell JA, Topp WC, Rifkin DB, Moreau PE (1980): Proc Natl Acad Sci USA 77:3978
5. Lusky M and Botchan M (1981): Nature 293:79
6. Mes A-M, Hassell JA (1982): J Virol 42:621
7. Prasad L, Zouzias D, Basilico C (1976): J Virol 18:436
8. Tooze J, ed (1980): DNA Tumor Viruses, Part 2, Cold Spring Harbor NY: Cold Spring Harbor Laboratory
9. Treisman R, Novak V, Favaloro J, Kamen R (1981): Nature 292:595

Gene Transfer and Cancer, edited by M. L. Pearson
and N. L. Sternberg. Raven Press, New York © 1984.

Homologous Recombination Between Segments of the Herpes Simplex Virus Thymidine Kinase Gene in Mouse L Cells

Fwu-Lai Lin and Nat Sternberg

Cancer Biology Program, National Cancer Institute, Frederick Cancer Research Facility, Frederick, Maryland 21701

ABSTRACT. We have constructed a vector consisting of two defective herpes simplex virus (HSV) thymidine kinase (tk) genes cloned in bacteriophage λ DNA (λtk^2) to measure homologous recombination after calcium phosphate-mediated DNA transfer into TK$^-$ mouse L (LMtk$^-$) cells. The appearance of Tk$^+$-transformed colonies was used as an assay for recombination; the colonies presumably would arise after an intact tk gene is reconstructed by recombination between the two defective genes. We found that transformation to Tk$^+$ can be stimulated 50-fold by cutting the λtk^2 DNA between the two defective tk genes. Southern gel analysis of five transformants obtained with the cut DNA indicated that they all had undergone the expected recombination event. We conclude that homologous recombination can occur efficiently in mouse L cells.

INTRODUCTION

Analysis of the mechanism of homologous recombination in somatic cells has proven to be a difficult task compared to similar analyses in bacteria and yeast because of the size and complexity of the eucaryotic genome and because of the lack of both suitable genetic markers and easy methods for scoring recombinants. One approach for partially overcoming these difficulties is to study recombination of a simpler genome, such as that of a virus. Results obtained with the simian virus 40 and adenovirus model systems have indicated that homologous recombination occurs efficiently (4,8,9,14), is dependent of viral replication (10), and occurs through intermediates similar to those involved in procaryotic recombination (13).

We chose to study homologous recombination in mouse L cells using gene transfer techniques with a defined DNA substrate, the HSV tk gene. The use of this gene allows us to detect rare recombination events easily and to probe the molecular nature of those events without isolating the products of recombination. Our studies indicate that this system can be used both to detect recombination and to elucidate some of its substrate requirements.

RESULTS

Our original λtk vector consists of the 3.4-kb BamHI HSV tk fragment (2) cloned in bacteriophage λ DNA at map coordinate 71.3. When mouse

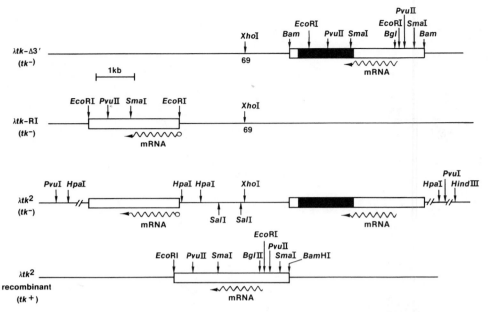

FIGURE 1. DNA substrates used to measure homologous recombination in mouse L cells. Lines represent λ DNA, open bars are DNA from the 3.4-kb BamHI HSV tk fragment (2), closed bars are deleted DNA, and wavy lines below bars are tk mRNA. The circle at the 5' end of mRNA indicates that transcription is inefficient from this DNA. The numbers below the line indicate λ map coordinates and the arrows above the lines and bars indicate restriction sites.

TABLE 1. Relative transformation efficiency with λtk[2] DNA[a]

DNA	Restriction enzyme treatment	Relative transformation efficiency
λtk-Δ3'	–	0
λtk-RI	–	0.02
λtk[2]	–	0.03
λtk[2]	XhoI	1.00
λtk-RI	XhoI	0.01
λtk[2]	SalI	1.19
λtk[2]	PvuI	0.03
λtk[2]	HindIII	0.03

[a] The DNA-mediated gene transfer procedure used is essentially that described by Graham and Van der Eb (3). All of the transformations were carried out with 20 μg of LMtk⁻ carrier DNA. The efficiency of transformation with λtk DNA containing an intact tk gene is 1 transformant per 0.1 ng of λtk DNA per 10[6] cells. The standardized transformation efficiency of 1.00 is 4% of that value. The cell line used in these experiments is the mouse LMtk⁻A⁻ line described in reference 12.

LMtk⁻ cells are transformed with this DNA using the calcium phosphate method (3), one transformant is obtained per 0.1 ng of λtk DNA per 10⁶ cells (see legend to Table 1). The tk substrates used to study recombination are described in Figure 1. The first substrate is a spontaneous deletion derivative of λtk designated λtk-Δ3' that was isolated during the growth of this phage in Escherichia coli. The deletion mutation removes the 3' end of the tk structural gene and, consequently, abolishes the ability of λtk-Δ3' to transform Tk⁻ cells to Tk⁺ (Table 1). The second substrate is designated λtkRI and consists of the EcoRI HSV tk fragment cloned in λ at map coordinate 65.4. This fragment contains the entire tk structural gene and the tk promoter "TATA" sequence but does not contain another important promoter control region, the "CAT" sequence, located between the right EcoRI and PvuII sites of the tk BamHI fragment (Figure 1). λtkRI transforms LMtk⁻ cells inefficiently. We observed a transformation frequency of about 0.1% that of λtk (Table 1), which is 20 times lower than that observed by McKnight et al. (5). We believe this variability is caused by differences in the DNA flanking the EcoRI site into which the fragment is cloned (N. Sternberg and F. L. Lin, manuscript in preparation). The last substrate, which we have used to study recombination, was made by cleaving both λtk-Δ3' and λtk-RI at the single XhoI site in λ DNA at map coordinate 69 and ligating the fragments. One of the products of that ligation, designated λtk², contains two defective tk genes oriented in the same direction relative to each other such that recombination in a 1.0-kb region of tk homology shared by the two defective genes reconstructs a functional tk gene.

The frequency of transformation with λtk² DNA is not significantly higher than the frequency of λtk-RI transformation (Table 1). However, when the λtk² DNA is cleaved with either XhoI or SalI before transformation, enzymes that cut the DNA only in the λ sequences between the two defective tk genes, the transformation efficiency increases from 0.1 to 4%. We can think of two possible explanations of this result: a) recombination between homologous tk segments is stimulated by the presence of ends between the segments, or b) the cleaved λtk² DNA is an efficient substrate for the ligation of carrier DNA sequences on the 5' side of the λtk-RI fragment. Those sequences might substitute for the missing tk "CAT" element, resulting in enhanced tk expression and transformation. Ligase activity capable of sealing both blunt and cohesive ends is high in somatic cells (1). The second explanation is ruled out by the observation that cutting λtk-RI DNA at the XhoI site does not stimulate transformation (Table 1). To determine whether the increased frequency of transformation detected with XhoI-cleaved DNA is caused by recombination, we examined the arrangement of tk sequences in transformed cells by Southern hybridization analysis. The DNAs from five transformants obtained with XhoI-cleaved DNA (series I transformants) and from four transformants obtained with uncleaved DNA (series II transformants) were analyzed using the restriction enzymes SmaI and PvuII (N. Sternberg and F.L. Lin, manuscript in preparation). If the intact tk gene is reconstructed by recombination between the two defective genes, the transformants should contain a 1.7-kb SmaI and a 2-kb PvuII tk fragment (Figure 1). Neither of these fragments is present in λtk-Δ3', λtk-RI, or λtk² DNA. The results of this analysis indicate that all five series I transformants contain the 1.7-kb SmaI tk fragment, but only two of them contain the 2-kb PvuII tk fragment. The copy number of the SmaI fragment in all of the transformants is 1 to 2 per cell genome. The 3' terminus of the tk gene is located 20 bp to the 3' side of the left SmaI site of the BamHI tk fragment (11) (Figure 1). Thus only a small portion of the 620-bp SmaI-PvuII fragment that contains the 3' end of the tk gene is needed for tk gene integrity. Nevertheless the fact that sequences just beyond the 3' end of the gene are frequently rearranged is surprising. Whether those rearrangements are associated with the recombination event is still unclear.

These results are quite different from those obtained with the four series II transformants in which the major SmaI fragment detected in gels is 5.7 kb. It is present in 40-100 copies per genome. The size of this fragment is exactly that expected for unrecombined λtk^2 DNA. Besides the major 5.7-kb SmaI fragment, all four series II transformants also contain a whole spectrum of SmaI fragments that hybridize to tk DNA and that range in size from less than 1 kb to more than 5.7 kb. Because of the large number of fragments, the determination of whether any of the transformants contain a recombined 1.7-kb SmaI fragment is difficult.

The simplest interpretation of these results is that, in the series I transformants, a functional tk gene has been reconstructed by recombination, whereas in the series II transformants, it has not. The rare series II transformants (see Table 1) are presumably a consequence of the high copy number of the relatively inactive tk gene represented by the tk EcoRI fragment.

After determining that cutting the λtk^2 DNA between the two defective tk genes stimulates recombination, we wondered what effect cuts made in the λ DNA flanking the duplicated region would have on recombination. We cut λtk^2 with HindIII and PvuI, enzymes that only cut to one or both sides of the tk duplicated region (Figure 1), and used the DNA to transfect LMtk$^-$ cells. In both cases the frequency of transformation was not significantly higher than that of uncut DNA (Table 1). We conclude that homologous recombination is stimulated specifically by DNA ends between recombining segments.

DISCUSSION AND SUMMARY

We have constructed a DNA substrate, called λtk^2 (see Figure 1), to assess the efficiency of homologous recombination in mammalian cells. It consists of two HSV tk fragments, one defective in the 5' promoter region and the other defective in the 3' end of the gene; the fragments are oriented in the same direction and separated by 3 kb of phage λ DNA. Recombination in a 1.0-kb region of homology shared by the two defective genes should delete the λ DNA between them, should reconstruct the tk gene, and should permit transformation of LMtk$^-$ mouse cells to Tk$^+$. Contrary to our initial expectations, the λtk^2 DNA did not transform Tk$^-$ cells to Tk$^+$ by the calcium phosphate method more efficiently than did λ DNA containing just the promoter-defective tk fragment (Table 1). Furthermore, Southern hybridization analysis indicated that the rare Tk$^+$ transformants obtained with λtk^2 DNA did not reconstruct the tk gene by recombination. Rather they are Tk$^+$ because they contain many copies of the promoter-defective tk fragment.

When the λtk^2 DNA was cut in the λ sequences between the defective tk genes at either XhoI or SalI sites, the transformation efficiency increased 40-fold. We found that this increase is caused by homologous recombination between tk segments and that the tk copy number in these recombinant clones is low (1-2 per cell genome).

An intriguing observation made during the course of these studies is that most of the recombinants (3 of 5) do not retain the normal tk sequences just to the 3' side of the end of the gene. This segment of DNA is rich in stretches of G and C bases that could facilitate the formation of hairpin structures. If replication were required for recombination, such structures might impede replication forks, thereby producing the DNA rearrangements we found in this region.

The finding that DNA ends or single-stranded DNA regions can promote recombination has been observed in other recombination systems. In yeast, Orr-Weaver et al. (6) showed that by cutting transforming DNA within a gene, recombination between that gene and its chromosomal homology is stimulated by three orders of magnitude. In E. coli, the RecA protein has a strong affinity for single-stranded DNA and facilitates strand pairing (7). Indeed, one possible explanation for our results is that the cutting of λtk^2 DNA permits binding of a mammalian RecA-like protein to the DNA that promotes pairing between homologous tk segments. Alternatively, the DNA ends could be substrates for a cellular nuclease that would act to expose complimentary single strands in the two defective tk genes. Pairing between those strands and subsequent processing would reconstruct the tk gene. By varying the substrates we use in gene transfer experiments, we hope to distinguish between these and other recombination mechanisms. Although these results are still quite preliminary, we are encouraged by them and by the positive results reported by others in this volume (see Pomerantz et al.) to think that the tools for the unraveling of recombination pathways in somatic cells are at hand.

ACKNOWLEDGEMENTS

We thank Drs. R. Grafstrom and P. Strickland for their critical reading of this manuscript. The research was sponsored by the National Cancer Institute, DHHS, under contract No. NO-CO1-75380 with Litton Bionetics, Inc. The contents of this publication do not necessarily reflect the views or policies of the Department of Health and Human Services, nor does mention of trade names, commercial products, or organizations imply endorsement by the U.S. Government.

REFERENCES

1. Carbon J, Shenk TE, Berg P (1975): Proc Natl Acad Sci USA 72:1392
2. Enquist LW, Vande Woude GF, Wagner M, Smiley JR, Summers WC (1979): Gene 7:335
3. Graham FL, Van der Eb AJ (1973): Virology 52:456
4. Jackson DA (1980): In: Introduction of Macromolecules into Viable Mammalian Cells, (Baserga R, Croce C, Rovera G, eds.), New York: Alan R Liss, p. 65
5. McKnight SL, Gavais ER, Kingsbury R, Axel R (1981): Cell 25:385
6. Orr-Weaver TL, Szostak JW, Rothstein RJ (1981): Proc Natl Acad Sci USA 78:6358
7. Radding CM (1981): Cell 25:3
8. Upcroft P, Carter B, Kidson C (1980): Nucleic Acids Res 8:5835
9. Wake CT, Wilson JH (1979): Proc Natl Acad Sci USA 76:2876
10. Wake CT, Wilson JH (1980): Cell 21:141
11. Wagner MJ, Sharp JA, Summers WC (1981): Proc Natl Acad Sci USA 78:1441
12. Wigler M, Sweet R, Sim GK, Wold B, Pellicer A, Lacy E, Maniatis T, Silverstein S, Axel R (1979): Cell 16:777
13. Wolgemuth DJ, Hsu M-T (1981): Proc Natl Acad Sci USA 78:5076
14. Young CSH, Silverstein SJ (1980): Virology 101:503

Gene Transfer and Cancer, edited by M. L. Pearson and N. L. Sternberg. Raven Press, New York © 1984.

DNA-Mediated Transfer of Multidrug Resistance and Expression of P-Glycoprotein

V. Ling, N. Kartner, P. Debenham, A. Chase, L. Siminovitch, and J. R. Riordan

Ontario Cancer Institute, and Hospital for Sick Children, University of Toronto, Toronto, M4X 1K9 Canada

ABSTRACT. Resistance to multiple chemotherapeutic drugs has been reported in a variety of experimental tumors. Such a phenotype is observed in colchicine-resistant Chinese hamster ovary (CHO) cell mutants isolated previously in our laboratories. The mechanism of resistance appears to result from reduced drug permeability. An increased level of a 170-kd membrane glycoprotein (P-glycoprotein) is observed in these mutants. In the present study we have been able to confer both the multidrug resistant phenotype and expression of P-glycoprotein onto drug-sensitive mouse cells using DNA from hamster cell mutants. Such transformants are not observed with DNA from drug-sensitive cells. These results are completely consistent with a causal relationship between P-glycoprotein expression and the multidrug-resistance phenotype.

INTRODUCTION

We have observed previously that colchicine-resistant CH[R] mutants of CHO cells display a complex phenotype of resistance to diverse, unrelated drugs (2,12). This multidrug resistance appears to stem from a plasma membrane alteration resulting in reduced drug permeability to the compounds involved (4,7,12). Analysis of the membrane components of the mutant cells revealed the presence of a 170,000 dalton surface glycoprotein (P-glycoprotein) which is not detected in drug sensitive cells (7,14). The levels of P-glycoprotein expressed seem to be correlated with levels of resistance to the drug. Studies involving independent clonal isolates, cell:cell hybrids, and independent revertants all indicate that the multidrug-resistance phenotype results from the same mutation that confers colchicine resistance (1). Moreover, such studies also indicate that the expression of the P-glycoprotein is intimately associated with this phenotype.

The present study was undertaken with a 2-fold purpose. First we wished to investigate the genetics of multidrug resistance in more detail utilizing the approach of DNA-mediated gene transfer to ask whether the aforementioned properties thought to be associated with colchicine resistance are tightly linked and would be conferred concordantly on independent transformants. Second, as a long-range goal, we wished to develop

DNA-mediated transfer expertise in this system as a necessary first step in the identification and cloning of the gene(s) coding for multidrug resistance. In a separate publication, we presented results showing that DNA-mediated gene transfer of colchicine resistance can be achieved using L cells as recipients (6). Some general properties of this system are outlined in this paper.

RESULTS

DNA-mediated Transfer of Colchicine Resistance

Genomic DNAs from CHO cells were prepared with a procedure similar to that described by Pellicer et al. (13). Recipient mouse cells were either LMTk⁻ (murine L cells deficient in thymidine kinase) or LTA (L cells deficient in both thymidine kinase and adenosine phosphoribosyl transferase). Transformation of the mouse L cells was performed using the calcium phosphate procedure and treatment with dimethylsulfoxide (DMSO) as described by Srinivasan and Lewis (15). Usually 20 μg of DNA was applied per 100-mm tissue culture dish containing recipient cells seeded at 7×10^5 cells per dish 1 day earlier.

Since it had been reported previously that drug-resistant cells, phenotypically similar to membrane permeability mutants of CHO cells, could be isolated readily in mouse cells (5,9), the protocol worked out for selection of colchicine-resistant transformants was relatively stringent in order to prevent the isolation of such mutants. Thus it was important to utilize conditions where the colchicine concentration was high enough to give a negligible spontaneous mutation frequency but low enough to permit the growth of drug-resistant transformants. The conditions employed were as follows: 24 hr after DNA treatment, recipient cells were exposed to 0.1 μg/ml colchicine for 3 days; the medium was then changed to contain 0.3 μg/ml of colchicine and incubation continued for another 3 days; and finally the cells were exposed to 0.5 μg/ml of colchicine for the duration of the experiment.

Under these conditions, no colonies were observed in five different experiments where DNAs from colchicine-sensitive cells were used. The resultant estimated frequency of colchicine-resistant cells under these conditions was less than 3×10^{-8}. In contrast, in seven experiments where DNAs from colchicine-resistant cells were used, 38 colonies were observed, a frequency of 7×10^{-7}. In parallel control experiments using DNAs from both drug-resistant and drug-sensitive CHO cells, the frequencies of HAT-resistant colonies (transfer of Tk⁺ locus) ranged from $2\text{-}10 \times 10^{-6}$, which is similar to frequencies reported by others for transfer of this marker into L cells (10). Results from these control experiments provide assurance that both the cells and DNA preparations used were competent for DNA-mediated gene transfer. We believe that these results provide convincing evidence that the colchicine-resistant isolates of L cells resulted from the transfer of DNA from the donor colchicine-resistant CHO cells.

A number of independent transformants were picked and found to grow readily in the presence of the selecting drug concentration. When cultured in the absence of drug, the transformants lose their drug-resistance phenotype within a few weeks. Examination of the transformants also indicated that cotransfer of unlinked genes was infrequent. For example, when CHO cell genomic DNA bearing markers for colchicine resistance, HAT resistance, and ouabain resistance was used, transformants isolated for each of these markers expressed only the phenotype associated with the marker for which it was selected, and not the others.

Drug-resistance Properties of Transformants

Independent transformants all displayed a multidrug-resistance phenotype. As an example, one transformant line was 43-fold more resistant to
colchicine (i.e., requires 43-fold higher concentration of drug to kill
cells) than the recipient L cells, and at the same time, the line was 60-,
9-, 25-, and 11-fold more resistant to puromycin, actinomycin D, emetine,
and cytochalasin B, respectively. This pattern was fairly typical of
most transformants, although the actual degree of resistance varied.
Since both the colchicine-resistance and multidrug-resistance phenotypes
were concordantly transferred in independent transformants, it provides
strong support for the hypothesis that resistance to unrelated drugs in
the colchicine-resistant mutants is coded by a single gene (1). Furthermore, as mentioned above, unlinked genes are not cotransferred at a
detectable frequency in this system.

Expression of P-glycoprotein

We next examined the transformants for expression of the 170-kd surface
P-glycoprotein. Plasma membranes were isolated from transformants, and
proteins were fractionated by sodium dodecyl sulfate gel electrophoresis
(14). When the highly sensitive silver staining procedure of Switzer et
al. (16) was used, a faintly staining, diffuse band corresponding to the
P-glycoprotein could be detected. In order to characterize this component
more specifically, an antiserum raised against colchicine-resistant CHO
cell membranes was used to identify P-glycoprotein by radioimmune staining
in a replica Western blot procedure (17). With this approach, the presence of the P-glycoprotein was clearly distinguished in the transformants,
whereas such a component was not observed in recipient L cells or drug-
sensitive CHO cells. These results clearly demonstrate that the expression
of P-glycoprotein is associated with expression of multidrug resistance.
They support also the notion that this surface glycoprotein functions
directly in excluding a variety of drugs from mutant cells via molecular
mechanisms not yet understood.

The results obtained, however, do not provide conclusive evidence that
the P-glycoprotein detected in the tranformants was in fact of CHO cell
origin. In order to examine this aspect further, colchicine-resistant
L cell mutants were isolated after treatment with the mutagen ethylmethane
sulfonate. The mutants isolated displayed a multidrug-resistance phenotype
and were therefore likely to be permeability mutants. Analysis of their
membrane components indicated that these L cell mutants also contain a
170-kd component migrating at the same position as the P-glycoprotein of
the CHO cell mutants. Moreover, this component could be stained with the
antiserum raised against the CHO cell membranes. It thus appears that
the P-glycoproteins of hamster and mouse are very similar. This observation precludes drawing conclusions at this point as to whether it is in
fact the mouse or the hamster P-glycoprotein that is expressed in the
transformants. While our bias is that it is the CHO cell P-glycoprotein
that is expressed, we could not rule out the possibility that the transferred CHO cell DNA coded for an as yet unidentified function(s) which
mediates the expression of the mouse multidrug-resistance phenotype, including the expression of the mouse P-glycoprotein. Our success in
achieving DNA-mediated transfer of the colchicine resistance marker should
facilitate the molecular cloning of the CHO cell DNA responsible for this
phenotype. Subsequent characterization of this DNA should provide an
unequivocal answer to this question.

DISCUSSION

This study has provided strong evidence that expression of the surface P-glycoprotein is tightly associated with expression of the multidrug-resistance phenotype. How such a surface glycoprotein might function in limiting the cell membrane to diverse compounds is presently not known. However, a model has been proposed invoking a role for the P-glycoprotein as a modulator of membrane fluidity (7,11). Other models are, of course, possible. Further analysis of the genes involved in the DNA-mediated transfer of the multidrug-resistance phenotype could provide further insights to this question.

The fact that the P-glycoproteins of the mouse and hamster are so similar suggests that P-glycoprotein is a highly conserved protein that could be a functionally important constituent of the normal mammalian cell plasma membrane. One can speculate that overproduction of this gene product leads to the generation of drug-resistant cells of the multidrug-resistance phenotype. Evidence in support of this speculation stems from two sources. First, as mentioned earlier, in mutants selected in multi-step for increased colchicine resistance, an increased expression of the P-glycoprotein is observed (7,14). Second, along the same vein, transformants selected for ability to grow in increased drug concentrations also display an increased level of P-glycoprotein. Significantly, in such transformants extrachromosomal DNA-containing particles similar to double minutes are also observed to increase in number concordantly (S. Robertson, V. Ling, and C.P. Stanners, unpublished observation). Double minutes are characteristic of gene amplification in other drug-resistant systems (8). Thus, this system may lend itself to the study of control of gene expression and possibly to gene amplification.

Many of the drugs to which the colchicine-resistant mutants are resistant are used widely in the treatment of cancer. It is possible that nonresponse to treatment with combination chemotherapy results from the emergence of a drug-resistant tumor cell subpopulation bearing the membrane impermeability, multidrug-resistance phenotype (3). In this respect, study of the colchicine-resistance phenotype is of relevance to cancer chemotherapy.

ACKNOWLEDGEMENT

This work was supported by grants from the Ontario Cancer Treatment and Research Foundation, the National Cancer Institute of Canada, and the Medical Research Council of Canada. P. Debenham was a recipient of an MRC postdoctoral fellowship.

REFERENCES

1. Baker RM, Ling V (1978): In: Methods in Membrane Biology (Korn ED, ed), New York: Plenum Press, Vol. 9, pp 337
2. Bech-Hansen NT, Till JE, Ling V (1976): J. Cell Physiol 88:23
3. Bech-Hansen NT, Sarangi F, Sutherland DJA, Ling V (1977): J Natl Cancer Inst 59:21
4. Carlsen SA, Till JE, Ling V (1976): Biochim Biophys Acta 455:900
5. Crichley V, Mager D, Bernstein A (1980): J Cell Physiol 102:63
6. Debenham P, Kartner N, Siminovitch L, Riordan JR, Ling V (1982): Molec Cell Biol 2:881.
7. Juliano RL, Ling V (1976): Biochim Biophys Acta 455:152
8. Kaufman RJ, Brown PC, Schimke RJ (1979): Proc Natl Acad Sci USA 76:5669

9. Kessel D, Bosmann HB (1970): Cancer Res 30:2695

10. Lewis WH, Srinivasan PR, Stokoe N, Siminovitch L (1980): Somatic Cell Genet 6:333

11. Ling V (1975): Can J Genetics and Cytology 17:503

12. Ling V, Thompson LH (1974): J Cell Physiol 83:103

13. Pellicer LA, Wigler M, Axel R, Silverstein S (1978): Cell 14:133

14. Riordan JR, Ling V (1979): J Biol Chem 254:12701

15. Srinivasan PR, Lewis HW (1980): In: Introduction of Macromolecules into Viable Mammalian Cells (Berga R, Croce C, Giovanni R, eds), New York: Alan R. Liss, vol. 1, pp 27-47

16. Switzer RC, Meril CR, Shifrin S (1979): Anal Biochem 98:231

17. Towbin H, Staehelin T, Gordon J (1979): Proc Natl Acad Sci USA 76: 4350

Gene Transfer and Cancer, edited by M. L. Pearson and N. L. Sternberg. Raven Press, New York © 1984.

Development of a Cloning System for the Gene for Asparagine Synthetase

Peter N. Ray, Irene L. Andrulis, and Louis Siminovitch

*Department of Genetics, Hospital for Sick Children,
Toronto, Ontario, M5G 1X8 Canada*

ABSTRACT. Asparagine synthetase, the sole enzyme responsible for the synthesis of asparagine, is regulated in CHO cells by the concentration of asparagine, as well as by the extent of tRNA aminoacylation. In order to obtain further understanding of the regulation of this enzyme and to develop a system whereby the gene for the enzyme could be transferred and possibly cloned, we initiated studies designed to select mutants altered in its structure or regulation. To this end, we have taken advantage of two susbtrate analogues, β-aspartyl-hydroxamate (β-AHA) and albizziin (Alb), which inhibit the enzyme in vitro.

Single-step mutants resistant to high levels of these drugs have been isolated. By training the Alb-resistant mutants, it was possible to derive amplified lines that greatly overproduce asparagine synthetase (300 times), some of which show a homogeneously staining region (HSR) in the karyotype. The trained β-AHA^R mutants owe their resistance to a structural change in the enzyme. Using the amplified lines as donors, we have been able to transfer the gene for asparagine synthetase into both CHO and simian COS-1 cell recipients.

Two independent methods are being used to clone the gene. In one, we are attempting to rescue the gene after transfer into the simian COS-1 cell line. In the other, a more traditional cDNA approach is being attempted using the amplified lines as a source of mRNA.

INTRODUCTION

Over the last few years, our laboratory has conducted several studies directed toward the development of an understanding of the structure and regulation of the gene for asparagine synthetase. To this end, mutants of CHO cells were selected that were resistant to either of two substrate analogues of the enzyme β-AHA and Alb (2,3), and studies have been conducted on the genetic and biochemical phenotype of such isolates. Although both recessive and dominant mutants were obtained in initial selections using β-AHA, we succeeded in isolating lines carrying two successive dominant mutations, which render the cells highly resistant to the drug. One such line was used as a donor to demonstrate successful DNA-mediated transfer of the gene to recipient CHO cells (1). Although the asparagine synthetase gene did not seem to be highly amplified in the donor doubly resistant line, such amplification was observed in transferent cells as indicated by elevated enzyme levels and the existence of an HSR (2).

The above results indicated that at least two methods might be available to clone the gene for asparagine synthetase. One method is based on DNA-mediated gene transfer. Such transfer followed by rescue of the donor DNA from the recipient has been used to isolate the genes for thymidine kinase (10) and adenine phosphoribosyl-transferase (7) as well as an oncogenic transforming gene (6).

An alternative method for cloning the asparagine synthetase gene is to take advantage of the increased level of expression offered by gene amplification. Recent developments in recombinant DNA technology have made it relatively easy to clone genes which express abundant mRNAs. Gene amplification is observed frequently during evolution of drug resistance, and its existence is usually signalled by increased levels of the target enzyme and an HSR of a chromosome (9,11,13). As indicated earlier, both of these latter phenotypes seemed to be present in our DNA transferents. However, for several reasons it would be preferable if amplification of the wild-type gene could be obtained. In this paper we describe experiments in which such dominantly acting isolates have been obtained using Alb for selection of the mutants. Such lines show an extensive increase in enzyme level and exhibit high frequencies in DNA-mediated gene transfer experiments. The methodology being used to clone the gene is also described.

RESULTS

Mutant Selection

For the selection of single-step mutants, CHO cells were mutagenized with 300 μg/ml ethyl methane sulfonate (EMS) and plated in complete αMEM (12) lacking asparagine and supplemented with 7% fetal calf serum and either 2 mM Alb or 100 μM β-AHA. After one month in selective medium, colonies were picked and recloned in complete medium minus drug.

Mutants with very high levels of resistance were obtained as follows (training). Cells resistant to albizziin were selected by plating 10^7 nonmutagenized parent cells in 2 mM drug. Colonies which grew in this concentration of drug were picked and subcultured into 4 mM Alb. The concentration of drug was then increased during each subsequent passage.

Highly resistant β-AHA mutants were selected in essentially the same way except that the parental line was a first-step EMS-induced dominant mutant (AH2).

Mutant Phenotypes

The degree of resistance of the mutants was determined from dose-response curves (Figure 1). First-step mutants resistant to Alb (e.g., Alb^R1) were approximately 20-fold more resistant than the parent line, while the first-step AH2 line resistant to β-AHA was only 2- to 3-fold more resistant than wild-type cells (3, Table 1). In both cases, as expected, the level of resistance of the lines increased as they were subcultured in higher doses of the respective drugs, and trained isolates were obtained which were as much as 100-fold more resistant than the parental line.

As a first step in examining the molecular nature of these mutations, we assayed the asparagine synthetase activity in crude extracts of the parent and mutant lines (Table 1). The first-step mutants resistant to either drug had increased specific activities of the enzyme, about 6-fold

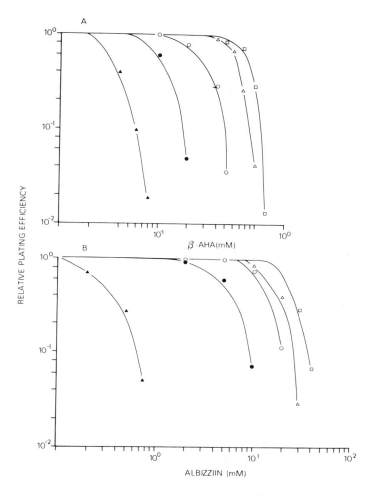

FIGURE 1. Dose response of parent and mutant lines to β-AHA and Alb.
A) Plating efficiency in β-AHA of wild-type cells, ▲-▲-▲; a
single-step EMS-induced mutant AH2, ●-●-●; and three trained derivatives
(AH2-3000, o-o-o; AH2-600, Δ-Δ-Δ; and AH2-800, □-□-□). B)
Plating efficiency in Alb of wild-type cells, ▲-▲-▲; a spontaneous
mutant Alb[R]42, ●-●-●; and three trained derivatives (Alb[R]42-10, o-o-o;
Alb[R]42-15, Δ-Δ-Δ; and Alb[R]42-30, □-□-□).

in β-AHA-resistant mutants and about 15-fold in Alb-resistant mutants.
However, the lines trained in β-AHA and Alb differed markedly in respect
to the changes in activity of the enzyme. Mutants trained in Alb showed
an increase in the specific activity of asparagine synthetase, which was
directly correlated with the degree of resistance achieved during the
training. Thus a 44- to 160-fold increase in resistance and a 300-fold
increase in enzyme activity was achieved in this system. There were no
changes observed in kinetic constants for asparagine synthetase in the
Alb-trained lines (Table 1). These data suggested that training in the
presence of Alb had resulted in amplification of the gene for asparagine

TABLE 1. Asparagine synthetase activity in wild-type, β-AHA^R, and Alb^R lines[a]

Cell line	D_{10} (μM β-AHA)	(mM Alb)	Relative asparagine synthetase activity	K_i (μM β-AHA)	(mM Alb)
wt	60	0.6	1	600	0.9
AH2 (EMS)	180		6	800	
AH2-300	460		9		
AH2-600	870		11	1640	
AH2-800	1160		11	2000	
Alb^R 1 (EMS)		14	13		1.6
Alb^{R}42		9.5	9		1.5
Alb^{R}42-10		20	15		
Alb^{R}42-15		27	71		
Alb^{R}42-30		37	150		1.5
Alb^{R}42-50			276		

[a] Enzyme activity and kinetic constants were determined as previously described (3).

synthetase and that a structural change in the enzyme was not involved in the lesion in these cells. As indicated earlier, another important indication of gene amplification is the presence of HSRs. We therefore analyzed the karyotype of the highly resistant lines. All of them exhibited an HSR not present in the parent line (Figure 2). The evidence therefore is very strong that training of CHO cells in Alb results in amplification of the gene for asparagine synthetase.

In contrast to these results, the mutants trained in β-AHA did not show an increase in asparagine synthetase that correlated with the increase in resistance (Table 1). Although very high degrees of resistance to β-AHA could be achieved, we could not obtain lines with very high levels of the enzyme. This suggested that gene amplification was not the mechanism by which the cells trained in β-AHA became highly resistant. An alternate possibility was that the high resistance in this case was due to an alteration in the structural gene for the enzyme, resulting in a lowered affinity of the enzyme for the drug. To test this we determined the K_i of the enzyme for β-AHA at each step of the training

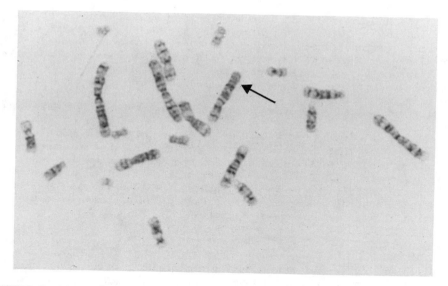

FIGURE 2. Trypsin-Giemsa banded spread of the chromosomes of the highly resistant alb⁻ trained line Alb42-30. The arrow indicates a large HSR not found in the parent line. The banding procedure has been previously described (14).

(Table 1). The first-step EMS-induced mutant (AH2) showed no significant change in Ki from the parent, but subsequent training resulted in an increased Ki at each step. Thus resistance to β-AHA was probably due to a structural change in the enzyme rather than gene amplification. This was supported by the fact that no HSRs could be found in any of the β-AHA-resistant mutants upon karyotypic analysis.

DNA-Mediated Gene Transfer

Both the Alb-resistant and the AH2 series of β-AHA-resistant mutants behave codominantly in somatic cell hybrids (2,3), and we have already shown that DNA-mediated gene transfer is feasible in CHO cells with one double β-AHA^R isolate (1). Therefore, it was of interest to determine whether the trained lines described earlier could also serve as efficient donors in gene transfer experiments.

Mutants highly resistant to either β-AHA or albizziin were therefore used as donors for DNA-mediated gene transfer using the calcium phosphate precipitation technique (1). The results summarized in Table 2 indicate that both the EMS-induced and subsequently trained β-AHA-resistant mutant, AH2 300, and the amplified Alb-resistant mutant, Alb^R-42-30, were efficient donors, giving transfer frequencies 10 times over background. Similar results were obtained when either wild-type CHO cells or SV40-transformed simian cells [cos-1 (5)] were used as a recipient.

Since the use of gene transfer for subsequent cloning requires ligation of a vector to the donor DNA prior to transfer, we tested several restriction enzymes to determine whether they cut the gene for asparagine synthetase.

Digestion of Alb^{R}42-30 DNA with HindIII had no effect on transfer activity (Table 2), indicating that the asparagine synthetase gene does not contain a HindIII restriction site and that this enzyme can be used in cloning experiments. Preliminary experiments with other restriction enzymes suggest that the gene is also insensitive to SalI and BglII but does not contain BamHI and EcoRI sites. Gel analysis showed that all enzymes gave substantial cleavage of the DNA.

DISCUSSION

Two different drugs and two selection protocols have been used to select mutations involving asparagine synthetase with the expectation that more than one type of mutant would be isolated. Our results confirm this expectation.

With β-AHA, subsequent training of single-step mutants yielded mutant cell lines with higher levels of resistance, due largely to an accumulation of structural changes in the enzyme that make it less sensitive to the drug.

In contrast to these findings, training with Alb resulted in highly resistant lines with greatly elevated asparagine synthetase activities and large HSRs in the karyotype. There is no evidence of structural changes in the enzyme in these lines.

These mutants have enabled us to initiate two independent methods for cloning the gene for asparagine synthetase. Both the structural gene mutants and the amplified mutants have been used as donors in DNA-mediated transfer, and analysis of the restriction sensitivity of the DNA has revealed at least one enzyme that does not cut the gene and is thus suita-

TABLE 2. DNA-mediated transfer of the gene for asparagine synthetase

Donor DNA	Recipient	Frequency (x 10^7)
wt	CHO	< 3
wt	cos-1	< 2
AH2-300	CHO	14
Alb^{R}42-30	CHO	16
Alb^{R}42-30	cos-1	40
Alb^{R}42-30 (HindIII)	CHO	21

ble for cloning. Work in our laboratory has indicated that plasmids containing DNA sequences adjacent to and containing the SV40 origin of replication can be transferred into cos-1 cells, maintained in a nonintegrated form by selection, and subsequently recovered intact from the Hirt supernatant (4). Since the cos-1 cell line can be used as a recipient for transfer of asparagine synthetase, we are attempting to use this system to clone the gene. A pBR322-SV40 hybrid plasmid (8) will be ligated to HindIII-digested Alb^R-42-30 DNA and transferred into the cos-1 cell line. We shall then attempt to select for β-AHA^R transferants. If our selection is successful, these will be picked and the plasmid containing the asparagine synthetase gene will be recovered. This approach presupposes that the ligation event will result in a plasmid in which the asparagine synthetase gene can be transcribed in cos-1 cells in the absence of integration.

Concurrently, as a second approach, we are constructing cDNA clones from mRNA isolated from the highly amplified Alb-resistant lines on the assumption that a 300-fold increase in enzyme activity is reflected in a comparable increase in mRNA. Clones specific for asparagine synthetase will be selected on the basis of differential hybridization using probes prepared from the amplified and nonamplified lines.

ACKNOWLEDGEMENTS

This work was supported by grants from the National Cancer Institute of Canada and the Medical Research Council. I.L.A. was the recipient of an NIH postdoctoral fellowship.

REFERENCES

1. Andrulis IL, Siminovitch L (1981): Proc Natl Acad Sci USA 78:5724
2. Andrulis IL, Siminovitch L (1982): In: Gene Amplification (Schimke RT, ed), Cold Spring Harbor NY: Cold Spring Harbor Laboratory, p 75
3. Andrulis IL, Siminovitch L (1982): Somatic Cell Genet 8:533
4. Breitman ML, Tsui L-C, Buchwald M, Siminovitch L (1982): Mol Cell Biol 2:966
5. Gluzman Y (1981): Cell 23:175
6. Goldfarb M, Shimizu K, Perucho M, Wigler M (1982): Nature 296:404
7. Lowy I, Pellicer A, Jackson JF, Sim G-K, Silverstein S, Axel R (1980): Cell 22:817
8. Mulligan RC, Berg P (1980): Science 209:1422
9. Nunberg JH, Kaufman RJ, Schimke RT, Urlaub G, Chasin L (1978): Proc Natl Acad Sci USA 75:5553
10. Perucho M, Hanahan D, Lipsich L, Wigler M (1980): Nature 285:207
11. Schimke RT, ed (1982): Gene Amplification, Cold Spring Harbor NY: Cold Spring Harbor Laboratory
12. Stanners C, Elicieri G, Green H (1971): Nature 230:52
13. Wahl GM, Vitto L, Padgett RA, Stark GR (1982): Mol Cell Biol 2:308
14. Worton RG, Duff C (1979): Methods Enzymol 58:322

Gene Transfer and Cancer, edited by M. L. Pearson
and N. L. Sternberg. Raven Press, New York © 1984.

DNA-Mediated Transfer of an RNA Polymerase II Gene

C. James Ingles, Jerry K-C. Wong, and Michael Shales

Banting and Best Department of Medical Research, University of Toronto, Toronto, M5G 1L6 Canada

ABSTRACT. Treatment of the temperature-sensitive mutant TsAF8 of Syrian hamster BHK21 cells with calcium phosphate precipitates of genomic Ts^+ DNAs from BHK21, Chinese hamster ovary (CHO) and human (Hela) cells permitted the selection of Ts^+ colonies at 40°C. Ts^+ transformation events were distinguished from spontaneous Ts^+ reversions by using α-amanitin sensitive (Ama^S) TsAF8 cells. Co-acquisition of the α-amanitin-resistance (Ama^R) phenotype was demonstrated. These Ts^+ transformed cell lines, when grown at 40°C, contained an Ama^R RNA polymerase II activity with a sensitivity to inhibition by α-amanitin characteristic of the particular DNA used to transform the Ts cells. At 34°C the same cells contain a mixture of donor Ama^R and recipient Ama^S polymerase II activities. Uptake of donor DNA sequences was further demonstrated by the transfer of marker DNA sequences. DNA of either two different plasmids ligated to Ama^R DNA before transformation or human AluI family DNA sequences were identified in Southern blot analyses of primary Ts^+ Ama^R transformants. These marker DNAs facilitate recombinant DNA cloning of this Ama^R polymerase II gene.

INTRODUCTION

The mechanisms that serve to regulate the activities of the mammalian DNA-dependent RNA polymerases are still in large part unknown. The availability of mutations with altered RNA polymerase activities can however provide a genetic approach for the study of RNA synthesis in mammalian cells. Mutations that alter the activity of RNA polymerase II, the enzyme responsible for the synthesis of messenger RNAs have been described. In our laboratory three different classes of RNA polymerase II mutations have been studied. These are mutations resulting in resistance to the inhibitor of RNA polymerase II α-amanitin (3,5,13), conditional-lethal Ts mutations (6,12) and second-site suppressor mutations that reverse the Ts effects on growth of a Ts polymerase II mutation (12). In order both to characterize these existing mutations and also to generate a wider range of altered RNA polymerase II phenotypes, we needed to isolate the mammalian RNA polymerase genes. We approached this goal by transferring DNA that introduces a selectable phenotype into appropriate recipient cells, and then rescuing the transforming DNA by recombinant DNA screening.

RESULTS

Resistance to α-amanitin is a codominantly expressed mutation. Cells with an Ama^R/Ama^S genotype are able to grow in the presence of α-amanitin. The DNA-mediated gene transfer of this selectable Ama^R phenotype was therefore one of the first transfers attempted, albeit unsuccessfully, in this and several other laboratories. The availability in our laboratory of the Syrian hamster BHK21 mutant cell line TsAF8 (10), a cell line with a Ts mutation in the same complementation group as the Ama^R polymerase II mutations (12), provided an alternative approach for DNA transfer of this polymerase II gene. Since TsAF8 cells do not grow at the nonpermissive temperature of 40°C, they were used as recipients for transfer of the dominant wild-type Ts^+ gene. A calcium phosphate-DNA precipitate of wild-type Ts^+ DNA from either CHO, BHK21 or human cell DNA was added to monolayer cultures of TsAF8 at 34°C. After 24 hr exposure to the DNA at 34°C, the medium was replaced and the cells were exposed to selection pressure and incubated at 40°C (for experimental details see ref. 7). In several experiments, the apparent frequency of Ts^+ transformation (the number of Ts^+ colonies per cell exposed to DNA) was variable, ranging from about 10^{-5} to 10^{-7}. Although the frequency of obtaining apparent Ts^+ transformants was normally higher than spontaneous reversion to the Ts^+ phenotype on control plates of TsAF8 cells not exposed to DNA, these initial experiments did not clearly distinguish between bona fide Ts^+ transformants and Ts^+ revertants.

To identify the Ts^+ transformants more readily, we therefore used DNA from CHO cell lines in which biochemically well-characterized mutant alleles for Ts^+ Ama^R polymerase II exist (5). Treatment of the Ts Ama^S cell line TsAF8 with DNA from the Ts^+ Ama^R CHO mutant cell line Ama1 also resulted in Ts^+ colonies able to grow at 40°C. These Ts^+ colonies were picked, grown up at 40°C, and tested in growth experiments for the presence of the transferred CHO gene, i.e., for a Ts^+ Ama^R phenotype. Not unexpectedly, a mixture of Ts^+ transformants (Ts^+ Ama^R at 40°C) and spontaneous revertants (Ts^+ and Ama^S at 40°C) was found (7).

To provide more stringent evidence for successful gene transfer, we next examined the nature of the RNA polymerase II activities in these Ts^+ Ama^R transformed cell lines. The recipient cell line TsAF8 contained an Ama^S polymerase II activity. The polymerase II activity in extracts of TsAF8 cells was inhibited by concentrations of α-amanitin that inhibit other wild-type mammalian polymerase II activities (Figure 1). In contrast the CHO mutant Ama1 contained an RNA polymerase II activity that was about 500-fold more resistant to inhibition by α-amanitin than the TsAF8 polymerase II. The RNA polymerase II activities in extracts of two independent Ts^+ Ama^R transformants also required much higher concentrations of α-amanitin for inhibition. The inhibition curves in fact revealed the presence of two distinctly different polymerase II activities. When grown at 40°C, about 10% of the activity had a sensitivity to α-amanitin inhibition like that of the Ama^S TsAF8 cells, whereas the remaining activity was like that of the Ama1 cells. When these cells were grown at 34°C, however, these same transformants had RNA polymerase II activities with titrations that were more clearly biphasic (Figure 1B). Both transformants had about one half their polymerase II with a sensitivity to α-amanitin inhibition like that of the Ama^S TsAF8 polymerase II and one half with a sensitivity only to inhibition by the higher concentrations of α-amanitin like that required to inhibit Ama1 polymerase II. It is quite clear that the expression of donor DNA sequences provided a new RNA polymerase II activity in these Ts^+ transformants of TsAF8.

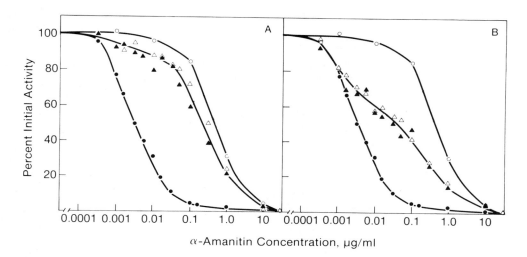

α-Amanitin Concentration, μg/ml

FIGURE 1. Inhibition of Ts and Ts⁺ transformed cell RNA polymerase II activities by α-amanitin. RNA polymerase II activities present in cell lysates of the recipient TsAF8 (●) and DNA donor Ama1 (o) cell lines and two independent Ts⁺ transformants (Δ, ▲) were assayed at 30°C in the presence of increasing concentrations of α-amanitin. The Ts⁺ transformants were grown up either at 40°C (panel A) or 34°C (panel B). Reprinted with permission from Ingles and Shales (7).

    The successful DNA-mediated transfer of this Ama^R polymerase II gene is the crucial step in setting up a viable approach to obtaining recombinant DNA clones of this gene. In order to isolate the polymerase II DNA, it will be necessary to identify the transferred DNA sequences that confer this Ama^R phenotype on recipient TsAF8 cells. To this end we have isolated three types of primary transformants that have acquired new Ama^R polymerase II activities. DNA of the donor CHO cell line Ama1 was partially cut with the restriction enzyme Mbo1 and ligated to marker Escherichia coli plasmid DNA sequences before gene transfer. In one case we ligated Ama1 DNA to DNA of the miniplasmid ph2(supF) cut with Sau3A which carries the suppressor tRNA gene supF (ph2(supF) was kindly provided by Dr. Brian Seed, Harvard University). We also ligated this partially cut Ama1 DNA to BamHI-cut pGA276 DNA (a derivative of pBR322 containing SV40 ori, Ecogpt and cos DNA, kindly provided by Dr. Gene An, Hospital for Sick Children, Toronto). A third type of DNA transfer containing marker DNA sequences was performed using DNA from the Ama^R human diploid fibroblast cell strain Ama1070 (1). The human AluI family repetitive elements can be readily distinguished from rodent sequences in DNA hybridization experiments. In each case putative transformants of TsAF8 with each of these DNAs were isolated. In addition to assessing the acquisition of new Ts⁺ or Ama^R polymerase II phenotypes and enzyme activities (as above), we confirmed that these transformants had indeed acquired donor DNA sequences.

    Genomic DNA from the three types of primary transformants was isolated, cut with EcoRI and probed in Southern blot experiments for the presence of the cotransferred marker DNA sequences; that is the presence of ph2(supF), pGA276 or human AluI family repetitive sequence DNAs. Using as probes nick-translated ph2(supF), pGA276, or BLUR8 (8) DNA, the

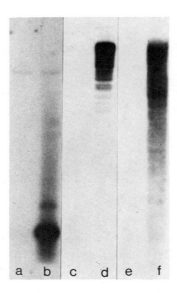

FIGURE 2. Presence of transferred marker DNA in primary transformants
of TsAF8 cells. 20 µg of genomic DNA from recipient TsAF8 cells
(lanes a,c and e) and from TsAF8 cells transformed with ph2-Ama1
(lane b), pGA276-Ama1 (lane d) and human Ama1070 (lane e) DNA were cut
with EcoRI, fractionated on a 1% agarose gel and probed in Southern blot
experiments with nick-translated ph2(supF) (lanes a,b), pGA276 (lanes
c,d) and BLUR8 (lanes e,f) DNAs.

TsAF8 cell lines transformed with ph2(supF)Ama1, pGA276-Ama1 and Ama1070
DNA were shown to contain respectively ph2(supF), pGA276 and human AluI
family DNA. TsAF8 DNA was shown in each case to contain no cross-hybri-
dizing DNA sequences (Figure 2). As in other gene transfer experiments,
uptake of multiple unlinked DNAs was apparent, for the primary transformants in each case contained an array of EcoRI fragments of different
sizes complementary to their respective probes. Using genomic DNA from
these primary transformants in a second round of Ts$^+$ Ama^R transformation
of TsAF8 cells, we have now been able to obtain some secondary transformants largely devoid of unwanted cotransferred marker DNA sequences.

DISCUSSION

In these studies we have shown that the gene for either hamster or
human RNA polymerase II, which determines sensitivity to inhibition by
α-amanitin, can be transferred to a Ts Syrian hamster BHK21 cell line.
By selection for survival at the nonpermissive temperature and assay for
the coacquisition of an Ama^R polymerase II activity, putative transformants can be readily distinguished from the all-too-frequent spontaneous
Ts$^+$ revertants of the recipient cell line TsAF8. TsAF8 is a Ts cell line
that was selected by 5-fluoro-2'-deoxyuridine killing of dividing cells
at a nonpermissive temperature (10). It arrests in the mid G1 phase of
the cell cycle (2). These gene transfer data provide unambiguous evidence
that the Ts function in TsAF8 cells is RNA polymerase II. Arrest at the

mid G1 phase of the cell cycle is probably due to an insufficiency in some other yet-unidentified cellular product whose synthesis is dependent on RNA polymerase II activity, i.e., mRNA synthesis. Thus this cell cycle mutant is unlikely to aid in any genetic dissection of mechanisms regulating cell cycle transition.

Isolation of the RNA polymerase II gene will be facilitated by these gene transfer experiments. The primary transformants described in this report have marker ph2(supF), pGA276, or human AluI DNA sequences in close proximity to the transferred Ts$^+$ Ama^R gene. This will enable rescue of the polymerase II DNA from a recombinant λ phage library of the DNA of secondary Ts$^+$ Ama^R transformants. For transformants with supF DNA, supF$^+$ phages can be readily identified on E. coli indicator strains (e.g., lacZ$^{(am)}$ or recA$^{(am)}$. Rescue of pGA276-containing phages can be accomplished by recombination in E. coli between the colE1 replicon of pGA276 and the supF miniplasmid πVX (Brian Seed, personal communication, see also ref. 9). Of course identification of the desired recombinant phage clones can also be achieved by screening λ plaques by hybridization with the appropriate radioactive probes.

The isolation of these recombinant clones of RNA polymerase II DNA will facilitate analysis of the regulatory mechanisms and mutations affecting RNA polymerase II. They may also lead to an understanding of the abnormalities in specific developmental pathways caused by mutation (4,11) of this same locus in other organisms such as Drosophila melanogaster.

ACKNOWLEDGEMENTS

We thank Lina Demirjian for technical assistance. This work was supported by a grant from the Medical Research Council of Canada.

REFERENCES

1. Buchwald M, Ingles CJ (1976): Somatic Cell Genet 2:225
2. Burstin SJ, Meiss HK, Basilico C (1974): J Cell Physiol 84:397
3. Chan VL, Whitmore GF, Siminovitch L (1972): Proc Natl Acad Sci USA 69:3119
4. Greenleaf AL, Weeks JR, Volker RA, Ohnishi S, Dickson B (1980): Cell 21:785
5. Ingles CJ, Guialis A, Lam J, Siminovitch L (1976): J Biol Chem 251:2729
6. Ingles CJ (1978): Proc Natl Acad Sci USA 75:405
7. Ingles CJ, Shales M (1982): Mol Cell Biol 2:666
8. Jelinek WR, Toomey TP, Leinwand L, Duncan CH, Biro PA, Choudary PV, Weissman SM, Rubin CM, Houck CM, Deininger PL, Schmidt CW (1980): Proc Natl Acad Sci USA 77:1398
9. Maniatis T, Fritsch EF, Sambrook J (1982): Molecular Cloning, Cold Spring Harbor, NY: Cold Spring Harbor Laboratory
10. Meiss HK, Basilico C (1972): Nature (London) New Biol. 239:66
11. Mortin MA, Lefevre G Jr. (1981): Chromosoma 82:237
12. Shales M, Bergsagel J, Ingles CJ (1980): J Cell Physiol 105:527
13. Somers DG, Pearson ML, Ingles CJ (1975): J Biol Chem 250:4825

Gene Transfer and Cancer, edited by M. L. Pearson and N. L. Sternberg. Raven Press, New York © 1984.

Gene Transfer of an RNA Polymerase II Mutation that Affects Muscle Differentiation

Clyde W. Shearman, Pamela Benfield, Robert Zivin, David Graf, and Mark L. Pearson

Cancer Biology Program, National Cancer Institute, Frederick Cancer Research Facility, Frederick, Maryland 21701

ABSTRACT. We have used DNA-mediated gene transfer to analyze the developmental defect in an ethylmethane sulfonate-induced, α–amanitin-resistant (Ama^R) RNA polymerase II mutant, Ama27, of the rat myoblast line L6. In the absence of amanitin, Ama27 fuses normally; in its presence, fusion and the associated increase in creatine kinase activity is delayed. Therefore, Ama27 has an amanitin-conditional, myogenic-defective phenotype, designated as Myo(ama).

To test whether the RNA polymerase II mutation itself and not some other unlinked mutation is responsible for this differentiation defect, we used CaPO$_4$-DNA gene transfer to transform wild-type L6 D$_O$ cells to the Ama^R phenotype using DNA from the mutant clone, Ama27. The Myo phenotype of three unstable transfectants were compared to that of the Ama27 donor and of the D$_O$ recipient myoblasts. Assays for myotube formation and creatine kinase and measurements of muscle creatine kinase mRNA levels indicated that the Ama^R transfectants acquired the conditional Myo(ama) phenotype characteristic of the donor, Ama27. These observations support the hypothesis that the Ama27 mutation to α–amanitin resistance in RNA polymerase II is directly responsible for the developmental defect in the myogenic pathway in Ama27.

INTRODUCTION

We have been studying the molecular mechanisms that control gene expression during muscle development in the L6 rat myoblast cell line. This cell line is able to undergo the terminal stages of myogenic development in cell culture, including the formation of myotubes (17,24) and the increase in the levels of several muscle-characteristic proteins such as actin, myosin and creatine kinase (1,7,17,18).

Our experimental approach to the study of developmental regulation of gene expression in this system was to isolate and characterize mutants defective in cellular functions presumed to be essential for myogenesis. One such function is RNA polymerase II, a key cellular enzyme required for proper mRNA synthesis. In bacteria, mutations in RNA polymerase are known that interfere with normal transcriptional control of genes required for sporulation (21) or for bacteriophage development (8,9). We wondered if similar mutations could be found in more complex cells that could specifically impair development, in this case muscle differentiation. Therefore, we set out to isolate and characterize a series of mutants in L6 myoblasts, using α-amanitin, a specific inhibitor of RNA polymerase II (12), as the selective agent (19).

We isolated Ama[R] L6 mutants and showed that they possess an altered form of RNA polymerase II unable to bind α-amanitin as readily as the wild-type enzyme (5,6,19). These ama[R] mutations are codominant in diploid and tetraploid L6 cells (6). When the mutants are grown in the presence of amanitin, the wild-type form of the enzyme is inactivated, whereas the mutant form is produced in greater amounts to compensate for the loss of the sensitive RNA polymerase II (6,20). Many of these Ama[R] mutants were subsequently found to be defective in myogenesis (Myo[−]) as assayed by their ability to form myotubes in culture and to show the associated increase in muscle creatine kinase (15). A subset of these mutants exhibited an amanitin-conditional Myo[−] phenotype; fusion was normal in the absence of amanitin but not in its presence, even though growth in amanitin was unimpaired. The existence of these Myo(ama) conditional mutants suggests that some Ama[R] mutations result in a pleiotropic defect in myogenesis because of altered patterns of transcription by the mutant form of RNA polymerase II. This interpretation has been strengthened by the determination of the pattern of muscle proteins synthesized by these mutants in the presence and absence of amanitin (15).

In this report, we describe experiments that further support this pleiotropy hypothesis, based on DNA-mediated gene transfer of the ama27 mutation and subsequent measurements of the expression of the gene encoding the muscle isozyme of creatine kinase (CKM).

RESULTS

DNA-mediated Gene Transfer of the Ama[R] Phenotype

To examine the hypothesis that certain mutations in RNA polymerase II might be directly responsible for the altered myogenic phenotype of the L6 Myo(ama) mutants, DNA-mediated gene transfer studies were performed to test for the simultaneous transfer of the ama[R] gene and the defect in myogenesis. Such a simultaneous transfer would be unlikely to occur if the defect in myogenesis was due to some gene other than the ama[R] gene, unless the other gene was very closely linked to ama[R]. Table 1 presents the results of this experiment using the parent wild-type D_O rat myoblast as the recipient cell. The donor DNAs were extracted from either Ama27, a conditionally defective Ama[R], Myo(ama) mutant, or from D_O, the Ama[S], Myo[+] parent. The transfer of amanitin resistance from the Ama27 DNA to the D_O cell was relatively efficient (0.15 Ama[R] transformants/μg of Ama27 DNA), nearly 150-fold above the spontaneous mutation frequency to the Ama[R] phenotype. Three independent Ama[R] transformant clones were further characterized.

Stability of the Transferred Ama[R] Phenotype

The stability of the Ama[R] putative transformants was examined in order to demonstrate that their Ama[R] phenotypes were the result of gene transfer and not of spontaneous mutations. The relative plating efficiency, expressed as the ratio of plating efficiency in the presence of amanitin to that in its absence, was measured after growth in nonselective medium (lacking α-amanitin). The Ama[R] phenotype of the transformants was unstable, showing a progressive loss of amanitin resistance when grown in nonselective medium. Their relative plating efficiencies decreased

TABLE 1. Transformation of L6 Rat Myoblasts to Amanitin Resistance[a]

Clone	Donor DNA Phenotype	Ama^R transformants/µg DNA
Ama27	Ama^R, Myo(ama)	0.150
D_o	Ama^S, Myo^+	<0.001

[a] Wild-type L6 rat myoblasts (clone D_o) were maintained in Dulbecco's modified Eagle's medium containing gentamicin and 10% fetal calf serum. Twenty-four hours after seeding 5×10^5 cells on 100-mm plates, the cultures were transfected with 20 µg of donor DNA according to the method of Graham and van der Eb (11) as modified by Corsaro and Pearson (4). After 6 days expression time at 37°C, the transfected cultures were shifted into medium containing 2 µg/ml α-amanitin. Colonies were isolated after 3–4 weeks for further analysis. The number of Ama^R transformants was determined by counting colonies both before and after fixing them in methanol and staining them with 0.2% methylene blue. Surviving colonies were tested for their Ama^R phenotype by replating in the presence of α-amanitin.

approximately 50% during the first 2 wk and stabilized at about 20% by 6–8 wk. Such phenotypic instability usually indicates a trait acquired during gene transfer but not yet stably integrated in the genome (23). In contrast, the Ama27 donor and the one spontaneous new Ama^R mutant tested were stable as expected.

Transfer of the Myo(ama) Phenotype

Having transferred the ama27 gene to a wild-type myoblast recipient, we tested for simultaneous transfer of the myogenic defect. Several factors of myogenesis were studied: the kinetics of myotube formation; changes in the level of CKM activity; and changes in the transcription of the muscle-specific creatine kinase gene, ckm.

Figure 1 shows the morphological changes characteristic of the conditional Myo(ama) phenotype exhibited by the Ama27 donor. In this study, day 0 was defined as the time when the cultures became confluent and were shifted into fusion medium (1% fetal calf serum, 5 µg/ml insulin) (14). By day 2, the myoblasts had aligned in preparation for fusion both in the absence and presence of amanitin. On day 3, cells grown in the absence of amanitin had formed myotubes, whereas cells grown in its presence had not. By day 4, cultures grown in the absence of amanitin had already begun to denegrate (a characteristic of L6 cultures). In contrast, the Ama27 mutant grown in the presence of amanitin was just beginning to form myotubes. Also, the myotubes appeared to be much smaller in the presence of amanitin. This amanitin-dependent delay in myogenesis characteristic of the parent donor Ama27 was also found in each of the three independent transformants examined.

Since the kinetics of fusion is at best a semiquantitative indicator of differentiation, we examined a biochemical marker of myogenesis, CKM.

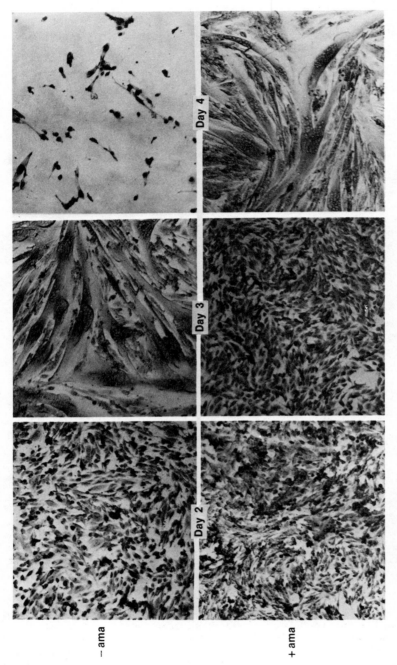

FIGURE 1. Morphology of the Myo(ama) phenotype of Ama27. Ama27 myoblasts were maintained in Dulbecco's modified Eagle's medium containing gentamicin and 10% fetal calf serum with or without 2 μg/ml α-amanitin for several generations before use. The cells were plated on 60-mm dishes at a density of 2 x 10^5 cells/dish in medium with or without amanitin. When the cultures reached confluence, the medium was changed to fusion medium (DME containing 1% fetal calf serum and 5 μg/ml insulin) again with or without 2 μg/ml amanitin (day 0). Plates are removed at 24-hr periods, fixed in methanol and stained with 0.015% w/v Geimsa in methanol.

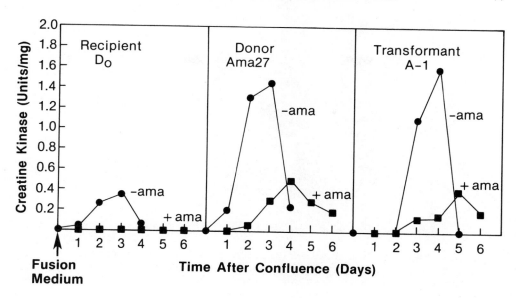

FIGURE 2. Creatine kinase specific activities during development of wild-type recipient (D_O), mutant donor (Ama27) and transformant (A-1) myoblast cultures. At daily intervals after reaching confluence and shifting into fusion medium, a sample of cells was washed with 10mM Tris-acetate, pH 6.8, 25 mM magnesium acetate, 0.5 mM dithiothreitol, 10% glycerol and then harvested by scraping from the tissue culture dish into the same buffer containing 0.2% Nonidet-P40, 0.1 mM phenyl-methylsulfonyl fluoride, 2 µg/ml leupeptin and 1 µg/ml pepstatin. Cells were disrupted by freezing and thawing them twice and then passing them through a 27-gauge needle. Samples were stored frozen at -20°C. Creatine kinase was assayed by determining creatine formation from crea-tine phosphate during a 20-minute incubation, using the fluorometric method of Zalin (25). Protein was estimated by the method of Bradford (2). A unit of creatine kinase is defined as the amount needed to cata-lyse the formation of 1 µmol creatine/min at 37°C.

Figure 2 shows the specific activity of CKM as a function of time after the cultures reached confluence and were changed to fusion medium. In the absence of amanitin, the D_O recipient cells showed a rise in CKM activity coinciding with the formation of myotubes. In the presence of amanitin, the D_O cells died. In the absence of amanitin, the donor Ama27 cells also showed CKM activity that peaked during myogenesis. For reasons we do not understand, this peak CKM activity in fusing Ama27 showed a charac-teristic elevation compared to that observed in D_O cells. In Ama27 cells in the presence of amanitin, there was both a delay and a decrease in the peak CKM activity. Like the Ama27 donor, the transformant A-1 also ex-hibited the Myo(ama) phenotype with both a delay and a decresase in peak CKM activity in the presence of amanitin. In the absence of amanitin, the A-1 transformant also showed an increase in peak CKM activity similar to that of the Ama27 donor. Other independent transformants had CKM profiles similar to A-1 and Ama27.

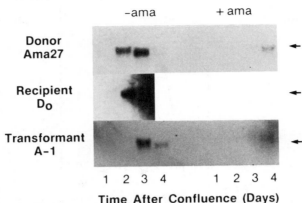

Time After Confluence (Days)

FIGURE 3. Temporal appearance of muscle creatine kinase transcripts in wild-type recipient (D_O), mutant donor (Ama27) and transformant (A-1) myoblast cultures. Myoblasts were grown to confluence in 100-mm dishes in the absence or presence of 2 µg/ml α-amanitin. At confluence, the growth medium was replaced with fusion media, again with or without α-amanitin. Two plates of each cell line, one with and one without α-amanitin, were harvested each day after confluence for 4 days. Cells were harvested by replacement of the fusion medium with 2.5 ml of 4 M guanidinium thiocyanate, containing 50 mM sodium citrate, pH 6.5; 0.7% v/v β-mercaptoethanol, and w/v 0.5% Sarkosyl NL97 (3). The resulting material was pipetted repeatedly to reduce its viscosity, loaded atop a CsCl shelf in an ultracentrifuge tube and processed to prepare RNA. The denatured RNA samples were run on a 1% agarose-formaldehyde gel (15 µg RNA/well) (10) and transferred to nitrocellulose filters for Northern blot analysis (22). Each filter was probed with [^{32}P]-pckm-1, a muscle creatine kinase cDNA clone labeled by nick translation, to detect muscle creatine kinase-specific RNA sequences. This probe contains a ckm cDNA insert of 700 bp that includes the active site of CKM, corresponding roughly to half the total coding sequence of the 1.5 kb ckm mRNA.

The decrease and delay in peak CKM specific activity in the presence of amanitin associated with the myogenic defect has been assumed to reflect an altered pattern of ckm transcription. Figure 3 shows that this assumption is correct, as shown by Northern blot hybridization analyses of the accumulation of muscle-specific creatine kinase mRNA as a function of time after confluence, both in the absence and presence of amanitin. The probe used to assay ckm transcripts is specific for the muscle isozyme of creatine kinase as shown by hybrid selection for mRNA translatable into CKM in vitro and by direct nucleotide sequence analysis (R.A. Zivin et al., in preparation). The size of mature rat ckm mRNA is about 1.5 kb, the same as that of chicken ckm mRNA (13). Generally, the steady-state level of ckm mRNA paralleled the CKM activity, and in the presence of amanitin, transcription was delayed. In the Ama27 donor, ckm mRNA appeared on day 2 and reached a peak on day 3 in the absence of amanitin. In the presence of amanitin, ckm mRNA appeared on day 4 and was lower in concentration. This is the same pattern found for CKM activity. The Ama^R transformants, illustrated here by A-1, showed a similar profile with a decrease and delay in ckm mRNA in the presence of amanitin.

DISCUSSION

The results presented here strongly support the hypothesis that some ama^R RNA polymerase II mutants result in a pleiotropic defect in myogenesis because of altered patters of muscle-specific gene transcription by the mutant form of RNA polymerase II.

Because Ama27 is a mutant induced by ethylmethane sulfonate treatment, the possibility existed that the Ama^R and Myo(ama) phenotypes were the result of independent mutations. However, the high frequency of association of these two phenotypes in independently derived mutants noted previously (15) and the results of the DNA mediated gene transfer experiments reported here indicate that this possibility is very unlikely. Even though competent mammalian cells can acquire up to 1,000 kb of exogenous DNA in typical $CaPO_4$-DNA transfer experiments (16), the probability of a competent cell taking up two separate unlinked genes would be approximately 10^{-6} – 10^{-8}. Therefore, only 1 out of every 1,000–10,000 Ama^R tranformants would be expected to have acquired the Myo(ama) phenotype as well. The possibility that these two phenotypes are due to two closely linked genes, however, cannot be formally excluded until the $ama27$ gene is cloned.

Studies have shown that the Ama^R phenotype of Ama27 results from a mutation of RNA polymerase II (15). Preliminary data with crude extracts of independent Ama^R transformants indicate that these transformants also contain Ama^R RNA polymerase II. The levels of mutant RNA polymerase II expressed in these transformants is under investigation.

The increase in creatine kinase activity and the isoenzyme switch from brain to muscle CKM has been shown to be associated with myogenesis (14, 17). In these studies, we found that the Myo(ama) phenotype is characterized by a delay in myotube formation which coincides with the delay in both peak creatine kinase activity and the transcription of ckm genes. These results suggest that the mutant RNA polymerase II is defective in its ability to transcribe genes necessary for myogenesis, possibly because of altered interactions with effector molecules signaling differentiation. Further analysis may provide insight into the molecular processes involved in transcriptional regulation of muscle-specific gene expression during normal muscle development.

ACKNOWLEDGEMENTS

Research sponsored by the National Cancer Institute under Contract No. NO1-CO-75380 with Litton Bionetics, Inc.

REFERENCES

1. Benoff S, Nadal-Ginard B (1979): Biochemistry 18:494
2. Bradford MM (1976): Anal Biochem 72:248
3. Chirgwin JM, Przybyla AE, MacDonald RJ, Rutter WJ (1979): Biochemistry 18:5294
4. Corsaro CM, Pearson ML (1981): Somatic Cell Genet 7:603
5. Crerar MM, Andrews SJ, David ES, Somers DG, Mandel J-L, Pearson ML (1977): J Mol Biol 112:317
6. Crerar MM, Pearson ML (1977): J Mol Biol 112:331
7. Delain D, Meienhofer MC, Proux D, Schapira F (1973): Differentiation 1:249
8. Georgopoulos CP (1971): Proc Natl Acad Sci USA 68:2977
9. Ghysen A, Pironio M (1972): J Mol Biol 65:259
10. Goldberg DA (1980): Proc Natl Acad Sci USA 77:5794

11. Graham FL, Van der Eb AJ (1973):   Virology 52:456
12. Lindell TJ, Weinberg F, Morris PW, Roeder RG, Rutter WJ (1970):
     Science 170:447
13. MacLeod AR (1981):   Nucleic Acids Res 9:2675
14. Mandel J-L, Pearson ML (1974):   Nature 251:618
15. Pearson ML, Crerar MM (in press):   In: Molecular and Cellular Control
     (Pearson ML, Epstein HF, eds), Cold Spring Harbor NY: Cold Spring
     Harbor Laboratory
16. Perucho M, Hanahan D, Wigler M (1980):   Cell 22:309
17. Shainberg A, Yagil G, Yaffe D (1971):   Dev Biol 25:1
18. Shani M, Zevinsonkin D, Saxel O, Carmon Y, Katcoff D, Nudel Y,
     Yaffe D (1981):   Dev Biol 86:483
19. Somers DG, Pearson ML, Ingles CH (1975):   J Biol Chem 250:4825
20. Somers DG, Pearson ML, Ingles CH (1975):   Nature 253:372
21. Sonenshein AL, Cami B, Brevet J, Cote R (1974):   J Bacteriol 120:253
22. Thomas P (1980):   Proc Natl Acad Sci USA 77:5201
23. Wigler M, Pellicer A, Silverstein S, Axel R, Urlaub G, Chasin L
     (1979):   Proc Natl Acad Sci USA 76:1373
24. Yaffe D (1968):   Proc Natl Acad Sci USA 61:477
25. Zalin RI (1973):   Exp Cell Res 78:152

Gene Transfer and Cancer, edited by M. L. Pearson
and N. L. Sternberg. Raven Press, New York © 1984.

Bovine Papillomavirus/pML2 Hybrid Vector: A Dual Host Replicon

Nava Sarver, Stella Mitrani-Rosenbaum, Ming-Fan Law,
Janet C. Byrne, and Peter M. Howley

Laboratory of Pathology, National Cancer Institute, Bethesda, Maryland 20205

ABSTRACT. The utility of the subgenomic transforming segment of the bovine papillomavirus type 1 (BPV-1) genome as a eucaryotic cloning vector has been previously described (18,19). One limitation of this vector system has been the marked reduction in the transformation efficiency of the cloned BPV-1 DNA or the cloned 69% subgenomic transforming fragment (BPV$_{69T}$) when it is covalently linked to pBR322 DNA. We have examined the ability of the BPV-1 genome and the BPV$_{69T}$ to transform mouse cells when cloned into pML2 (15), a deletion derivative of pBR322. The complete BPV genome cloned into pML2 is highly efficient in transforming mouse cells whether or not the BPV-1 sequences have been separated from the procaryotic sequences. The hybrid DNA is maintained as an extrachromosomal plasmid and in most instances there are no detectable rearrangements. Plasmids indistinguishable from the input DNA can be rescued by transformation of bacteria with the cellular DNA.

The 69% transforming segment of BPV-1 cloned in pML2 is, however, approximately 100-fold less efficient in its transforming ability when not physically separated from the procaryotic sequences. DiMaio et al. (2) have recently shown that a BPV$_{69T}$-pML2 hybrid DNA containing a 7.6-kb human β-globin gene fragment can efficiently transform mouse cells without the removal of the procaryotic sequences. We have identified three additional defined eucaryotic genomic fragments which provide a similar transformation enhancement when inserted into the BPV$_{69T}$-pML hybrid DNA.

INTRODUCTION

Vectors derived from several animal viruses are presently being utilyzed for the introduction of foreign genes into eucaryotic cells. These include SV40 (6,16), the retroviruses (3,11,24), and the human adenoviruses (21). The 69% subgenomic transforming fragment of BPV-1 DNA (BPV$_{69T}$) has been used as a eucaryotic cloning vector for the rat preproinsulin gene (18,19).

BPV-1 transformed cells contain multiple copies of viral DNA existing exclusively as unintegrated extrachromosomal plasmids (13). Since integration is not necessary for transformation by BPV-1, the physical contiguity the of linked foreign gene is preserved. Moreover, the extrachromosomal state provides a homogeneous sequence environment for each of the multiple copies of the inserted gene, thereby making subsequent analysis

of normal and mutant gene expression feasible. The extrachromosomal
plasmid state of BPV-1 linked DNAs should also permit the shuttling of
genes between eucaryotic and procaryotic cells provided the BPV-1 hybrid
DNA contains a bacterial plasmid origin of replication and a selective
marker for bacteria (2). Earlier studies (10,14) have indicated that
BPV DNA transformation of mouse cells is markedly inhibited when it is
covalently linked to pBR322 DNA. Thus, for efficient transformation of
mouse cells by BPV-1 DNA or by BPV_{69T}, the BPV sequences must be cleaved
from the pBR322 sequences, a step which has precluded the sequential
rescue of the hybrid DNA back into bacteria.

Covalently linked pBR322 DNA sequences have been shown to inhibit
SV40 DNA replication in simian cells (1,7,15). A deletion derivative of
pBR322 (pML2) has been described that lacks the specific sequence that
is cis-inhibitory to SV40 DNA replication in simian cells (15). To test
whether the specific pBR322 sequence that inhibits SV40 DNA replication
in monkey cells also inhibits BPV-1 DNA-mediated transformation of mouse
cells, we examined the transformation efficiency of linked BPV/pML2 hybrid DNAs.

RESULTS AND DISCUSSION

The cis-inhibition of BPV-1 DNA transformation by a specific pBR322
sequence was examined by transformation assay (4,5) on mouse C127 cells
with recombinant DNAs that were either separated from the procaryotic
sequences by restriction endonuclease cleavage or left covalently linked
to pBR322. BPV-1 DNA cloned in pBR322 at the BamHI site [pBPV-1 (8-2)]
transforms very poorly, inducing only 2 colonies per μg DNA (Table 1).
BamHI digestion of this hybrid DNA into its BPV-1 and pBR322 components
results in a 100-fold increase in transformation efficiency. Gel-puri-
fied, linearized cloned BPV-1 DNA transforms with the same efficiency as
the BamHI digestion mixture containing linearized BPV and pBR322 DNA
components, indicating that the inhibition by pBR322 is cis-acting
(Table 1). The cis-inhibition of BPV-1 DNA-mediated transformation was
not specific to one orientation in that a BPV/pBR322 hybrid DNA [pBPV-1
(79-2)] with the BPV-1 genome inserted at the BamHI site in the opposite
orientation was also very inefficient for transformation (Table 1).
Also, BPV/pBR322 hybrid DNA with the BPV-1 genome inserted at the HindIII
site [pBPV-1 (9-1)] was also inhibited in its transformation efficiency
by covalently linked pBR322 sequences (Table 1).

The ability of the pBR322 deletion derivative pML2 to permit efficient
replication of SV40 DNA in simian cells suggested that it may also permit
transformation of mouse cells by the intact hybrid DNA if the cis-inhibition were due to an inhibition of the replication of BPV-1 plasmid DNA.
The full BPV-1 genome was therefore cloned into a derivative of pML2 at
the BamHI site (Figure 1), and the hybrid DNA was assayed for its capacity to transform mouse cells. In contrast to the low transformation
levels observed with pBR322/BPV hybrids, intact pML2/BPV DNA transformed
with the same efficiency as the cleaved pML2/BPV molecule (approximately
200 foci/μg BPV-1 DNA, Table 1) indicating that the specific pBR322
sequence that inhibits SV40 DNA replication in monkey cells also blocks
efficient BPV DNA transformation of mouse cells.

The structure of the recombinant pML2-BPV hybrid in the transformed
cell lines was next examined. Low-molecular-weight DNA was extracted by
differential salt precipitation (9) and analyzed by restriction endonuclease digestion, gel electrophoresis, and DNA blotting. Analysis of
uncleaved DNA from each of these lined indicated that the DNA was present

TABLE 1. Transformation of mouse cells by BPV hybrid DNAs

DNA	BPV segment[a]	Vector	Cloning site	Treatment	Transformants/ μg BPV DNA/ 10^6 cells[b]
8-2	BPV	pBR322	BamHI	BamHI	246
8-2	BPV	pBR322	BamHI	Uncleaved	2
8-2	BPV	pBR322	BamHI	BamHI purified fragment[c], linear	176
8-2	BPV	pBR322	BamHI	BamHI purified fragment[c], re-circularized[d]	882
79-2	BPV	pBR322	BamHI[e]	Uncleaved	1
9-1	BPV	pBR322	HindIII	HindIII	183
9-1	BPV	pBR322	HindIII	Uncleaved	1
142-6	BPV	pML2	BamHI	BamHI	200
142-6	BPV	pML2	BamHI	Uncleaved	198
17-6	BPV$_{69T}$	pBR322	BamHI/HindIII	BamHI/HindIII	116
17-6	BPV$_{69T}$	pBR322	BamHI/HindIII	Uncleaved	1
54-2	BPV$_{69T}$	pML2	BamHI[f]	BamHI	126
54-2	BPV$_{69T}$	pML2	BamHI[f]	Uncleaved	0
54-2	BPV$_{69T}$	pML2	BamHI[f]	BamHI purified fragment[c], linear	95
54-2	BPV$_{69T}$	pML2	BamHI[f]	BamHI purified fragment[c], re-circularized[d]	65

[a] BPV = 7.95 kb; BPV$_{69T}$ = 5.45 kb.

[b] Transformants/μg/10^6 cells = $\dfrac{\text{No. of foci}}{\text{μg of plasmid DNA}} \times \dfrac{\text{size of plasmid (kb)}}{\text{size of BPV DNA (kb)}}$

[c] DNA fragment was purified in agarose gel and recovered by electroelution.

[d] Recircularization of the purified DNA fragment was achieved with T4 ligase under dilute DNA concentration.

[e] The BamHI linear genome of BPV-1 is inserted in pBR322 in an orientation opposite to that of 8-2 DNA.

[f] The HindIII site of BPV$_{69T}$ was converted to a BamHI site with synthetic linkers (Collaborative Research). BamHI cleavage thus generates a BPV$_{69T}$ segment with complementary cohesive ends.

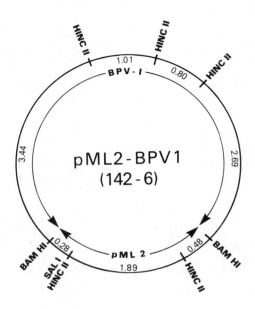

FIGURE 1.   Physical map of pML2-BPV hybrid DNA.   pML2 was derived from
pJYM (11), a pBR322/SV40 hybrid molecule containing a deletion from 1095
to 2485 on the pBR322 map (M. Lusky and M. Botchan, personal communication).   This deletion removes the sequence inhibitory to pBR322/SV40
replication in simian cells.   The small fragment extending from the
BamHI to HindIII site in pML2 was removed and the HindIII site was converted to a BamHI recognition site with synthetic BamHI linkers generating a 2.65-kb pML2 molecule that is 0.35 kb smaller than the original
pML2.   Full-length BPV DNA, isolated from pBR322/BPV (8-2) by BamHI
cleavage, was inserted at the BamHI site of pML2 (2.65 kb).   The resulting pML2/BPV hybrid is designated as 142-6.   The 5' orientation of pML2
extends in a clockwise direction on the map and that of BPV is in a
counterclockwise direction.

as a 10.6-kb plasmid which could be detected as supercoiled form I DNA
and nicked monomeric circular form II DNA (data not shown).   After
cleavage with BamHI to separate the plasmid into its BPV-1 and pML2 components, the DNA was transferred bidirectionally (20,21) to produce two
identical templates, one of which was probed with ^{32}P-labeled BPV-1 DNA
and the other with ^{32}P-labeled pBR322 DNA.   As shown in Figure 2, the
7.95-kb BPV-specific segment and the 2.65-kb pML2 fragment each comigrated with the appropriate fragment from the input plasmid (142-6) in
seven independent lines analyzed.   Analysis of total cellular DNA from
these lines indicated a copy number per diploid genome of 5 to 100,
which is in the range of that found in cells transformed by BPV-1 virus,
cloned viral DNA, or BPV[69T] DNA (13).   Thus, the pML2/BPV-1 hybrid DNA
is capable of transforming mouse cells as an intact plasmid and can
replicate efficiently as an extrachromosomal plasmid in the transformed
cells.   In one of these lines, NS142-6U-3, in addition to the 10.6-kb
monomeric circular forms, we also observed a slower migrating circular
DNA form which hybridized to both BPV and pML2 DNAs (not shown).   This
line thus harbors two species of extrachromosomal DNA, one similar to

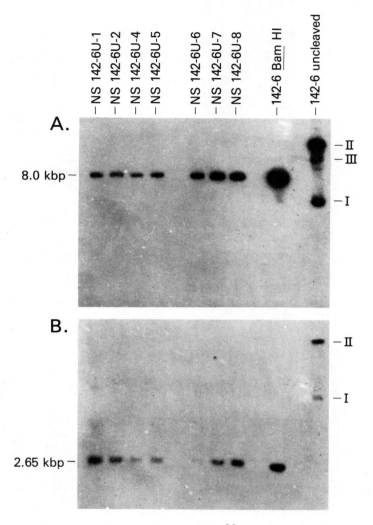

FIGURE 2. Southern blot hybridization of ^{32}P-labeled BPV-1 DNA and ^{32}P-labeled pBR322 DNA to low-molecular-weight DNAs prepared from mouse cells transformed by intact pML2/BPV-1 (142-6). Low-molecular-weight DNAs extracted from transformed cell lines were fractionated through a 0.6% agarose gel, partially depurinated and denatured in situ (23), and transferred bidirectionally (20,21) to nitrocellulose filters to produce two identical templates. The immobilized DNAs were then hybridized to 5 x 10^6 (1 x 10^8 cpm/μg DNA) of nick-translated (16) denatured ^{32}P-labeled BPV DNA or ^{32}P-labeled pBR322 DNA. The filters were exposed to X-ray film for 24 hr at -70°C with intensifying screens. The transformed cell lines, derived from isolated transformed foci, are indicated above each lane. Migration positions of uncleaved and BamHI cleaved fragments of 142-6 DNA are indicated. Panel A, ^{32}P-labeled BPV probe; Panel B, ^{32}P-labeled pBR322 probe.

the input plasmid and the other a rearranged plasmid molecule containing duplicated or acquired DNA sequences.

Low-molecular-weight DNA from three representative cell lines was used to transform competent bacterial C600 cells to ampicillin resistance. One percent of the Hirt supernatant from a 75-cm^2 flask yielded 2 to 20 ampicillin-resistant colonies under conditions which yielded 5×10^6 colonies per µg pBR322 DNA. Analysis of the bacterial plasmid with several multiple-cut restriction endonucleases for the pML2/BPV-1 DNA hybrid demonstrated that the recovered recombinant DNAs were indistinguishable from the input plasmid DNA (not shown). These recovered DNAs were tested for their ability to retransform mouse cells and found to have specific transformation activities similar to that of the original pML2/BPV plasmid (approximately 200 transformants per µg of BPV-1 DNA).

The effect of pBR322 and pML2 on the transforming ability of the subgenomic transforming region of BPV (BPV_{69T}) was also examined. As was the case with the pBR322/BPV hybrids, the $pBR322/BPV_{69T}$ DNA transformed mouse cells with high efficiency (100 foci/µg DNA) only following cleavage of the BPV_{69T} from the pBR322 sequences (Table 1). Surprisingly, the $pML2/BPV_{69T}$ hybrid DNA also had to be separated into its BPV_{69T} and pML2 components to effect efficient transformation of mouse cells with the transforming activity of the intact $pML2/BPV_{69T}$ hybrid approximately 100-fold lower than that of the cleaved molecule (Table 1). Thus, although the full BPV-1 genome can transform mouse cells efficiently when cloned into pML2, the subgenomic transforming segment cannot.

The linear BPV_{69T} is consistently less efficient than linear full-length BPV-1 DNA in transforming mouse cells (14, Table 1). Conversion of the HindIII site of BPV_{69T} to a BamHI site with synthetic linkers to permit simple circularization of the input DNA within the cells does not increase the specific transformation activity of the fragment (Table 1). The reduced activity of the fragment is therefore not simply a result of the physical constraint imparted by the presence of nonhomologous ends impairing circularization. In addition, although the purified, circularized full BPV-1 DNA is 4- to 5-fold more efficient in transforming mouse cells than its linear counterpart, the circularized BPV_{69T} molecule with BamHI ends is slightly lower in its transforming capacity (Table 1). These experiments in toto indicate that the 31% segment of BPV (BPV_{31NT}), not essential for transformation, has a specific facilitative role in BPV-1 DNA-mediated transformation.

Although the precise mechanism by which BPV_{31NT} facilitates transformation is still not known, we do not believe that BPV_{31NT} encodes a protein that mediates this effect since the bodies of each of the transcripts detected in BPV-1 transformed cells map within BPV_{69T} (8). We are currently entertaining the possibility that a transcriptional promoter sequence normally active in BPV-1 transformed cells may be located within BPV_{31NT}. We have initiated experiments to determine whether the facilitative effect is cis- or trans-acting and to define mutants in BPV_{31NT} which affect the function.

Recently DiMaio et al. (2) reported that plasmids consisting of BPV_{69T} and a 7.6-kb fragment of the human β-globin gene cloned into a pBR322 variant similar to pML2, are capable of effectively transforming mouse cells. The parental hybrid molecule $pBRd/BPV_{69T}$ lacking the globin fragment was 500-fold less efficient in transforming mouse cells. Evidently, the human β-globin DNA can also facilitate the transformation by BPV_{69T} and as such, can functionally complement BPV_{31NT}.

We have identified three additional eucaryotic sequences that can facilitate transformation by $pML2/BPV_{69T}$. These include a 5.3-kb frag-

TABLE 2. Transformation of mouse C127 cells with intact recombinant plasmid DNAs containing different eucaryotic DNA sequences

		BPV		Foci/µg of BPV DNA/10^6 cells[a,b]	
DNA	Vector	Segment	DNA Insert	uncleaved	cleaved
54-2	pML2	BPV$_{69T}$	None	4	111
143-1	pBRd[c]	BPV$_{69T}$	Human growth hormone, (2.6 kb)	338	NT[d]
212-3	pML2	BPV$_{69T}$	Rat prepro-insulin 1, (5.3 kb)	639	NT[d]
62-3	pBR322	BPV$_{69T}$	Rat prepro-insulin 1, (5.3 kb)	10	NT[d]
148-4	pBRd[c]	BPV$_{69T}$	Rat intergen-ic segment, (7.3 kb)	532	NT[d]
146-4	pBRd[c]	BPV$_{69T}$	Mouse metalo-thionine, (3.0 kb)	4	NT[d]
58-1	pML2	BPV$_{69T}$	PvuII/Bam seg-ment of pSV2gpt (1.65 kb)	1	NT[d]
142-6	pML2	Full genome	None	229	250
--	pML2	--	--	0	0

[a] $\text{Foci/µg} = \dfrac{\text{No. of foci}}{\text{µg of plasmid DNA}} \times \dfrac{\text{size of plasmid (kb)}}{\text{size of BPV specific DNA (kb)}}$

[b] BPV$_{69T}$ = 5.45 kb; BPV-1 = 7.95 kb

[c] pML2 is that described in legend to Figure 1

[d] NT = not tested

ment of the rat preproinsulin gene, a 2.6-kb fragment of the human growth hormone gene, and a 7.3-kb fragment of rat intergenic DNA (Table 2). In addition, many DNA segments do not provide this function, but apparently eucaryotic DNA segments that can facilitate transformation by pML2/BPV$_{69T}$ are ubiquitous. Although the mechanism underlying this enhancement of transformation efficiency may be similar to that of BPV$_{31NT}$, it is also possible that these fragments facilitate transformation by a different mode.

In these studies we have demonstrated the capacity of a BPV hybrid DNA to function as a vector for the shuttling of genes between animal cells and bacteria. This should allow the selection of a specific gene from a DNA library by virtue of the phenotypic changes imparted on the host cell and permit the subsequent recovery of the selected gene in bacteria.

Other studies in this laboratory have demonstrated the use of other dominant selective markers linked to BPV$_{69T}$ (12). Experiments are now in progress to test the feasibility of using dominant selective markers in conjunction with a pML2/BPV shuttle vector. This could expand the host range of cells susceptible to transformation and allow the development of a papillomavirus-derived vector that does not utilize the malignant phenotype as a selective marker.

ACKNOWLEDGEMENTS

We are grateful to Ms. Susan Hostler for her assistance in the preparation of this manuscript.

REFERENCES

1. Benoist C, Chambon P (1980): Proc Natl Acad Sci USA 77:3865
2. DiMaio D, Treisman R, Maniatis T (1982): Submitted
3. Doehmer J, Barinaga M, Vale W, Rosenfeld MG, Verma IM, Evans RM (1982): Proc Natl Acad Sci USA 79:2268
4. Frost E, Williams J. (1978): Virology 91:39
5. Graham FL, van der Eb AJ (1973): Virology 52:456
6. Gruss P, Khoury G (1981): Proc Natl Acad Sci USA 78:133
7. Hanahan D, Lane D, Lipsich L, Wigler M, Botchan M (1980): Cell 21: 127
8. Heilman CA, Engel LW, Lowy DR, Howley PM (1982): Virology 119:22
9. Hirt B (1969): J Molec Biol 40:141
10. Howley PM. Law M-F, Heilman C, Engel L, Alonso MC, Lancaster WD, Israel MA, Lowy DR (1980): In: Viruses in Naturally Occurring Cancers (Essex M, et al, eds), New York: Cold Spring Harbor NY: Cold Spring Harbor Laboratory, p 233
11. Joyner A, Yamamoto Y, Bernstein A (1981): In: Developmental Biology Using Purified Genes, ICN-UCLA Symposia on Molecular and Cellular Biology (Brown DD, Fox CF, eds), New York: Academic Press, p 535
12. Law M-F, Howard B, Sarver N, Howley PM (1982): In: Viral Vectors, Cold Spring Harbor NY: Cold Spring Harbor Laboratory
13. Law M-F, Lowy DR, Dvoretzky I, Howley PM (1981): Proc Natl Acad Sci USA 78:2727
14. Lowy DR, Dvoretzky I, Shober R, Law M-F, Engel L, Howley PM (1980): Nature 287:72
15. Lusky M, Botchan M (1981): Nature 293:79
16. Mulligan RC, Berg P (1980): Science 209:1423
17. Rigby P, Rhodes D, Dieckmann M, Berg P (1977): J Mol Biol 113:237
18. Sarver N, Gruss P, Law M-F, Khoury G, Howley PM (1981): Mol Cell Biol 1:486
19. Sarver N, Gruss P, Law M-F, Khoury G, Howley PM (1981): In: Developmental Biology Using Purified Genes, ICN-UCLA Symposia on Molecular and Cellular Biology (Brown DD, Fox CF), New York: Academic Press, p 547
20. Smith GE, Summers MD (1980): Anal Biochem 109:123
21. Southern EM (1975): J Mol Biol 98:503
22. Thummel C, Tjian R, Grodzicker T (1981): Cell 23:825
23. Wahl GM, Stern M, Start GR (1979): Proc Natl Acad Sci USA 76:3683
24. Wei C-M, Gibson M, Spear P, Scolnick E (1981): J Virol 39:935

Gene Transfer and Cancer, edited by M. L. Pearson and N. L. Sternberg. Raven Press, New York © 1984.

Development of Friend Spleen Focus-Forming Virus as a Mammalian Gene Transfer Vector

Alexandra L. Joyner and Alan Bernstein

Ontario Cancer Institute, and Department of Medical Biophysics, University of Toronto, Toronto, M4X 1K9 Canada

ABSTRACT. Friend spleen focus-forming virus (SFFV), an erythroleu-kemia-inducing murine retrovirus, can be used as a high efficiency gene transfer vector in mammalian cells. Recombinants between molecular clones of the integrated form of SFFV, containing both the 5' and 3' long terminal repeats (LTR), and the herpes simplex virus (HSV) thymi-dine kinase (tk) gene have been constructed. These clones can be res-cued and propagated as infectious tk retroviruses by cotransfection with a molecular clone of Moloney murine leukemia virus helper DNA. Infec-tious tk vectors have also been created starting with a subgenomic SFFV fragment containing only the SFFV 5' LTR and SFFV-derived gag sequences into which has been cloned the tk gene. These LTR-TK clones can be efficiently rescued and packaged as an infectious tk virus provided the tk gene has not been inserted into SFFV sequences close to the 5' LTR. The ability to generate an infectious retrovirus from the LTR-TK clones indicates that recombination between the LTR-TK constructs and the helper virus genome must take place to generate a transmissible retrovirus. These studies should facilitate the construction of other retrovirus vectors carrying heterologous sequences and suggest novel strategies for high-efficiency transfer and recovery of selectable cellular genes.

INTRODUCTION

The introduction of purified DNA segments into mammalian cells in vitro and in vivo provides a functional approach to the elucidation of the factors that regulate gene expression; moreover, the ability to transfer functionally active genes into cells has provided several strat-egies for the molecular cloning of selectable cellular genes (reviewed in 20). Hence, the development of techniques that either increase the efficiency of gene transfer or expand the range of useful recipient cells should facilitate our understanding of the mammalian genome. In bacteria, transducing viruses such as bacteriophage λ have been widely used for analyzing individual bacterial genes. Acquisition of cellular genes by phage λ results from the integration and subsequent abnormal excision of the integrated prophage from the bacterial chromosome (2); viruses resulting from these rare nonhomologous recombination events can be enriched biologically under selective growth conditions.

Based on the demonstrated usefulness of transducing phages as gene transfer vectors, animal viruses have been used as vehicles for introducing purified DNA segments into animal cells in culture. Several of these host-vector systems are discussed elsewhere in this volume. Here, we summarize recent experiments from this laboratory on the development of a murine erythroleukemia-inducing retrovirus, Friend SFFV, as a high-efficiency gene transfer vector.

Neoplastic transformation by rapidly transforming retroviruses appears to result from the presence of specific sequences on the viral genome that have been acquired from homologous cellular sequences of the host (for review, see refs. 1,18). Thus, these viruses, like phage λ, appear to be naturally occurring transducing agents that can transfer genetic information between cells of the same or different species. Retroviruses have many properties in common with the bacterial transducing viruses, a fact that makes them ideal transfer vectors. First, because integration into the host chromosome is a natural part of the retrovirus life cycle, the viral genomes are replicated along with the host genome and thus remain stably associated in the chromosomes of the recipient cell. Second, productive infection by retroviruses almost never kills the host cell. Third, host genes that are transduced by retroviruses usually come under the transcriptional control of viral promoter regions, or, as shown here, they remain under their own transcriptional control. Fourth, these viruses can very efficiently infect a wide range of recipient cell types, both in vitro and in vivo. Fifth, like phage λ, which appears to pick up cellular genes by a process of integration following by nonhomologous recombination during excision, recent evidence (see Discussion) suggests that retroviruses can also acquire heterologous sequences by a two-step process of integration followed by nonhomologous recombination.

In this paper, we describe the construction and rescue of molecular clones containing all or portions of the Friend SFFV genome into which has been inserted the purified HSV tk gene. Several central features of this host-vector system are discussed, including the effects of site and transcriptional orientation of the tk gene on rescue efficiency, evidence of recombination between SFFV-tk and helper virus genomes, and the prospects of utilizing SFFV as a vector to introduce DNA segments into hematopoietic progenitor cells.

RESULTS

Construction of SFFV-TK Vectors

Numerous retroviruses have been used as vectors for the HSV tk gene, including avian spleen necrosis virus (15), Harvey sarcoma virus (19), Moloney murine leukemia virus (16), and Friend SFFV (8). We chose SFFV as vector because a highly leukemogenic clone of the integrated form of this virus was available (21). This clone is colinear with the viral RNA genome and contains two LTR at the host-provirus junctions (Figure 1). Moreover, infection of susceptible mice with SFFV induces macroscopic spleen foci resulting from the rapid proliferation of erythroid progenitor cells. SFFV also induces malignant transformation of hematopoietic target cells 1 to 2 months after infection in vivo (11,12) or in long-term culture (3). Thus, SFFV might be a suitable vector for gene transfer into hematopoietic cells.

Figure 1 shows the structure of four parental SFFV clones that have been used as vectors for the tk gene. pSFFV502 contains the entire SFFV genome plus adjacent host rat cellular sequences cloned into the EcoRI

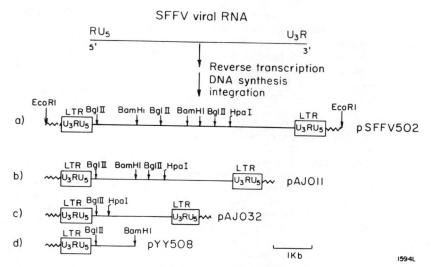

FIGURE 1. Schematic representation of the SFFV parental molecules used as vectors for the HSV tk gene. a) pSFFV502 is the full length molecular clone of the integrated form of SFFV and adjacent rat flanking sequences (indicated by the saw-tooth lines; b) pAJO11 is a deletion mutant lacking sequences between the two extreme BamHI restriction enzyme recognition sites of pSFFV502; c) pAJO32 is a deletion mutant lacking sequences between the two extreme BglII restriction enzyme recognition sites of pSFFV502; d) pYY508 contains the SFFV 5' LTR and 1.2 kb of adjacent gag sequences (9). Abbreviations: U_5, R, and U_3 are the unique (U) and repetitive (R) sequences located at the 5' and 3' ends of the viral RNA genome.

site of pBR322 (7a,21). This molecule can induce all of the cellular changes characteristic of the polycythemic variant of Friend SFFV in susceptible mice (21). Because SFFV is replication defective, the biological activity of this virus can only be demonstrated after rescue with either a replication-competent helper virus or cloned helper virus DNA. To facilitate cloning into the SFFV vector and to overcome any possible problems in packaging large genomes into virions, we first constructed deleted SFFV vectors containing unique restriction enzyme sites useful for cloning. The plasmids pAJO11 and pAJO32 contain deletions of the SFFV genome extending from the two extreme BamHI or BglII sites, respectively. The resulting viral genomes contain unique restriction enzyme recognition sites for BamHI (pAJO11) or BglII (pAJO32). The functionally active HSV tk gene, contained on a 3.4-kb BamHI fragment, was inserted into the BglII and BamHI sites of pAJO32 and pAJO11, respectively. Similarly, a 2.0-kb PvuII fragment containing the functionally active HSV tk gene was inserted into the HpaI site of pSFFV502.

Rescue of SFFV-TK Vectors

To rescue the SFFV-TK clones described above as infectious retroviruses, we used two protocols. The first protocol was identical to the one previously used to rescue the defective SFFV genome (21). This method involves DNA-mediated gene transfer with the calcium phosphate precipitation technique (6) into NIH/3T3 cells followed by superinfection of these cells with replication-competent Friend murine leukemia virus. In the second protocol, SFFV-TK molecules were cotransfected into NIH/3T3 cells along with pMOV-3, a highly infectious clone of the integrated form of Moloney murine leukemia virus (7). A schematic of this procedure is shown in Figure 2. Virus harvested from either rescue procedure was then tested for its titer of tk transducing virus by virus infection of TK⁻ 3T3 cells under selective conditions (HAT medium) that only allow the growth of TK⁺ cells. The rescued virus was tested also for its ability to induce spleen foci in susceptible mice.

Although the first procedure involving superinfection of transfected cells with helper virus successfully results in the recovery of infectious SFFV genomes (21), we were repeatedly unable to detect biologically infectious virus (as measured by either the tk assay in vitro or the spleen focus assay in vivo after transfection of various SFFV-TK recombinants. Rescue of SFFV-TK vectors by cotransfection with pMOV-3 did, however, result in the recovery of infectious tk retrovirus. The results of these experiments are summarized in Table 1. By analogy with similar terminology in bacterial systems, virus harvested from the initial co-transfection procedure is referred to as low-frequency transducing (LFT). Virus harvested from the TK⁺ transformants after infection with a LFT is referred to in Table 1 as high-frequency transducing (HFT).

With the exception of those recombinants that contained the tk gene

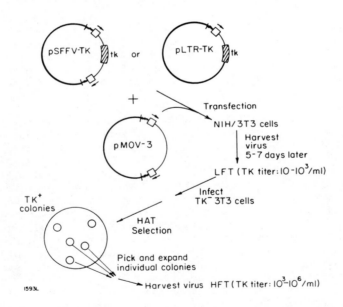

FIGURE 2. Cotransfection protocol used to generate LFT and HFT prepara-tions of tk virus. 5 µg of pMOV-3 and either pSFFV-TK or pLTR-TK were cotransfected into NIH/3T3 cells by the calcium phosphate procedure (6). Five to seven days later, the cell culture medium was harvested, filtered and tested for its titre of tk virus by infection of TK⁻ 3T3 cells. The number of TK⁺ transformants that survived in the HAT selective medium indicates the initial titre of the LFT virus. Some of these TK⁺ colon-ies were subcultured and the virus produced by these transformants (the HFT) was titered for its tk transforming activity.

inserted 0.2 kb downstream from the 5' LTR at a BglII site, all of the SFFV-TK constructs could be rescued as tk virus by cotransfection with pMOV-3. The initial titers of tk virus varied significantly depending on the site of insertion of the tk sequences but did not depend markedly on the transcriptional orientation of tk sequences relative to the SFFV vector. To determine whether the initial LFT titers of tk virus could be increased, HFT preparation of virus was made by harvesting virus produced by the infected TK⁻ 3T3 cells growing under selective HAT medium conditions (Figure 2). Titers of the recycled HFT virus were generally 10^2- to 10^3-fold higher when assayed on TK⁻ 3T3 cells (Table 1) than titers of the original LFT virus.

The LFT and HFT viruses described in Table 1 were also assayed for their ability to induce spleen foci in susceptible DBA02J mice. Interestingly, although low but significant spleen focus-forming virus was detected in the LFT viruses that had tk⁺ activity, no spleen foci were induced with the HFT viruses - even those that showed high tk activity. The observation that the LFT viruses, but not the HFT viruses, contained spleen focus-forming ability suggested that segregation takes place between the tk and spleen focus-inducing markers.

Construction and Rescue of LTR-TK Clones

The observation presented above suggests that recombination between the SFFV-TK constructs and the Moloney murine leukemia helper virus may occur at high frequency. As a means of testing and taking advantage of this possibility, we attempted to rescue infectious tk virus starting with molecular clones containing just the SFFV 5' LTR, some adjacent gag

TABLE 1. Effect of cloning site and transcriptional orientation on generation of SFFV-TK virus[a]

SFFV vector	Cloning site for tk fragment[b]	Transcriptional orientation of tk gene relative to 5' LTR	Virus titer[c]	
			LFT	HFT
pSFFV502	HpaI	same	10^3	10^4–10^5
		opposite	–	–
pAJ011	BamHI	same	5–10	> 10^3
		opposite		> 10^3
pAJ032	BglII	same	0	–
		opposite	0	–

[a] 5 μg of each SFFV-TK plasmid DNA and 5 μg of pMOV-3 DNA was mixed with 20 μg of carrier DNA and used to transform NIH/3T3 cells.
[b] The HSV PvuII tk fragment was cloned into the HpaI site of pSFFV502. The BamHI tk fragment was inserted into the unique BamHI and BglII sites of pAJ011 and pAJ032, respectively.
[c] The virus titer was determined as the number of TK⁺ colonies surviving 1 wk in HAT medium after infection of 2×10^5 TK⁻ 3T3 cells with 1 ml of virus stock.

sequences and the tk gene, but lacking 3' SFFV sequences and the 3' LTR. The construction of these molecules, starting with the clone pYY508 (Figure 1) has been described previously (9). As determined by calcium phosphate-mediated gene transfer, all of the LTR-TK constructs contain a functionally active tk gene (9), including a construct in which just the tk coding sequences (contained on a BglII-BamHI fragment) were cloned into the BglII site of pYY508 (Table 2).

The experiments summarized in Table 2 demonstrate that infectious tk virus can be generated after cotransfection of NIH/3T3 with pMOV-3 and chimeric molecules in which the tk gene is inserted at the BamHI site of 1.2 kb downstream from the 5' LTR. However, no infectious tk virus could be detected with constructs in which the tk gene had been inserted at the BglII site located 0.2 kb downstream from the 5' LTR.

DISCUSSION

The results summarized in this study indicate that SFFV, like other retroviruses (15,16,19), can be used as a gene transfer vector for the tk gene of HSV. Using similar techniques, one should be able to use SFFV as a vector for other selectable or nonselectable genes. Because SFFV replicates to high titers in the hematopoietic tissues of susceptible adult mice, this virus should also be a useful vector for the introduction of foreign genes into hematopoietic progenitor cells.

The DNA segment containing the tk gene contains both a functional promoter region for the tk coding sequence as well as polyadenylation/termination signals for transcription (13,18). Clones in which the tk gene is inserted into the SFFV vector in either transcriptional orientation can be recovered as infectious tk virus with equal efficiency, suggesting that the presence of these transcriptional control signals neither inhibits nor enhances the production of SFFV-TK virus.

Although the transcriptional orientation of the tk gene relative to the SFFV LTR does not seem to affect the recovery of SFFV-TK virus, the site of insertion of the tk gene has a marked effect on recovery of infectious virus. In particular, insertion of the tk gene very close to the 5' LTR resulted in the failure to recover any infectious SFFV-TK

TABLE 2.   Generation of transmissible retrovirus from
SFFV 5' LTR fragment[a]

SFFV vector	Cloning site for tk fragment[b]	Transcriptional orientation of tk gene relative to 5' LTR	Virus titer[c]	
			LFT	HFT
pYY508	BamHI	same	5-10	–
		opposite	5-10	> 10³
pYY508	BglII	same	0	0

a NIH/3T3 cells were transfected as described in Table 1.
b The HSV BamHI tk fragment was inserted into the BamHI site of pYY508. The BglII/BamHI tk fragment was inserted into the BglII site of pYY508.
c The virus titer was determined as described in footnote c of Table 1.

virus. The failure to recover infectious tk virus is not due to inhibition by the LTR of tk gene expression nor conversely was it due to inhibition of the functional promoter contained within the SFFV LTR by the tk insert: we have shown that these clones contain both functional tk and viral promoters as determined by their ability to transform TK⁻ mouse cells to TK⁺ with high efficiency after DNA-mediated gene transfer (7a,8,9). Our results are consistent with the conclusion that there are cis-acting sequences, located close to the 5' LTR, that are required for the production of infectious retrovirus. Linial (10) has described a mutant of Rouse sarcoma virus that is defective in the packaging of its own genomic RNA into virus. The mutation appears to be caused by a large deletion located between 300 and 600 base pairs downstream from the 5' LTR (14). Based on the properties of this mutant, and similar deletion mutants constructed in vitro in the spleen necrosis virus genome with the endonuclease Bal31 (S. Watanabe and H. Temin, personal communication), we suggest that the failure to rescue SFFV-TK clones constructed from the vector pAJ032 is due to the deletion of viral recognition sequences involved in the encapsidation or packaging of retrovirus genomes into nascent virus particles. Similarly, the failure to rescue infectious tk virus from LTR-TK clones in which the tk gene is inserted 0.2-kb downstream from the 5' LTR may be due to disruption of these viral packaging sequences.

Our results suggest that recombination events between the vector and helper virus genomes are taking place at relatively high frequency. Restriction enzyme and Southern gel analysis of TK⁺ transformants after infection with LFT and HFT viruses is currently in progress to verify that the biological segregation between the tk gene and the spleen focus-forming function observed during the preparation of the HFT viruses is reflected in the predicted molecular changes in the structure of the emerging SFFV-TK virus. We have made use of this recombination between vector and helper virus to generate complete infectious retrovirus starting with cloned DNA molecules containing only the 5' LTR, gag sequences and the tk gene. Our results extend previous observations by others that cells transformed with subgenomic fragments of either Harvey (5), Abelson (4), or Moloney (D. G. Blair and G. F. Vande Woude, personal communication) virus that include the 5' end of the viral genome but are missing 3' sequences, nevertheless contain a rescuable transforming virus. In these latter cases, the generation of infectious transforming virus presumably involves packaging of these subgenomic transcripts followed by recombination between the helper and transforming virus genomes during reverse transcription in cells coinfected by both viruses. In the experiments described in the present study involving the LTR-TK clones, the production of a complete infectious SFFV-tk virus must also involve recombination between the LTR-tk constructs and the helper virus genome. This recombination event could either occur between the input DNA molecules during the initial DNA transfection, or as noted above during reverse transcription in subsequent rounds of infection.

The generation of infectious retrovirus starting with just LTR and adjacent gag sequences has two general implications. First, it suggests, as does the earlier in vivo work cited above, that defective but infectious retroviruses containing heterologous sequences can be efficiently generated by one or more recombination events with a helper virus genome. The generation of strongly transforming retroviruses may also involve the acquisition of potential cellular oncogenes (c-onc) by similar recombination events. Thus, further molecular studies on the generation of tk virus may provide insight into the origins of these transforming viruses. Second, the ability to generate highly infectious retroviruses containing heterologous sequences by simply ligating these sequences at a convenient site downstream from the 5' LTR suggests a novel strategy for the detection and recovery of single-copy, selectable cellular genes. Experiments designed to determine the constraints of this strategy are currently in progress.

ACKNOWLEDGEMENTS

We thank Dr. R. Jaenisch for providing us with pMOV-3, the Moloney murine leukemia virus clone. The excellent technical assistance of G. Cheong is gratefully acknowledged. This work was supported by grants from the Medical Research Council and National Cancer Institute of Canada. A. Joyner is the recipient of a studentship from the Medical Research Council of Canada.

REFERENCES

1. Bishop JM (1981): Cell 23:5
2. Cambell AM (1969): In: Episomes, New York: Harper and Row
3. Dexter TM, Allen TD, Testa NG, Scolnick EM: (1981): J Exp Med 154:594
4. Goff SP, Tabin CJ, Wang JY-J, Weinberg RA, Baltimore D (1981): J Virol 41:271
5. Goldfarb MP, Weinberg RA (1981): J Virol 41:271
6. Graham FL, van der Eb AJ (1973): Virology 52:456
7. Harbers K, Schnieke A, Stuhlmann H, Jahner D, Jaenisch R (1981): Proc Natl Acad Sci USA 78:7609
7a. Joyner A, Bernstein A (in press): Mol Cell Biol
8. Joyner A, Yamamoto Y, Bernstein A (1981): In: Developmental Biology Using Purified Genes (Brown DD, ed), New York: Academic Press, p 535
9. Joyner AL, Yamamoto Y, Bernstein A (1982): Proc Natl Acad Sci USA 79:1573
10. Linial M, Medeiros E, Hayward WS (1978): Cell 15:1371
11. Mager D, MacDonald ME, Robson IB, Mak TW, Bernstein A (1981): Mol Cell Biol 1:721
12. Mager D, Mak TW, Bernstein A (1981): Proc Natl Acad Sci USA 78:1703
13. McKnight SL (1980): Nucleic Acids Res 8:5959
14. Shank PR, Linial M (1980): J Virol 36:450
15. Shimotohno K, Temin H (1981): Cell 26:67
16. Tabin CJ, Hoffmann JW, Goff SP, Weinberg RA (1982: Mol Cell Biol 2:426
17. Viral Oncogenes (1979): In: Cold Spring Harbor Symp Quant Biol: 40
18. Wagner JM, Shart JA, Summers WC (1981): Proc Natl Acad Sci USA 78:1441
19. Wei C-M, Gibson M, Spear PG, Scolnick EM (1981): J Virol 39:935
20. Weinberg RA, (1981): Biochim Biophys Acta 651:25
21. Yamamoto Y, Gamble CL, Clark SP, Joyner A, Shibuya T, MacDonald ME, Mager D, Bernstein A, Mak TW (1981): Proc Natl Acad Sci USA 78:6893

Gene Transfer and Cancer, edited by M. L. Pearson and N. L. Sternberg. Raven Press, New York © 1984.

Construction of a Small Retrovirus Cloning Vector and Splicing of Genomic Mouse α-Globin DNA Inserted in this Vector

[1]Shinichi Watanabe, [1]Kunitada Shimotohno, and Howard M. Temin

McArdle Laboratory for Cancer Research, University of Wisconsin, Madison, Wisconsin

ABSTRACT. The minimum cis-acting DNA segments other than the long terminal repeat (LTR) that is required for formation of an infectious retrovirus cloning vector was determined using spleen necrosis virus (SNV)-herpes simplex virus (HSV) type I thymidine kinase (TK) recombinants. The 3' end of the spleen necrosis virus sequence was removed up to 40 base pairs from the 3' LTR with only a 2-fold effect on the recovery of infectious recombinant virus. Viral sequences adjacent to the 5' LTR were removed starting from an XbaI site at position 1017 bp by Bal31 digestion. The extent of deletion was determined by DNA sequencing, and the efficiency of recovery of infectious recombinant virus was determined by infectivity assay and formation of unintegrated viral DNA. The recovery of infectious virus was reduced by deletions near the SalI site at 860 bp Therefore, the region between the LTR and approximately 900 bp (gag starts at 980 bp) is required for encapsidation. We call this region E.

Mouse genomic α-globin DNA with the polyA addition sequences removed was inserted into an SNV-TK vector and infectious progeny virus were recovered. The size of these viruses was smaller than the original viral construct, a result consistent with removal of intervening sequences from the α-globin DNA and RNA.

INTRODUCTION

Several methods to introduce foreign DNA into living cells have been developed to study the function of the foreign DNA. Viral vectors seem more advantageous than other methods such as DNA-mediated gene transfer. In particular, retroviruses are naturally occurring viral vectors, since many retroviruses contain DNA substitutions with transforming genes (onc genes) and can introduce these onc genes into cells by infection (7).

RESULTS AND DISCUSSION

Previously it was shown that the HSV-TK gene without its polyadenylation signal (TKΔter) could be maintained stably in a replication-

---

[1]Present addresses: National Cancer Institute, Bethesda, Maryland (SW); National Cancer Center Research Institute, Tokyo, Japan (KS).

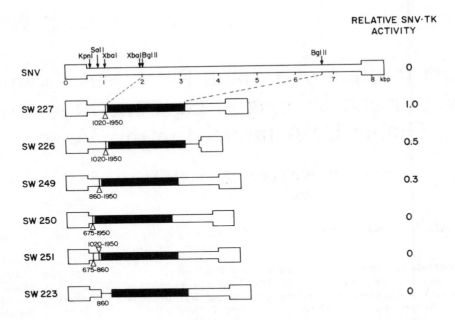

FIGURE 1. Relative recovery of infectious, transforming SNV-TK virus.
The HSV-TK gene lacking the terminal sequences for mRNA was inserted
between the two BglII sites at 2.0 and 6.7 kbp in SNV DNA (TK23a). A
0.9-kbp fragment between two XbaI sites at 1.02 and 1.95 kbp was removed
from TK23a resulting in SW227. The SNV sequences remaining at the 3'
end of SW227 up to 40 bp from the LTR were replaced by a pBR322 EcoRI-
BamHI fragment of 375bp (SW226). SNV sequences from the SalI (860 bp)
to XbaI (1017 bp), KpnI (675 bp) to XbaI (1020 bp), or KpnI (675 bp) to
SalI (860 bp) cleavage sites were removed from SW227 resulting in SW249,
SW250, and SW251, respectively. SW223 contains the 275-bp BamHI-SalI
fragment of pBR322 between 860 bp and 2 kbp of SW227. Symbols: Hatched
area indicates HSV-TKΔterR gene; open area is SNV DNA; large boxes
at the ends of SNV DNA are the LTR; open triangles represent deletions
given in bp of SNV. Virus was recovered 5 days after cotransfection
with DNA of helper virus, reticuloendotheliosis virus strain A, and
assayed using BRL TK cells (4).

defective avian retrovirus, SNV-TK (4-6). Using SNV-TK, we now have
determined the minimum SNV sequences outside the LTR required for formation of infectious recombinant virus. Figure 1 illustrates some structures of DNA recombinant viruses and the relative recovery of these
viruses as infectious SNV-TK recombinant virus. A 930-bp fragment
between 1017 bp and 1950 bp on the SNV map was removed from a recombinant
SNV-TKΔterR virus that contains the TKΔter sequence between the
two BglII sites of the SNV genome, resulting in SW227. Infectious recombinant virus was recovered after chicken embryo fibroblast cells were
transfected with SNV-TKΔterR DNA and helper virus DNA, reticuloendotheliosis virus strain A (REV-A). The infectivity of the SNV-TKΔterR
recombinant virus was determined by infecting TK⁻ BRL or chicken cells
followed by selection in HAT medium. The amount of recombinant virus
and helper virus was also determined by infecting chicken cells with the

recovered virus followed by preparation of unintegrated viral DNA. DNA was then separated by electrophoresis in an agarose gel, was transferred to a nitrocellulose filter, and was hybridized with either a ^{32}P-labeled SNV probe or a TK probe.

The 3' SNV sequences, up to 40 bp from the LTR, were substituted by the 375-bp EcoRI-BamHI fragment of pBR322 (SW226). The relative recovery of SW226 was half of SW227. Therefore, most of the 3' SNV sequences can be removed without a large loss of recovery of infectious virus.

5' SNV sequences in SW227 were removed in various ways. When the SNV sequences between the SalI site (860 bp) and the XbaI site (1950 bp) were removed (SW249), the relative recovery of infectious virus was reduced to 30% that of SW227. However, when the sequences between the KpnI site (675 bp) and the XbaI site (1950 bp) were removed (SW250), infectious recombinant virus was not recovered. The importance of the sequence between the KpnI (675 bp) and SalI sites (860 bp) was shown by deleting the KpnI-SalI fragment from SW227 (SW251). SW251 failed to produce infectious recombinant virus. Substitution between the SalI site (860 bp) and the BglII site (2kbp) by the 275-bp SalI-BamH1 fragment of pBR322 (SW223) caused a large decrease in the recovery of infectious virus. In addition, various other deletions between the SalI site (860 bp) and the XbaI site (1920 bp) were made from the XbaI site of SW227 by digesting with exonuclease Bal31, resulting in small decreases in recovery of SNV-TK. A summary of the results with all constructions is shown in Figure 2.

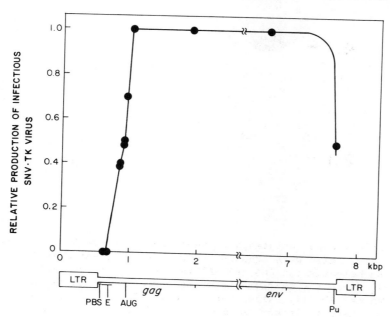

FIGURE 2. Summary of relative recovery of transforming, infectious SNV-TK virus. The relative recovery of infectious, transforming recombinant viruses is compared to SW227. Each point is plotted at the 3' end of SNV sequences at the left end of the deletion or at the 5' end of SNV sequences at the right end of the deletions. The left ends of the two deletions closest to the left LTR are located at the KpnI site and 6 bp 3' to the SalI site, respectively.

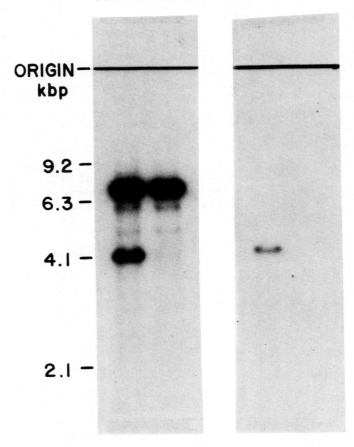

FIGURE 3. Production of unintegrated recombinant SNV-TK DNA. Chicken embryo fibroblast cells were transfected with recombinant DNAs (SW227 and SW223) and helper virus DNA (REV-A) in the presence of carrier DNA (10 µg/ml) using the calcium-phosphate coprecipitation method of Graham and Van der Eb (1). Virus was harvested 5 days after transfection and was used to infect chicken embryo fibroblast cells. Unintegrated viral DNA was harvested 3 days after infection by the procedure of Hirt (2). DNA was fractionated by electrophoresis in a 1% agarose gel, transferred to a nitrocellulose filter, and hybridized to either a ^{32}P-labeled SNV probe or a labeled TK probe. The numbers on the left side of the figure indicate the position of the size markers. Maps of SW227 and SW223 are shown in Figure 1. REV-A is the helper virus.

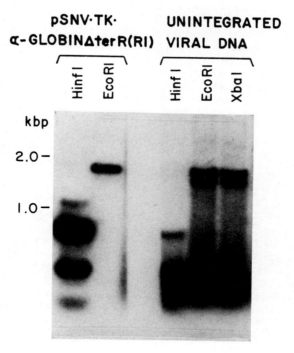

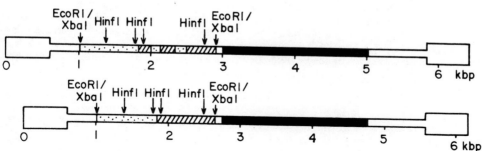

FIGURE 4. Production of unintegrated recombinant SNV-TK-α-globin-ΔterR(R1) viral DNA. pSNV-TK-α-globinΔterR(R1) and helper virus (REV-A) DNAs were used to transfect chicken embryo fibroblasts cells. Unintegrated recombinant viral DNA was isolated as described in the legend to Figure 3. DNA was digested with HinfI, EcoRI, or XbaI. DNA fragments were fractionated by electrophoresis in a 1.3% agarose gel, transferred to a nitrocellulose filter, and hybridized to a ^{32}P-labeled-α-globin probe (right three lanes). The left two lanes show a control experiment carried out with DNA of pSNV-TK- α-globinΔterR(R1) digested with HinfI or EcoRI. The maps at the bottom indicate the structure of viral DNA synthesized from unspliced RNA (top) and spliced RNA (bottom). The filled area is the TK gene; hatched areas are the α-globin exons; shaded areas are the α-globin noncoding region; open areas are SNV; vertical lines in exons 1 and 3 indicate the ends of protein coding sequences.

The reduction in recovery of SNV-TKΔterR seen here results from a failure of encapsidation of viral RNA. Virion RNA containing TK sequences was not detected by hybridization to labeled TK DNA in the supernatant medium of cells transfected by SW250 and REV-A DNA (data not shown, 8). Transcription is most likely normal in these cells (8). Therefore, the block in the production of infectious recombinant virus from SW250, SW251, and SW223 appears to be in packaging of viral RNA. This block was confirmed by the absence of unintegrated viral TK DNA in cells infected with a virus stock prepared from chicken cells transfected with SW223 and REV-A DNA (Figure 3). The results presented in Figure 3 also show that there is no gross change in the size of SNV-TKΔterR viral DNA and that the amount of SNV-TKΔterR viral DNA made in infected cells is approximately as great as the amount of helper virus DNA.

The SNV-TKΔterR vector was also used to study the rate and accuracy of production of cDNA by removal of intervening sequences from genomic DNA. Mouse α-globin genomic DNA contains two intervening sequences and was sequenced previously (3). We prepared α-globinΔterR as we did for TKΔterR (4). After both ends of an EcoRI fragment containing α-globinΔterR were filled by DNA polymerase, the fragment was inserted into the XbaI site of SW227 previously filled by T4 DNA polymerase (Figure 4, upper map). Recombinant virus was recovered from chicken cells transfected with SNV-TK-α-globinΔterR(R1) DNA. EcoRI and XbaI digestion produced two bands that hybridized to an α-globin probe. The difference in molecular size of these bands is consistent with the absence of the intervening sequences from α-globinΔterR (Figure 4, lower map). The result with HinfI digestion was similar to that with EcoRI and XbaI digestion.

α-globin DNA from unintegrated viral DNA was molecularly cloned and DNA sequences around the splicing sites were determined (data not shown). The sequencing demonstrated that precise splicing occurred in the progeny recombinant virus. Splicing must have occurred in viral genomic RNA to generate new smaller genomic RNA lacking intervening sequences, since the absence of the α-globin promoter did not affect these results (data not shown, 9).

CONCLUSION

The minimum cis-acting sequences other than the LTR required for the formation of an infectious retrovirus cloning vector are small. The 3' viral sequences can be removed up to 40 bp from the 3' LTR with only a 2-fold effect on the recovery of infectious recombinant virus. Sequences near the 5' LTR are involved in encapsidation of viral RNA. Deletion between the KpnI site (675 bp) and the SalI site (860 bp) abolished formation of infectious virus. This region is called E (8). E is removed from subgenomic env mRNA by splicing from genomic RNA (K. Whilhelmsen, personal communication, 10). Therefore, env mRNA is not encapsidated.

Mouse genomic α-globin DNA with the termination sequences removed was inserted in an SNV-TK vector and infectious virus was recovered. Recovered virus lost intervening sequences as shown by the DNA sequence around the splice sites in a DNA clone of progeny virus (9). Thus, cDNA genes can be made by insertion of genomic DNA into a retrovirus vector.

ACKNOWLEDGEMENTS

This work was supported by PHS grants CA-22113 and CA-07175. S.W. is a trainee supported by PHS grant CA-22443. H.M.T. is an American Cancer Society Research Professor.

REFERENCES

1. Graham FL, Van der Eb AJ (1973): Virology 52:456
2. Hirt B (1967): J Mol Biol 26:365
3. Nishioka Y, Leder P (1979): Cell 18:875
4. Shimotohno K, Temin HM (1981): Cell 26:67
5. Tabin CJ, Hoffmann JW, Goff SP, Weinberg RA (1982): Mol Cell Biol 2:426
6. Wei C-M, Gibson M, Spear PG, Scolnick EM (1981): J Virol 39:935
7. Weiss RA, Teich N, Varmus HE, Coffin JM, eds (1982): The Molecular Biology of Tumor Viruses. Part III. RNA Tumor Viruses, Cold Spring Harbor, NY: Cold Spring Harbor Laboratory
8. Watanabe S, Temin HM (1982): Proc Natl Acad Sci USA 79:5986
9. Shimotohno K, Temin HM (1982): Nature 299:265
10. Watanabe S, Temin HM (in press): Mol Cell Biol

Gene Transfer and Cancer, edited by M. L. Pearson and N. L. Sternberg. Raven Press, New York © 1984.

Defective Virus Vectors (Amplicons) Derived from Herpes Simplex Viruses

Niza Frenkel, Louis P. Deiss, Ann D. Kwong, and [1]Richard R. Spaete

Department of Biology, The University of Chicago, Chicago, Illinois 60637

ABSTRACT. We have employed subsets of herpes simplex virus (HSV) DNA sequences to derive cloning/amplifying vectors (amplicons) which can replicate in eucaryotic cells in the presence of standard HSV helper viruses. The HSV amplicon system can be used to study cis replication functions of HSV DNA and to introduce relatively large stretches of foreign DNA sequences into replication-defective virus genomes which can be stably propagated in virus stocks. Using amplicons cloned in bacteria we have mapped three replication origins in HSV DNA. Two of these origins (ori 1 and ori 1') are present in the inverted repeat sequences of the S component within map coordinates 0.952 to 0.963 and 0.860 to 0.871. The third origin (ori 2) has been localized to the U_L sequences bounded by map coordinates 0.413 to 0.423.

In addition to a replication origin, the seed amplicons must contain sequences from the end of the S component of HSV DNA necessary for cleavage of viral DNA concatemers and the packaging of viral DNA into structural virions. Using a cloned amplicon containing ori 2, we have introduced a 12-kb DNA segment containing the chicken ovalbumin gene (derived by O'Malley and coworkers) and an 11.7-kb segment containing the α subunit of the human chorionic gonadotropin gene (cloned by Fiddes and Goodman) into replication-defective HSV genomes. In addition to defective genomes containing reiterations of the input chimeric seed amplicons, the derivative virus populations have been shown to contain genomes in which segments of the cloned genes have been deleted. Although it is as yet unclear whether the inserted foreign eucaryotic DNA sequences can be expressed in cells infected with the derivative virus stocks, previous studies have shown that the inclusion of viral genes within defective genome repeat units results in abundant expression of the amplified genes.

INTRODUCTION

This paper summarizes our recent studies concerning defective virus cloning amplifying vectors (amplicons) derived from HSV. The rationale for undertaking these studies was 2-fold. First, defective HSV genomes have been shown to contain only limited subsets of the standard virus DNA sequences and to utilize the HSV-specific replication functions

---

[1]Present address: Department of Medical Microbiology, Stanford University School of Medicine, Palo Alto, California 94305

supplied in trans by their standard helper virus counterparts (reviewed in 3). Therefore, they are potentially useful reagents for studies of HSV DNA cis replication signals, including replication origin(s), site(s) specifying DNA maturation-cleavage and packaging, and sequences mediating the inversions and duplications known to constitute structural features of the complex standard HSV genome (reviewed in 14). The bacterially cloned HSV amplicons facilitate the introduction of specific alterations in these replication signals so as to establish their functional domains.

The second reason underlying our studies concerns the potential use of defective HSV-derived vectors for cloning and amplifying foreign genes. Specifically, the HSV virion can accomodate relatively large (approximately 150 kb) DNA molecules (14). As reviewed elsewhere (3), defective virus DNA molecules that are present in mature cytoplasmic virions within cells infected with serially passaged virus stocks are indistinguishable in their overall size from their standard virus counterparts. However, they consist of multiple reiterations of sequences (repeat units) arranged in a head-to-tail tandem array, with repeat unit sizes ranging from 3 to 30 kb. Furthermore, full-length defective HSV genomes containing multiple head-to-tail repeat units can be regenerated from individual monomeric repeats, following cotransfection of cells with helper virus DNA (18). The regenerated concatemers are packaged into structural virions and can be stably propagated in serially passaged virus stocks (18,19). These features provide the basis for the potential derivation of chimeric defective genomes composed of uniform head-to-tail reiterations of seed repeat units constructed to contain foreign DNA sequences linked to cis replication functions of HSV DNA.

RESULTS AND DISCUSSION

Derivation of Defective Genomes Containing Foreign DNA Sequences

The basic approach used in our studies is outlined in Figure 1. Specifically, subsets of HSV DNA sequences containing cis replication functions (derived either from defective virus genomes in serially passaged virus stocks, or from standard virus DNA) are cloned in bacteria. These cloned amplicons are transfected into animal cells in the presence of helper virus DNA and the resultant virus stocks are passaged serially to allow the accumulation of the replicated seed amplicons. Figure 2 shows the results of restriction enzyme analyses of ^{32}P-labeled DNA prepared from cells infected with passages 4 through 12 of a representative series derived by cotransfection of cells with helper HSV-1 (Justin) DNA and the cloned amplicon pP2-102 (16). As described elsewhere (16), the pP2-102 recombinant plasmid was constructed by inserting BglII cleaved repeat unit of defective genomes present in serially passaged HSV-1 (Patton) stocks (derived by B. Murray and coworkers) into the BglII site of the bacterial plasmid pKC7 (12). As seen in the figure, (and on the basis of additional analyses not shown), the cotransfection of cells with helper virus DNA and the seed cloned amplicon resulted in the generation of full-length (approximately 150 kb) chimeric defective genomes consisting of multiple head-to-tail reiterations of the input 9.6-kb cloned amplicon. Furthermore, the chimeric defective genomes containing the pKC7 DNA sequences were packaged into structural virions and were stably propagated in serially passaged virus stocks. As further described elsewhere (16), repeat units derived from replicated chimeric DNA molecules such as those shown in Figure 2 can be efficiently introduced into bacteria.

Studies of the HSV amplicon

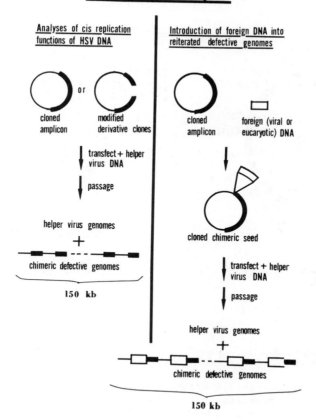

FIGURE 1. The general scheme used in the derivation of defective genomes from seed cloned amplicons. Left, mapping of cis replication functions by testing the ability of deleted derivatives of a functional cloned amplicon to generate concatemeric genomes which are stable during serial virus propagation. Right, construction of cloned chimeric seed repeats containing the additional foreign DNA sequences of interest. For experimental details, see refs. 16 and 18.

Thus, the pKC7-HSV recombinant amplicon can be conveniently shuttled between bacterial and eucaryotic cells.

Replication Functions of the HSV Amplicons

Previous studies concerning the replication of defective HSV genomes present in serially passaged virus populations and more recent studies utilizing constructed amplicons cloned in bacteria have revealed the following pertinent points:

a) Defective HSV genomes appear to be replicated primarily at late intervals post infection, as evident from comparison of the rate of accumulation of standard and defective virus DNA in serially passaged

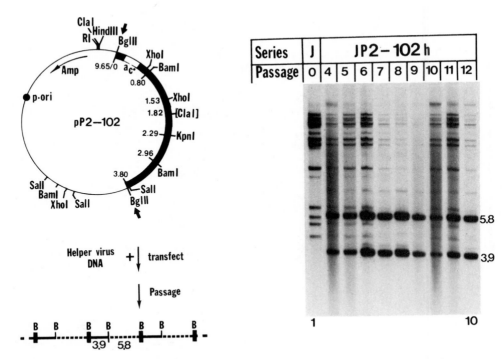

FIGURE 2. Propagation of defective genomes from the cloned amplicon pP2-102. Left, the structure of the pP2-102 cloned amplicon which was constructed by inserting a 3.9-kb BglII-cleaved repeat unit of class II defective HSV-1 (Patton) genomes (from a series derived by B. Murray and coworkers) into the BglII site of pKC7. The segment shown as ac* designates approximately 500 bp of sequences arising from the end of the S component. The remaining HSV DNA sequences in pP2-102 are derived from U_L. Bacterially cloned amplicons derived by us are designated by the letter p followed by the first letter of the HSV strain contributing the replication origin, the type of origin (1,1' or 2) and a number. Derivative virus series are designated by the first letter of the helper virus used in the derivation of the series followed by the cloned amplicon designation. Right, the BglII cleavage patter of ^{32}P-labeled DNA prepared from cells infected with plaque purified HSV-1 (Justin) (lane 1) or with passages 4 through 12 (lanes 2 through 10) of a series derived by cotransfection of rabbit skin cells with HSV-1 (Justin) helper virus DNA and the pP2-102 seed. The BglII bands of sizes 5.8 and 3.9 kb correspond to the pKC7 and HSV-1 DNA sequences (respectively) present in the repeat units of the generated concatemeric defective genomes. For further details see ref. 16.

virus-infected cells (18); replication requires the HSV-specified DNA polymerase (18), as evident from the inhibition of defective virus DNA replication by phosphonoacetate (PAA) treatment at concentrations known to affect the HSV-specified DNA polymerase (8). Furthermore, the replication of defective HSV genomes is inhibited at nonpermissive tempera-

ture in cells infected with virus stocks containing the HSV DNA replication T^S mutants C and D (11) as helper viruses (A.D. Kwong, N. Frenkel,
and P.A. Schaffer, unpublished results).

b) The full-length concatemeric defective HSV DNA molecules appear
to be generated by a rolling-circle replication of monomeric repeat
units, as evident from the head-to-tail organization of their repeat
units (reviewed in 3), from electron microscopy observations reported by
Becker et al. (1) and from the observation that individual monomeric
repeat units give rise to head-to-tail concatemeric progeny (18). Furthermore, cotransfection of cells with helper-virus DNA and a mixture of
different-sized repeat units resulted in the generation of homopolymers,
each containing stretches of identical repeat units within the same concatemeric DNA molecules. Thus, it is unlikely that concatemerization
arises by intermolecular recombinations.

c) There are two separate cis recognition sites required for the
successful propagation of defective virus genomes in HSV stocks. This
conclusion is based on our previous studies of the origin of DNA sequences contained within the two separate classes of defective HSV genomes accumulating in serially passaged virus populations (reviewed in
ref. 3). Furthermore, more recent studies (R.R. Spaete and N. Frenkel,
manuscript in preparation) have shown that two separate subsets of the
pP2-102 chimeric amplicon DNA sequences are required for its successful
propagation in virus stocks. The first recognition site is shared by
both classes (I and II) of defective HSV genomes and corresponds to the
DNA sequences located near the end of the S component of standard virus
DNA. Analyses of free and encapsidated defective virus DNA in serially
passaged virus-infected cells have shown that this site (designated as
clv) is required for the cleavage of viral DNA concatemers and for their
packaging into viral nucleocapsids (19). The second recognition site
corresponds most likely to a replication origin and is not shared by the
two classes of defective HSV genomes. Specifically, as reviewed elsewhere (3), the class I defective genomes contain DNA sequences, derived
exclusively from the S component. As seen in Figure 3 (and additional
data not shown), using the recombinant plasmid pRB373 constructed by
Mocarski and Roizman (9), we have recently mapped the class I replication origin within a 1-kb segment contained in the inverted repeat
sequence c of the S component (L.P. Deiss, E. Mocarski and N. Frenkel,
manuscript in preparation). These studies have thus defined two (similar if not identical) replication origins within the S component between
map coordinates 0.952 to 0.963 [origin (ori 1)] and coordinates 0.860 to
0.871 (ori 1') of standard virus DNA. Similar conclusions have recently
been reported by Stow and McMonagle (17) and by Mocarski and Roizman
(9). The class II defective HSV genomes (arising in serially passaged
virus stocks) consist of repeat units in which sequences from the U_L
region, providing the replication origin, are linked to sequences from
the end of S, providing the clv function (3,7,15). Using the pP2-102
recombinant amplicon, as well as deleted clones derived from it, we have
recently localized this second origin (ori 2) to a 1-kb segment within
map coordinates 0.413 to 0.423 of standard HSV-1 DNA (R.R. Spaete and N.
Frenkel, manuscript in preparation).

Introduction of Eucaryotic Cell DNA Sequences into
Defective HSV Amplicons

We have thus far attempted to introduce two different sets of eucaryotic DNA sequences into defective HSV genomes. The first corresponds to

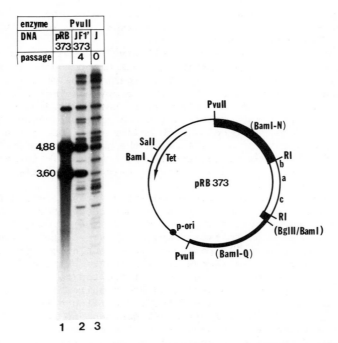

FIGURE 3. Propagation of defective genomes from the amplicon pRB373.
Right, representation of the pRB373 recombinant plasmid which was constructed by Mocarski and Roizman (9) to contain the α-tk gene, a 1.27-kb
segment constituting a bac type S-L junction and an EcoRI/PvuII segment
located at the left side of the BamI-N fragment of HSV-1(F) DNA. Left,
the PvuII restriction patterns of ³²P-labeled plasmid (pRB373) DNA
(lane 1), and DNA prepared from cells infected with plaque purified
HSV-1 (Justin) (lane 3), or with passage 4 of a series derived from the
cotransfection of cells with Justin helper virus DNA and the seed pRB373
amplicon (lane 2). The designation of this series as JF1'-373 follows
the nomenclature established in the legend to Figure 2. The 4.88- and
3.6-kb fragments represent the PvuII cleavage products of the generated
chimeric genomes. Data from L.P. Deiss, E. Mocarski and N. Frenkel
(manuscript in preparation).

the genomic copy of the chicken ovalbumin gene contained in the recombinant plasmid pOV12, constructed by O'Malley and coworkers (5). We
have introduced the 12-kb segment containing the gene and including also
its 5' and 3' flanking sequences into the HindIII site of the cloned
amplicon pP2-103, a derivative of pP2-102 (16). The resultant chimeric
plasmids pP2-501 and pP2-502 (overall size 19.7 kb, differing in the
orientation of the chicken DNA segment) were employed (A.D. Kwong and N.
Frenkel, unpublished results) in cotransfection experiments using two
different helper viruses, including a) wild-type HSV-1 (KOS) and b) the
mutant virus vhs-1 derived from HSV-1 (KOS) shown to be defective with
respect to its ability to turn off host polypeptide synthesis (13). Restriction enzyme and blot hybridization analyses of DNAs prepared from

cells infected with the transfection-derived virus stocks have revealed
(in some of the stocks) the presence of chimeric defective genomes containing the chicken ovalbumin DNA sequences. Although a certain proportion of the amplified chimeric genomes consisted of repeat units which
were indistinguishable from the input seed recombinant clones, a fraction of the chimeric defective virus DNA molecules consisted of repeats
in which portions of the chicken ovalbumin sequences as well as portions
of the HSV-1 amplicon sequences have been deleted (A.D. Kwong and N.
Frenkel, unpublished results). Studies currently in progress are designed to characterize in detail the structural features of these deleted
derivative genomes. Preliminary analyses, however, have indicated that
the deletions occur at specific locations because similarly deleted repeat units have been found to be present in virus stocks propagated from
independent transfections. Thus, the deletions might have arisen by re-
combination(s) through short stretches of homologous sequences.

The second set of eucaryotic cell DNA sequences which we have attempted to introduce into defective virus genomes corresponds to the genomic
copy of the α subunit of the human chorionic gonadotropin gene, cloned
and characterized by Fiddes and Goodman (2). In this case, an 11.7-kb
segment containing the gene was inserted into the BglII site of pP2-103
(L.P. Deiss and N. Frenkel, unpublished results). As seen in Figure 4,
virus populations derived from cotransfection of cells with the resultant pP2-401 clone and helper virus DNA contained substantial proportions
of the chimeric genomes consisting of the original input pP2-401 repeats,
as well as deleted derivative(s) thereof.

We conclude on the basis of these studies that relatively large segments of eucaryotic DNA sequences can be introduced into defective HSV
genomes and be stably propagated in virus stocks. Further studies currently in progress are designed to determine whether the tendency to delete sequences from amplicons containing large stretches of eucaryotic
DNA sequences reflects the existence of constraints on the size of defective genome repeat units or alternatively results from the presence
of short stretches of homologous sequences which render the chimeric
amplicons likely substrates for recombinational events.

Expression of Genes Residing Within Defective Genome Repeat Units

It is at present not clear whether the eucaryotic genes which have
been inserted into defective genomes under their authentic transcriptional promoters will indeed be expressed in cells infected with the
serially passaged virus stocks. There is, however, evidence to show
that the inclusion of viral genes in defective genome repeat units results in their efficient expression. Thus, as previously shown by us
and by others (3,4,10) the infected cell polypeptide (ICP) number 4 and
two additional polypeptides (MW 18,000 and 14,000) are greatly overproduced in cells infected with virus populations containing high proportions of defective genomes encoding these proteins. More recent studies
(U. Gompels, B. Norrild, N. Frenkel, and L. Pereira, in preparation)
have shown that the HSV-specified glycoprotein gE can also be efficiently expressed from defective genome repeat units. Similarly, the gene
encoding ICP 8, which resides within the U_L sequences contained in the
class II repeat units, is abundantly expressed in cells infected with
class II defective HSV stocks (3,7).

Analyses of viral transcription in serially passaged virus-infected
cells have revealed that the repeat unit DNA sequenes were preferentially transcribed (3, and H. Locker and N. Frenkel, unpublished results).

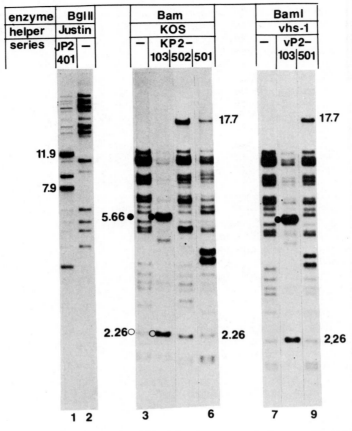

FIGURE 4. Derivation of defective genomes containing eucaryotic cell DNA inserts. Analyses of ^{33}P-labeled DNA from cells infected with plaque purified HSV-1 (Justin) (lane 2) or with serially passaged JP2-401 virus (lane 1). The JP2-401 series was derived by cotransfection of cells with Justin helper virus DNA and the pP2-401 seed. The pP2-401 recombinant clone was constructed by insertion of an 11.7-kb BglII fragment containing the gene specifying the α subunit of the human chorionic gonadotropin, originally cloned by Fiddes and Goodman (2), into the 7.9-kb pP2-103 amplicon. BamI digests of ^{32}P-labeled DNA from cells infected with plaque-purified HSV-1(KOS) (lane 3) or the vhs-1 mutant virus (ref. 13) (lane 8); the KP2-103 (lane 4) and vP2-103 (lane 8) series were derived by cotransfection of cells with the KOS or vhs-1 helper virus DNAs and the pP2-103 amplicon. The 5.66- and 2.26-kb fragments arise from defective genomes containing head-to-tail reiterations of the seed pP2-103 amplicon. The KP2-501 (lane 5), KP2-502 (lane 6), and vP2-501 (lane 9) series were derived following transfection of cells with KOS or vhs-1 helper viruses and the cloned seeds pP2-501 and pP2-502, each containing a 12-kb segment specifying the chicken ovalbumin gene, originally cloned by Lai et al. (5). The 17.7-kb and 2.26-kb fragments arise from concatemeric genomes containing reiterations of the input chimeric amplicons.

Furthermore, the expression of the overproduced viral polypeptides followed the regulatory scheme of viral gene expression in HSV infections as seen from the kinetics of their synthesis in the absence and presence of drugs (cycloheximide, canavanine, and PAA) known to differentially affect the various regulatory classes of HSV-specified polypeptides. Thus, it appears that the increase in gene dose of specific viral genes ultimately results in most abundant expression of these viral genes. As described above, further studies are currently in progress to extend these observations to genes of nonviral origin.

ACKNOWLEDGEMENTS

These studies were supported by U.S. Public Health Service Research Grants AI-15488 and CA-19264 from the National Cancer Institute and by National Science Foundation Grant PCM-8118303. L.P.D. and R.R.S. are predoctoral trainees supported by Training Grant PHS CA-09241.

REFERENCES

1. Becker Y, Asher Y, Weinberg-Zahlering E., Rabkin S. (1978): J Gen Virol 40:319
2. Fiddes JC, Goodman HM (1981): J Mol Appl Gen 1:3
3. Frenkel N (1981): In: The Human Herpesviruses - An Interdisciplinary Prospective (Nahmias AJ, Dowdle WR, Schinazy RS, eds), New York: Elsevier-North Holland, p 91
4. Frenkel N, Jacob RJ, Honess RW, Hayward GS, Locker H, Roizman B (1975): J Virol 16:153
5. Lai EC, Woo SLC, Bordelon-Riser ME, Fraser TH, O'Malley BW (1980): Proc Natl Acad Sci USA 77:244
6. Locker H, Frenkel N (1979): J Virol 29:1065
7. Locker H, Frenkel N, Halliburton I (1982): J Virol 43:574
8. Mao JC-H, Robishaw EE (1975): Biochemistry 14:5475
9. mocarski ES, Roizman B (1982): Proc Natl Acad Sci USA in press
10. Murray BK, Biswal N, Bookout JB, Lanford RE, Courtney RJ, Melnick JC (1975): Intervirology 5:173
11. Parris DS, Courtney RJ, Schaffer PA (1978): Virology 90:177
12. Rao R, Rogers SG (1979): Gene 7:79
13. Read GS, Frenkel N: (submitted)
14. Roizman B (1979): Cell 16:481
15. Schroder CH, Stegmann B, Lauppe HF, Kaerner HC (1975/76): Intervirology 6:270
16. Spaete RR, Frenkel N (1982): Cell 30:295
17. Stow ND, McMonagle EC (1982): In: Eukaryotic Viral Vectors (Gluzman Y, ed), Cold Spring Harbor, NY: Cold Spring Harbor Laboratory
18. Vlazny DA, Frenkel N (1981): Proc Natl Acad Sci USA 78:742
19. Vlazny DA, Kwong A, Frenkel N (1982): Proc Natl Acad Sci USA 79: 1423

Gene Transfer and Cancer, edited by M. L. Pearson and N. L. Sternberg. Raven Press, New York © 1984.

Structure of the Polyoma Virus Early Promoter: Sequences Required for Expression and Tumor Antigen Binding

Christopher Mueller, Anne-Marie Mes, Betsy Pomerantz, Mark Featherstone, Monica Naujokas, and John A. Hassell

Department of Microbiology and Immunology, McGill University, Montreal, Quebec H3A 2B4 Canada

ABSTRACT. Transcription of the polyoma virus early region is affected by cellular RNA polymerase II and is controlled by a product of this region, large tumor-antigen (T-antigen). To understand the mechanism of transcriptional regulation by large T-antigen requires knowledge of the spatial organization of the T-antigen-binding sites relative to the early promoter. We have performed experiments to define the sequences that comprise the polyoma virus early promoter and the T-antigen-binding sites. Using molecular cloning techniques and in vitro mutagenesis procedures, we constructed deletion mutants of recombinant plasmids with lesions in 5' noncoding sequences that bear the early transcription unit. The capacity of these mutant DNAs to transform cells in culture and to be transcribed in vitro was assessed. The results of our analyses reveal that at least three regions of the viral genome are required for efficient gene expression as measured by transformation. However, only one of these three sequence elements is required for transcription in vitro.

To map sites on polyoma virus DNA to which T-antigen binds, we used an immunoprecipitation assay. Using labelled restriction endonuclease fragments of both wild-type and mutant viral DNAs as substrates in binding assays with crude preparations of large T-antigen, we mapped two regions on the genome to which large T-antigen binds. The organization of these sites relative to the early promoter elements suggests that T-antigen retards initiation of transcription.

INTRODUCTION

The 5292-bp genome of polyoma virus encodes six proteins that are derived from two transcription units. During lytic infection of permissive mouse cells, the viral genome is expressed in two temporal phases described as early and late. The early phase begins soon after infection and is characterized by expression of the early transcription unit. Transcription of this part of the viral genome by the cell's RNA polymerase II yields nuclear RNA precursors that give rise to three coterminal mRNAs differing in internal sequences as a result of RNA splicing. Three T-antigens, designated large, middle, and small, are synthesized from the early mRNAs. The time of initiation of viral DNA replication defines the late phase of the lytic cycle. The late region of the viral genome is expressed to yield the structural proteins of the virus, VP1, VP2, and VP3. The transition from early to late phase is mediated by large T-antigen which is required to initiate each new round of viral DNA replication. During this time the number of transcripts arising from the early region is drastically reduced, when corrected for the number of genome copies per cell, in comparison to the early phase. Inhibition of early gene transcription at late times requires large T-antigen because mutants that encode a temperature-sensitive large T-antigen overproduce early gene products at the restrictive temperature. Therefore, large T-antigen plays a dual role during lytic infection: it initiates viral DNA replication and it regulates early gene transcription. It is thought that both of these processes require that T-antigen bind to the viral genome in close proximity to the initiation site for DNA replication and early transcription. The lytic cycle is generally completed 48-72 hrs post-infection and results in the death of the cell and the release of a new crop of virus particles.

Polyoma virus can also transform cells in which it does not replicate. Stable transformation is generally achieved when the viral genome is integrated into cellular DNA. In these cells, the early region is expressed but the late region is not and viral DNA replication does not occur. Although all the early proteins can be synthesized in transformed cells, only middle T-antigen is required to maintain the transformed state.

We are interested in the mechanism of transcription initiation and its control in mammalian cells and have chosen to utilize the early transcription unit of polyoma virus as a model. To understand the mechanism of transcriptional regulation by large T-antigen requires knowledge of the spatial organization of the large T-antigen-binding sites relative to the early promoter. These regulatory sequences have not been defined for polyoma virus. To position these sequences on the viral genome, we constructed deletion mutations in polyoma virus-plasmid recombinants and measured the capacity of the resulting mutants to be expressed in vivo and in vitro and to bind large T-antigen. Our results reveal that two and perhaps three upstream sequence elements are required for maximal gene expression in vivo as measured by transformation assays. Only one of the latter elements (element 3) that lies closest to the coding sequences and carries a TATA sequence is required for correct transcription initiation in vitro. Two independent T-antigen-binding regions have been mapped. One of these overlaps with the transcriptional element 3; the other lies farther upstream near the site of initiation of viral DNA replication. The location of the T-antigen-binding sites relative to the early promoter suggests that large T-antigen impairs transcription initiation during the late phase of infection.

RESULTS

The Structure Of The Polyoma Virus Early Promoter

To map the polyoma virus early promoter, we constructed mutants of recombinant plasmids that bear the transforming region of the virus. The fragment chosen for mutagenesis, the small BamHI to EcoRI fragment of polyoma virus DNA, carries all the genetic information necessary for maximal transformation of cell lines in culture (8). This fragment was cloned within the large BamHI to EcoRI fragment of the vector pBR322. Deletion mutations were introduced into the recombinant DNAs using standard procedures and were of two classes. One set of mutant carries deletions that begin at the BamHI site [polyoma virus nucleotide number 4632,

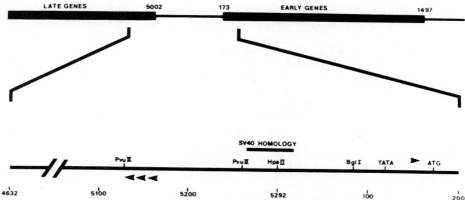

FIGURE 1. Physical map of the region near the 5' termini of the polyoma virus early and late transcription units. The > refer to the position where the abundant 5' termini of the early and late mRNAs map.

TABLE 1. Functional Assays of Mutant DNAs.[a]

DNA	Deletion boundaries	Transformation efficiency	Accurate initiation[b] in vitro
pPBR1	--	100	+
pBR520	4632–4782	50	ND
pPB510	4632–4827	36	ND
pPB505	4632–4834	29	+
pPB552	4632–4841	14	+
pPBP1	4632–5265	5	+
pPd1BgK	4632–93	1	+
pPSG4	4632–154	0.01	−
pPd1300	5130–5265	100	+
pPd1326	5126–5265	100	ND
pPd1304	5130–5277	50	+
pPd1310	5094–14	13	+
pPd11–8	1–149	50	−
pPdlPvuHph	5130–154	0.5	ND

[a] The nucleotide sequence about the deletion in each mutant DNA was determined by the chemical method of Maxam and Gilbert (5). Transformation efficiency was calculated by measuring the specific transforming activity of each mutant DNA by comparison to wt DNA in the same assay. The specific transforming activity of a given DNA was determined over a range of DNA concentrations, in triplicate, and the transforming activity calculated from the linear portion of the curve. In vitro transcription assays were performed with cell extracts prepared from Hela cells and radiolabeled GTP as a precursor. The DNA templates were cleaved with <u>Ava</u>I, and a total of 50 μg/ml of DNA was used in each assay.

[b] (+) denotes a run-off transcript of the same size as that synthesized from wt template. ND means that the DNA was not tested; (−) refers to the absence of a transcript of the same size as that transcribed from wt DNA.

or position -810 by reference to the 5' end of the early mRNAs (nucleotide 150)] and extend downstream (Figure 1). The 5' boundary of all of these deletions abut the same pBR322 sequences (viz. the BamHI site). The other class of mutants bear lesions internal to the sequences between positions 4632 to 150 (-810 to +1). After molecular cloning in Escherichia coli, each mutant DNA was characterized with restriction endonucleases to verify its mutant nature, screened for a phenotype by transformation of mammalian cells, and finally the primary structure of each mutant DNA around the mutation was determined by Maxam-Gilbert sequencing. We chose to measure the specific transforming activity of the DNAs by comparing them with the wild-type oncogene as an indirect indicator of in vivo gene expression because this method allows for quantitation of the relative efficiency of various forms of the promoter. In support of this contention McKnight et al. (7) have provided compelling evidence that there is an excellent correlation between the specific transforming activity of a DNA species (viz. the herpes simplex virus thymidine kinase gene) and its capacity to be transcribed in vivo during transient expression assays. Because not all mutants with upstream lesions that effect transformation need be altered in transcription, we also assayed the capacity of each mutant DNA to function as a template for transcription in vitro (4). The results of our analyses are presented in Table 1. Progressive deletion of upstream sequences from the BamHI site to downstream positions results in a decline of transforming activity until nucleotide position 154 (+4) is reached. Mutant DNAs with deletion that remove virtually all the upstream noncoding sequences (i.e. pPSG4) transform rat cells at very low but detectable frequencies (0.01% of wild type). Deletion mutations that extend into the coding regions completely abolish the transforming activity of the DNA (8). Careful examination of the phenotype of the various mutant DNAs reveals that a sharp decline in transforming activity (3-4 fold) occurs after removal of a short stretch of DNA (60 bp) between nucleotide positions 4782 and 4841 (-660 and -601). This suggests that these deletions impinge upon the 5' border of a sequence element important for transformation. In addition, if the deletion is extended to the BglI site at nucleotide number 93 (-57), the specific transforming activity of the DNA drops another 10- to 15-fold to 1.0% of wild-type levels, and a further 10-fold reduction in transforming activity results when all the 5' nontranscribed sequences are removed (Table 1). These observations suggested to us that multiple sequence elements important for transformation might reside between the upstream border of the promoter and the coding sequences of the early transcription unit. To determine if this was true we constructed additional mutants by deletion of sequences internal to the promoter region. We selected several conveniently located restriction endonuclease cleavage sites for mutagenesis. These included the PvuII sites at positions 5128 and 5262 and the BglI site at position 87. Deletion of the viral sequences between the PvuII sites yielded a mutant DNA pPd1300, that transforms cells at wild-type frequencies (Table 1). This implies that the region bounded by the PvuII sites is not required for gene expression as measured by transformation. Note however, that sequences farther upstream of the PvuII site at position 5128 are important for transformation (Table 1). Therefore, between the BamHI site (4632) and the PvuII site (5128), there lies a sequence which we have named element 1 that is required for maximal gene expression. To refine the downstream boundary of element 1, we extended the deletion present in pPd1300 with the Bal31 nuclease and derived three additional mutants (pPd1326, 304, and 310). Four bp were deleted from pPd1300 in the upstream direction only to create pPdl326. This mutant DNA transforms at wild-type frequencies. By contrast, 12 bp were deleted in only the downstream direction from the PvuII site in pPdl300 to create pPdl304, and its DNA transforms cells at nearly wild-type frequencies (50% of wild-type DNA). Finally, the mutant pPdl310 (this deletion extends 36 bp upstream and 41 bp downstream of the PvuII site in pPdl300) transforms cells at 13% the frequency of wild-type DNA. Its phenotype may be accounted for by deletion of sequences either in element 1 or in another element farther downstream.

Two mutants were characterized that bear deletions about the BglI site at position 87 (-63). One of these, pPdl1-8, carries a 148-bp deletion from position 1 to 149 (-149 to -1) and transforms cells at 50% the frequency of wild-type DNA. Another mutant pPdlPvuHph carries a 316-bp deletion that includes all the sequences deleted in pPdl1-8 plus another 162 bp upstream to position 5130 and another 5 bp downstream (position 154). This mutant DNA is drastically reduced in its capacity to transform cells (0.5% the frequency of wild-type DNA). The phenotype of these mutant DNAs can be accounted for if we postulate the existence of a second control sequence (element 2), located between positions 5265 and 1 (28 bp in length), that is required in concert with element 1 to elicit expression of the early region. This postulate can be justified not only by the phenotype of mutants pPdl1-8 and pPdlPvuHph but also by the phenotype of mutants pPBP1 and pPdlBgK. A 5-fold reduction in transformation efficiency results when sequences between nucleotide positions 5265 (-177) and 93 (-57) are removed from the transforming region, implying that an important control sequence has been deleted between these boundaries.

In Vitro Transcription of 5' Deleted DNAs

The mutant DNAs were individually assayed for their capacity to act as templates for transcription by incubation in extracts prepared from Hela cells with the appropriate substrates (4). The specificity of transcription was assessed by employing truncated templates and measuring the size of the resulting radiolabeled transcripts by comparison to those synthesized from wild-type DNA (the run-off assay). Transcription of AvaI cleaved wild-type DNA yields a run-off transcript 510 nucleotides long. This is the size expected if initiation were to occur near the in vivo start at nucleotide position 150 on the template. The results obtained after assay of many of the mutant DNAs are shown in Table 1. All deletion mutants that retain 57 or more base pairs of 5' upstream DNA, relative to nucleotide position 150 (+1), yield transcripts of identical size to the wild-type template. The DNA of two mutants, pPSG4 and pPdl1-8, do not support the synthesis of transcripts of appropriate size. The deletions borne by these mutant DNAs overlap between nucleotide position 93 and 149 (-57 and -1), thereby defining a 56-bp stretch of DNA required for accurate transcription initiation in vitro. Note that these sequences can be deleted from wild-type DNA with little consequence in vivo (pPdl1-8 transforms cells at 50% the frequency of wild-type DNA). However, an effect of this region on transformation can be measured when sequences upstream of nucleotide position 93 (-57) are removed from the DNA. Then, further deletion of sequences between position 93 and 154 leads to a 10-fold or more reduction in transformation efficiency (compare the transforming activity of pPdlBgK with that of pPSG4). On this basis, we define another control region (element 3) located between nucleotide positions 87 and 154.

Sequences to Which T-Antigen Binds

To map the sites on polyoma virus DNA to which T-antigen binds, we employed an immunoprecipitation assay (6). Radiolabeled fragments of viral DNA were reacted with crude nuclear extracts prepared from lytically infected 3T6 cells and the fragments bound by T-antigen immunoprecipitated with anti-T serum and formallin-fixed <u>Staphylococcus</u> <u>aureus</u>. The immunoprecipitated DNA was then analyzed by gel electrophoresis and

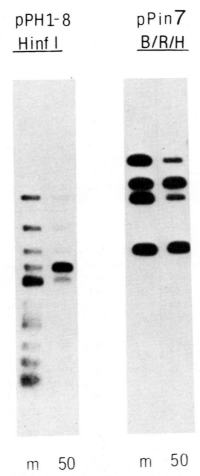

FIGURE 2. Immunoprecipitation of radiolabeled fragments of polyoma virus-plasmid DNAs by large T-antigen. The left panel represents an autoradiograph of pPH1-8 DNA cleaved with <u>Hinf</u>I that has been electrophoresed through a 1.4% (w/v) agarose gel after reaction with polyoma virus large T-antigen. The right panel represents an autoradiograph of pPin7 (a derivative of pPBR1, see Table 1, that carries a <u>Hin</u>dIII linker in place of the <u>Bgl</u>I site in the viral genome that has been digested with <u>Bam</u>HI, <u>Eco</u>RI, and <u>Hin</u>dIII and reacted with T-antigen. M refers to the unreacted fragments, whereas 50 refers to the same fragments that have been immunoprecipitated after reaction with 50 µl of a T-antigen preparation.

autoradiography. An example of such an autoradiograph is shown in Figure 2. HinfI digestion of pPH1-8 DNA (the HindIII -1 fragment of polyoma virus DNA cloned within pBR322 DNA at its HindIII site) yields a number of fragments, only one of which is immunoprecipitated when reacted with a crude T-antigen preparation. This fragment spans the region from which DNA replication initiates (nucleotide position 5073 to 385). The other panel shown in Figure 2 shows that there exist two regions within polyoma virus DNA to which T-antigen binds. One of these lies downstream and the other upstream of the BglI site (nucleotide position 87) in polyoma virus DNA (see Figure 1). To map the T-antigen-binding sites on the viral genome more precisely, we used various restriction endonucleases to generate defined fragments of both wild-type and mutant recombinant plasmid DNAs (Table 1) in assays of the type described above. The results of many such reactions are summarized at the bottom of Figure 3. Polyoma virus large T-antigen binds independently to two regions on the viral genome. The farthest upstream region maps approximately between nucleotide positions 14 and 87, whereas the other is located between positions 87 and 162. The latter T-antigen-binding region overlaps the transcriptional element 3 and the site from which transcription initiates in vivo.

DISCUSSION

Analysis of the sequences required for expression of the polyoma virus early region revealed an unexpected complexity. Three sets of sequences were identified that are required for efficient transformation of cells in culture. Only one of these is necessary for accurate transcription initiation in vitro. The 5' border of the farthest upstream sequence (element 1) is located near nucleotide position 4827 some 660 bp from the site where the 5' termini of the early mRNAs map. This sequence may be as long as 300 bp and overlaps with a stretch of DNA that encodes one of the structural proteins of the virus (VP2). Preliminary results from our laboratory indicate that element 1 acts as an enhancer of gene expression and in this regard is analogous in function to the 72-bp repeat of SV40 (1). Element 1 is incapable of eliciting expression of the early region unless other control sequences are also present before the gene. Element 2 and/or 3 can serve in this capacity. Element 2 is located 150 bp upstream of the start site for transcription. This sequence is approximately

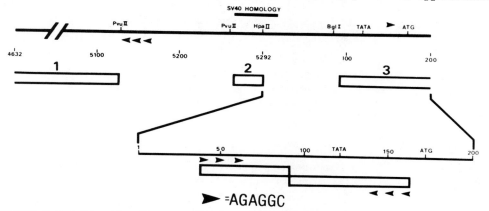

FIGURE 3. Schematic diagram showing the boundaries of the transcriptional elements and the large T-antigen binding regions of the polyoma virus genome.

30 bp long and is homologous to the region in SV40 DNA where early transcription initiates. In SV40 DNA, the TATA sequence as well as the 5' termini of the early mRNA map in this area. The existence of element 2 is most readily demonstrated by comparison of the phenotypes of mutants pPdl1-8 and pPdPvuHph (Table 1). Both of these mutant DNAs lack element 3 (the sequence that carries the polyoma virus early TATA box). However, only pPd13-14 is drastically reduced in its transforming efficiency (0.5% of wild-type). It is possible that a sequence within element 2, related to the TATA sequence, can substitute for element 3 when it is deleted from the viral genome. Whether element 2 is required in conjunction with both element 1 and 3 for maximal gene expression requires isolation and characterization of additional mutants with lesions in element 2 only. Element 3, the sequence closest to the coding sequences, is required for accurate transcription initiation in vitro. Its requirement for in vivo expression can only be demonstrated when all the other upstream elements have been deleted from the transforming region (Table 1: compare pPdlBgK with pPSG4). The 5' border of this element maps near nucleotide number 93 (-57). Its 3' boundary has not been mapped. This stretch of DNA contains sequences homologous and in similar positions to those found before other genes. They include the pentameric sequence GATCC at positions -50 to -45, the TATA box at positions -30 to -20, and the cap box PyCATTCPy located very near to the mRNA start site (for a review, see 7). There is no CCAAT sequence near position -70 to -80 before the early transcription unit of polyoma virus, although a related sequence can be found near -80 to -90. In any event this conserved sequence is apparently not required for accurate initiation in vitro.

Two T-antigen-binding regions have been localized on the polyoma virus DNA molelcule. One of these regions maps near the site from which DNA replication initiates, (site 2) whereas the other encompasses the site from which transcription initiates (site 1). Polyoma virus T-antigen interacts independently with both regions, and under standard reaction conditions binds equally tightly to both sites. The sequence AGAGGC or the pentamer GAGGC is repeated three times, always separated by 4 to 6 bp, on the L-strand (the DNA strand homologous to early mRNA) near nucleotide position 40, 50, and 60 and on the E-strand (the DNA strand homologous to late mRNA) in the opposite orientation at nucleotide number 140, 150, and 160. The two sets of repeats are separated from each other by 100 to 120 bp (Figure 2). T-antigen-binding site 1 (nucleotide position 90 to 165) is not required in cis for DNA replication, whereas no viable virus mutants have been isolated that lack binding site 2 (2; Muller and Hassell, unpublished), implying but not proving that site 2 is required for initiation of viral DNA replication. From the position of T-antigen-binding site 1 and the phenotype of virus mutants that delete this site (2), we infer that it is required for efficient repression of E-strand transcription at late times. However, definitive proof of this hypothesis must await experiments in which the effect of polyoma virus large T-antigen on transcription can be measured in vitro.

ACKNOWLEDGEMENTS

This research was supported by funds from the Medical Research Council and the National Cancer Institute of Canada. J.A.H. is a research scholar of the National Cancer Institute, and A.M.M. and M.F. are research students of the National Cancer Institute. G.M. is a research student of the Natural Sciences and Engineering Research Council of Canada.

REFERENCES

1. Banerji J, Rusconi S, Schaffner, W (1981): Cell 27:299
2. Bendig MM, Thomas T, Folk WR (1980): Cell 20:401
3. Hassell JA, Topp WC, Rifkin DB, Moreau PE (1980): Proc Natl Acad Sci USA 77:3978
4. Manley JL, Fire A, Cano A, Sharp PA, Gefter ML (1980): Proc. Natl Acad Sci USA 77:3855
5. Maxam A, Gilbert W (1980): Meth Enzymol 65:499
6. McKay RDG (1981): J Mol Biol 145:471
7. McKnight SL, Gavis ER, Kingsbury R (1981): Cell 25:385
8. Mes A-M, Hassell JA (1982): J Virol 42:621
9. Tooze J (ed) (1980): DNA Tumor Viruses, Part 2, Cold Spring Harbor Laboratory: Cold Spring Harbor, NY

Gene Transfer and Cancer, edited by M. L. Pearson
and N. L. Sternberg. Raven Press, New York © 1984.

Human Papilloma Virus Type 1 RNA Transcription and Processing in COS-1 Cells

Louise T. Chow and Thomas R. Broker

Cold Spring Harbor Laboratory, Cold Spring Harbor, New York 11724

ABSTRACT. Papilloma viruses cannot be propagated in cell culture in amounts sufficient for recovery of DNA, RNA, or proteins for molecular analysis. It has been necessary to clone them in bacterial plasmids. We are studying the structures of human papilloma virus (HPV) type-1 mRNAs made after transfection of SV40-transformed monkey CV-1 cells (COS cells) with HPV-1 DNA cloned in the shuttle vectors pSV08 and pSV010 which contain the SV40 origin of DNA replication. The vectors were linked in both orientations to various full-length circular permutations of the HPV DNA sequences. RNA isolated 48 hr post-transfection was hybridized with HPV-1 DNA and analyzed by electron microscopy. One clone (D2) gave rise to two different spliced RNA transcripts that have the same 5' ends derived from SV40 sequences in the vector, but they have different 3' ends. The short species has two spliced segments and spans 40% of the HPV DNA while the longer has three segments and spans 76% of the HPV genome. Spliced RNAs produced from other clones have the same conserved HPV-specific sequences as those from clone D2, but they have different 5' leader segments originating from the SV40 early promoter in the vector. The HPV RNAs have been correlated with the recently published DNA sequence (5). The main bodies of the conserved HPV sequences correspond to one of two early region open reading frames and one of two late region open reading frames, and both 3' ends map near AATAAA signals in the DNA.

INTRODUCTION

Papilloma viruses have been classified, together with the well-studied SV40 and polyoma viruses, as papovaviruses on the basis of their icosahedral capsids and circular, double-stranded DNA chromosomes. But that is where the similarities end. The many types of human papilloma viruses cause various types of warts of keratinized and mucosal epithelia. They establish long-term infections of basal cells, in which the viral DNA is maintained as low-copy-number, extrachromosomal plasmids (1,17,19,31,39). They proliferate only in the terminally differentiated, upper keratinocyte layers of the skin. The viruses can transform cultured cells but undergo full lytic expression in cell culture systems presently available (39). Until recently, studies of the wart viruses have been limited largely to epidemiology. Papilloma viral DNAs from human, cow, and rabbit have since been cloned in bacterial vectors. Comparisons of these by hybridization analysis and restriction mapping have shown there to be

many different types of viruses, sharing various extents of sequence
homologies [6,10,15,18,26,27,29,30,32,35,36,38; and our own unpublished
electron microscopical (EM) heteroduplex analyses]. What emerges is a
close association of particular viruses with specific manifestations of
epidermal infections (13,37). For instance, human papilloma virus
types 1 and 4, viruses with very little sequence homology (15), are
associated with deep plantar warts (10). HPV-2 causes benign common
warts that tend to afflict children and young adults (26). HPV-3, rather
closely related to HPV-2 based on our EM analysis of DNA:DNA heteroduplexes, is responsible for flat warts associated with one type of epidermodysplasia verruciformis (e.v.) (27). HPV-5, which does not establish
heteroduplexes with HPV-3 or HPV-2, causes flat reddish warts associated
with another type of e.v. (27). About 25% of the patients with HPV-5
develop malignancies showing a distinct familial pattern of incidence
(28), possibly related to deficient cell-mediated immunity (33). A
common and serious venereal disease, condyloma acuminata, is caused by
HPV-6 or HPV-11 (6,7,36). Some genital infections progress to carcinomas
(22,34). Juvenile laryngeal papillomatosis (j.l.p.) is caused primarily
by HPV-11 and has been correlated with mothers exhibiting condylomas,
suggesting that infection occurs in utero or during parturition (40).
HPV-7 is implicated in the common warts of meat handlers (29,30). Many
more types of HPV have been identified or cloned from other cases of
epidermodysplasia verruciformis.

Although large amounts of cloned papilloma virus DNAs are now available for molecular characterization, we still do not know how the genomes
of the human papilloma viruses are expressed. In this aspect, bovine
papilloma viruses (BPV) present an advantage because one can obtain large
amounts of wart tissue from infected animals. BPV-1 can also propagate
in connective tissues (1) and transform fibroblast cells in culture (17,
19). Recently, studies of BPV-1 gene expression in tumors or in transformed cells in culture have shown that only one DNA strand of the viral
genome is transcribed and that it gives rise to multiple, overlapping
mRNA species (16). The question arises whether HPV-1 is also organized
in a similar manner.

                        RESULTS AND DISCUSSION

We have begun to investigate the genomic organization of human papilloma viruses by utilizing shuttle vectors that can replicate in both
bacterial and mammalian cells. The strategy is to prepare large amounts
of the HPV-containing recombinant plasmids from bacteria and, using the
calcium phosphate precipitate method (8,12), transfect them into mammalian cells in which they can replicate to high copy numbers. The expectation is that even low levels of expression by the amplified plasmids
might provide enough RNA for molecular analysis.

The two vectors, pSV08 and pSV010 (24,25), that we used contain about
half of pBR322, including the bacterial replication origin and the ampicillin-resistance gene. The tetracycline-resistance gene and the poison
sequences which hamper plasmid replication in mammalian cells (21) have
been removed. In their place, a 229-bp segment of SV40 spanning the origin of replication, the early promoter, and the coding sequences for the
5' ends of the early and some minor late RNAs has been inserted. Neither
plasmid contains the SV40 72-bp enhancer sequences responsible for efficient early RNA transcription (2,3,14) nor the sequences encoding the
major 5' ends of late mRNAs (9). These vectors have been useful in
studying transcription of cloned genes without significant interference

from viral promoters (23). The two vectors differ by the presence, in pSV010, of a poly-linker (constructed by Brian Seed and Tom Maniatis) consisting of many restriction endonuclease recognition sites useful for cloning. Both can replicate in COS-1 cells (11), which are monkey CV-1 cells transformed by SV40 that can provide the SV40 T-antigen necessary for plasmid DNA replication from an SV40 origin.

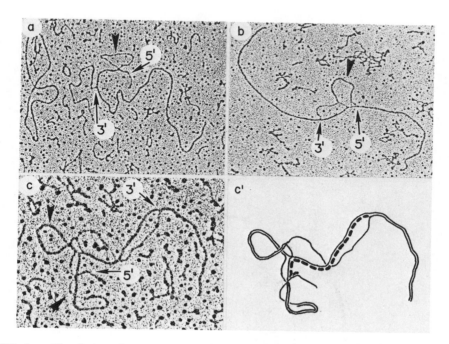

FIGURE 1. Electron micrographs of RNA transcripts of HPV-1 initiated from a late promoter of SV40. (a) Total cytoplasmic RNA was isolated 48 hr post-transfection of COS-1 cells with HPV-1:pSV08 plasmid D2 (see Figure 2A). It was annealed to plasmid 6.3 DNA, which consists of HPV-1 DNA opened at the <u>Bgl</u>II site at nucleotide 4868 and inserted into the pSV010 <u>Bgl</u>II site in the poly-linker (Figure 2B). Plasmid 6.3 was lin-earized prior to R-loop formation at its <u>Cla</u>I site in the poly-linker on the side of the vector (near nucleotide 7100 in Figure 2B). The RNA is annealed to a terminal fork in the partially denatured DNA. (b) RNA from the same preparation was annealed to plasmid 55.2 DNA, which con-sists of HPV-1 DNA opened at the <u>Bgl</u>II site at HPV-1 nucleotide 2041 and inserted into the pSV010 <u>Bgl</u>II site in the poly-linker in the same orientation as plasmid 6.3 (Figure 2B). Plasmid 55.2 was linearized at the <u>Cla</u>I site in the poly-linker prior to R-loop formation. The 5' and 3' ends of the RNAs are labeled with arrows and the DNA deletion loop corresponding to the single intervening sequence in each RNA is marked with a large arrowhead. (c) and (c') RNA from the same COS cell extract was annealed to plasmid 6.3 DNA, as in panel (a). The RNA termini and the two DNA deletion loops corresponding to the two intervening sequences removed from the RNA are indicated as in panels (a) and (b). In the in-terpretive tracing, RNA is depicted with the dashed line. The locations of the 5' ends of both species of RNA, as shown in Figure 2A, suggests they were initiated from an SV40 late promoter in the vector.

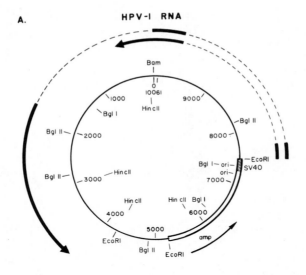

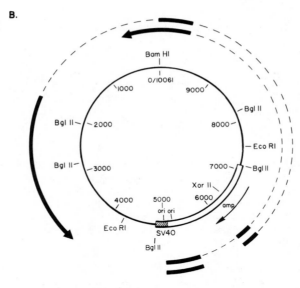

FIGURE 2. HPV-1 RNA transcripts synthesized by shuttle vectors in COS-1 cells. (A) Graphic representation of RNAs generated from an SV40 late promoter in plasmid D2 (see Figure 1). (B) RNAs generated from the SV40 early promoter in plasmid 6.3 (see Figure 3). Identical RNAs were observed in COS-1 cells transfected with B38 plasmid. HPV-1 in B38 was cloned at the same EcoRI site as in plasmid D2 and in the same orientation as that in clone 6.3. Note the use of cryptic donor and acceptor splice sites derived from the pBR322 sequences in the vector, and also the identity of the conserved HPV RNA sequences produced from the two plasmids.

Because we did not know where and how many transcription units are expressed from the HPV-1 genome, we linearized the HPV-1 viral DNA extracted from a single plantar wart by partial digestion with EcoRI, BamHI, or BglII restriction endonuclease, and we cloned each of the resulting circular permutations of the entire viral DNA into one of the two vectors. Irrespective of the number and location of the transcription units, each is expected to be intact in at least one of the recombinant plasmids.

Several cloned DNAs were individually transfected into COS-1 cells and total cytoplasmic RNA was isolated 48 hr later. In dot-blot analyses of these RNA preparations, using nick-translated ^{32}P-HPV-1 DNA as a probe, we found that all samples gave positive results. They were then examined by electron microscopy after R-loop formation with two different HPV-1: vector recombinant plasmids, each linearized with a single-cut restriction endonuclease. (The use of two plasmid DNAs, cloned in different circular permutations, allowed unambiguous orientation and mapping of the RNA.) The preparations contained very low levels of HPV-1-specific RNA (probably less than 0.001% of all poly(A)-containing RNA). One of the clones, D2, (Figure 2A) produced mainly two RNA species (Figures 1 and 2A). The 5' ends of both RNAs mapped essentially at the cloning site, close to where the SV40 minor, 5' cap sequences on late RNA can be encoded. (The major SV40 cap sites are deleted in these plasmids). The major species consisted of a leader of 210 nucleotides spliced 1950 nucleotides downstream to a main body of 920 nucleotides. The less frequent species had the same 5' leader spliced 1950 nucleotides to a second segment of only 400 nucleotides, which constitutes the 5' portion of the main body of the major RNA species just described, and is then spliced 1900 nucleotides further downstream to a third segment about 2000 nucleotides long. From these lengths, it is clear that the RNA covers 76% of

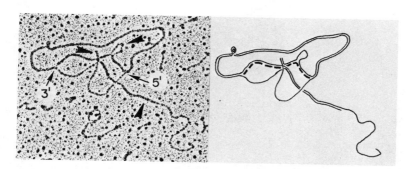

FIGURE 3. Electron micrographs of RNA transcripts of HPV-1 initiated from the early promoter of SV40. Total cytoplasmic RNA isolated 48 hr post-transfection of COS-1 cells with HPV-1:pSV010 plasmid B38 (see Figure 2B) was annealed to plasmid 6.3 DNA (see legend to Figure 1a) to form R-loops. The DNA deletion loop corresponding to the first intervening sequence (IVS) encoded by the pSV010 vector is indicated with an arrowhead. The DNA was linearized at the XorII site in the vector, which is within the second IVS, as reflected by the short and long duplex DNA tails, also marked by large arrowheads. In the interpretive tracing, RNA is depicted with the dashed line. (See Figure 2B for a graphic representation). Identical RNAs were also found in cells transfected with plasmid 6.3, the structure of which is shown in Figure 2B.

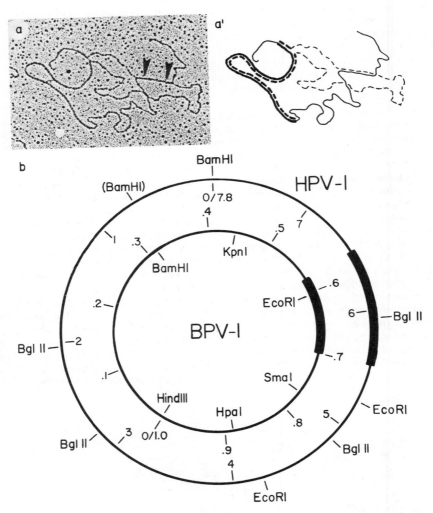

FIGURE 4. Alignment of HPV-1 and BPV-1 Genomes. (a) and (a'): Electron micrograph of a heteroduplex formed between HPV-1 and BPV-1 DNAs. (Both plasmids were cloned by P.M. Howley and colleagues). The HPV-1a DNA was cloned at its single <u>Bam</u>HI site in pBR322 and linearized at the <u>Cla</u>I site in pBR322. The BPV-1 was cloned at its single <u>Hind</u>III site in pBR322 and linearized at its <u>Hpa</u>I site. An interpretive tracing is included; the arrowheads point to the papilloma viral DNA segments with partial homology. The BPV-1 sequence is represented by a thin continuous line and the HPV-1 sequence with a dashed line. The pBR322 sequences are shown with bold lines. (b): Alignment of the HPV-1 and BPV-1 restriction maps based on EM heteroduplex analysis. The HPV scale is in kilobase pairs and the BPV scale in decimal map units. (While this manuscript was in press, a similar EM heteroduplex comparison of HPV-1 and BPV-1 DNA homology was reported by Croissant et al. (35).

the HPV-1 genome; therefore probably only one strand is transcribed, as is the case with BPV-1.

To distinguish whether the RNA species originated from an HPV-1 promoter located very close to the cloning site in the D2 plasmid or whether they were indeed derived from an SV40 late promoter, RNA was prepared from cells transfected with either of two other clones. In plasmid B38, HPV-1 is opened at the same EcoRI site as in plasmid D2, but it is inserted into the vector in the opposite orientation. Plasmid 6.3 has HPV-1 opened at the BglII site at nucleotide 4868 and inserted into the vector in the same orientation as plasmid B38 (Figure 2B). If the RNAs produced by the D2 plasmid originated from an HPV-2 promoter, then the same RNA species should also be generated from plasmids B38 and 6.3. These RNA preparations were examined by electron microscopy as described before. Again, both clones produced very low amounts of, predominantly, two HPV-2 RNA species. The 3' segments of both were the same as those produced by plasmid D2. However, the two 5' leaders were clearly derived from the cap site(s) of early SV40 RNAs and from pBR322 sequences (Figures 2B and 3). These results reinforce the likelihood that the D2 RNAs originated from the SV40 late promoter. We conclude that 1) the promoter(s) of HPV-1 are extremely weak or nonfunctional in the COS cells; 2) both the early and the minor late promoters of SV40 can serve as surrogate promoters for the HPV transcripts; and 3) the donor and acceptor splice sites and polyadenylation sites in HPV-1 are reproducible irrespective of the 5' promoter used and the sequences of the 5' ends of the RNA. Therefore, these sites are probably bona fide and reflect signals utilized in the natural HPV-1 transcripts.

Our conclusions are in agreement with recent mapping data on BPV-1 RNAs. Sequence homology between HPVs and BPV-1 DNA has been reported by Law et al. (18) using the Southern blotting technique. We have aligned the genomes of HPV-1 and BPV-1 more precisely using EM heteroduplex analyses (Figure 4). The region with the most extensive partial homology under our conditions of hybridization and sample preparation falls within the genetic interval necessary for BPV-1 transformation of mouse cells (18,20). Recently, a number of overlapping RNAs from cultured mouse cells transformed by BPV-1 were mapped by S1 nuclease analysis to have coterminal, 3' ends near map unit 0.34 in the BPV-1 genome (16). They have different 5' ends extending various distances clockwise towards the HindIII site. The possibility of spliced segments at the 5' ends of these BPV-1 RNAs was not excluded. Taking into account our EM alignment of the HPV-1 and BPV-1 chromosomes, the main body of the major BPV-1 RNA is equivalent in position and length to the shorter of the two HPV-1 RNA species that we mapped. In addition, the mRNA for the major capsid protein of BPV-1 has been assigned to a 2-kb RNA species occupying a genome position (L. Engel, C. Heilman and P. Howley, personal communication) equivalent to the longer of the two HPV-1 RNA species shown in Figures 1C and 2.

Our RNA mapping results are also consistent with the HPV-1 DNA sequence which has subsequently been published (4,5). The RNAs coincide with major open reading frames, and there are polyadenylation signals (AAUAAA) at both sites where the 3' ends of the RNAs were mapped. Therefore, in the hybrid transcription system described here, the HPV-1 DNA is expressed from SV40 promoters, but the RNA terminates and is spliced at what appear to be appropriate sites. The structures of minor RNA species that might utilize the other open reading frames and the location of the HPV-1 promoter remain to be determined.

ACKNOWLEDGEMENTS

This research was sponsored by American Cancer Society Research Grant MV-144 to L.T.C. and by an NIH/NCI Cancer Program Project grant to Cold Spring Harbor Laboratory. We thank Robert LaPorta and Lorne Taichman for providing HPV-1, Richard Myers and Bob Tjian for sending pSV08 and pSV010, Yakov Gluzman for the COS-1 cells, Joe Sambrook and Pamela Mellon for helpful suggestions, Peter Howley for communicating unpublished results and for the BPV-1 cloned and for the HPV-1 cloned in pBR322.

REFERENCES

1. Amtmann E, Müller H, Sauer G (1980): J Virol 35:962
2. Banerji J, Rusconi S, Schaffner W (1981): Cell 27:299
3. Benoist C, Chambon P (1981): Nature 290:304
4. Clad A, Gissmann L, Meier B, Freese UK, Schwarz E (1982): Virol 118:254
5. Danos O, Katinka M, Yaniv M (1982): EMBO J 1:231
6. deVilliers E-M, Gissmann L, zur Hausen H (1981): J Virol 40:932
7. Ferenczy A, Braun L, Shah KV (1981): Am J Surg Pathol 5:661
8. Frost E, Williams J (1978): Virol 91:39
9. Ghosh PK, Reddy VB, Swinscoe J, Lebowitz P, Weissman SM (1978): J Mol Biol 126:813
10. Gissmann L, Pfister H, zur Hausen H (1977): Virol 76:569
11. Gluzman Y (1981): Cell 23:175
12. Graham FL, van der Eb AJ (1973): Virol 52:456
13. Gross C, Pfister H, Hagedorn M, Gissmann L (1982): J Invest Dermatol 78:160
14. Gruss P, Dhar R, Khoury G (1981): Proc Natl Acad Sci USA 78:943
15. Heilman CA, Law MA, Israel MA, Howley PM (1980): J Virol 36:395
16. Heilman CA, Engel L, Lowy DR, Howley PM (1982): Virol 119:22
17. Lancaster WD (1981): Virol 108:251
18. Law M-F, Lancaster WD, Howley PM (1979): J Virol 32:199
19. Law M-F, Lowy DR, Dvoretzky I, Howley PM (1981): Proc Natl Acad Sci USA 78:2727
20. Lowy DR, Dvoretzky I, Shober R, Law M-F, Engel, Howley PM (1980): Nature 287:72
21. Lusky M, Botchan M (1981): Nature 293:79
22. Medical World News. Papilloma virus seen as a key culprit in cervical dysplasia. March 29, 1982, pp 8-9
23. Mellon P, Parker V, Gluzman Y, Maniatis T (1981): Cell 27:279
24. Myers RM, Rio DC, Robbins AK, Tjian R (1981): Cell 25:373
25. Myers RM, Tjian R (1980): Proc Natl Acad Sci USA 77:6491
26. Orth G, Favre M, Croissant O (1977): J Virol 24:108
27. Orth G, Jablonska S, Favre M, Croissant O, Jarzabek-Chorzelska M, Rzesa G (1978): Proc Natl Acad Sci USA 75:1537
28. Orth G, Jablonska S, Jarzabek-Chorzelska M, Obalek S, Rzesa G, Favre M, Croissant O (1979): Cancer Res 39:1074
29. Orth G, Jablonska S, Favre M, Croissant O, Obalek S, Jarzabek-Chorzelska M, Jibard N (1981): J Invest Dermatol 76:97
30. Ostrow RS, Krzyzek R, Pass F, Faras AJ (1981): Virol 108:21
31. Pfister H, Fink B, Thomas C (1981): Virol 115:414
32. Pfister H, Nürnberger F, Gissman L, zur Hausen H (1981): Int J Cancer 27:645
33. Prawer JE, Pass F, Vance JC, Greenberg GJ, Yunis EJ, Zelickson AS (1977): Dermatol 113:495

34. zur Hausen H (1977): In: Current Topics in Microbiology and Immunology 78 (Arber W et al., eds), pp 1-30
35. Croissant O, Testaniére, Orth G (1982): Compte Rendu Acad Sci (Paris) 294:581
36. Gissmann L, Diehl V, Schultz-Coulon H-J, zur Hausen H (1982): J Virol 44:400
37. Howley PM (1982): Arch Pathol Lab Med 106:429
38. Kremsdorf D, Jablonska S, Favre M, Orth G (1982): J Virol 43:436
39. LaPorta RF, Taichman LB (1982): Proc Natl Acad Sci USA 79:3393
40. Quick CA, Faras AJ, Krzyzek R (1978): Laryngoscope 88:1789

Gene Transfer and Cancer, edited by M. L. Pearson
and N. L. Sternberg. Raven Press, New York © 1984.

Identification of an Adenovirus Function Required for Initiation of Cell Transformation Possibly at the Level of DNA Integration

*D. T. Rowe, †M. Ruben, †S. Bacchetti, and *,† F. L. Graham

*Departments of *Biology and †Pathology, McMaster University, Hamilton, Ontario, L8S 4J9 Canada*

ABSTRACT. During transformation of mammalian cells by purified DNA, DNA fragments are probably taken up and integrated into the cellular chromosome by purely cellular mechanisms. In transformation by most tumor viruses, integration of the viral genome probably involves the action of one or more viral functions. In the human adenovirus-rodent cell transformation system there are several lines of evidence suggesting that integration of the viral genome may occur by a specific mechanism controlled at least in part by a viral function. First, in cells trans- formed under stringent nonpermissive conditions, the entire viral genome is frequently found integrated colinearly into the host chromosome even though only the left end of the genome is needed for the maintenance of transformation. Second, in semipermissive cells transformed by adeno- viruses, in which deletion or rearrangement of cytotoxic viral genes might be a requisite for cell survival, both the left and right ends of the viral genome are frequently retained. These observations suggest a specific integration mechanism involving the ends of the adenovirus DNA molecule. Third, studies involving transformation-defective mutants of adenovirus type 5 have identified a viral protein that is needed for transformation of rodent cells by virions but not by viral DNA and which is not required for maintenance of transformation. This protein is a likely candidate for a function involved in integration of viral DNA.

INTRODUCTION

Transformation of mammalian cells by human adenovirus type 5 (Ad5) requires integration and expression of only a subset of the viral DNA sequences corresponding to the left-most 12% of the viral genome and comprising the early transcriptional region 1 (E1). The evidence for this is based on the observation that E1 sequences are always present and expressed in transformed cells, usually in the absence of other viral sequences (8,11), and on the fact that only E1 sequences are neces- sary and sufficient for DNA-mediated cell transformation (13,15,33).

Several studies have demonstrated that the E1 region comprises two nonoverlapping, independently promoted transcription units: E1A (1.5-4.5 map units) and E1B (4.5-11 map units), each specifying 3 mRNAs (13S, 12S and 9S in E1A, and 22S, 13S and 9S in E1B) (3,5,19,35). In both cases,

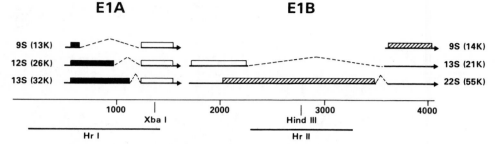

FIGURE 1. Ad5 mRNA species and polypeptides encoded by the E1 transforming region (1.5-11 map units). The Ad5 DNA sequences corresponding
to early region E1 are represented by the continuous line where numbers
indicate bp and vertical lines the cleavage sites of the restriction
endonucleases XbaI and HindIII. The location of the group I and II hr
mutants is delineated by the two horizontal lines beneath the DNA. mRNA
species within E1A and E1B are represented above the DNA molecule: the
solid portion of each line referring to the exons and the dashed portion
to the introns that are apliced out of the final messages. The direction
of translation is indicated by the arrows. Proteins are represented by
solid, open, or shaded blocks depending upon their reading frames. Size
of transcripts (in Svedbergs) and predicted molecular weight of translated products (in kd) are given beside each message. References are
listed in the text.

the 9S messages appear to specify late, and not early, proteins which are
generally not expressed in transformed cells (30,31,36); thus the gene
products relevant for transformation must be among those translated from
one or more of the other mRNAs. On the basis of the DNA sequence of the
E1 region and the size and structure of the E1 transcripts, it has been
predicted that proteins of 32 kd and 26 kd, respectively, can be encoded
by the 13S and 12S E1A mRNAs (24,34). Similarly, within E1B, the 22S
mRNA is predicted to encode both a 55-kd and a 21-kd polypeptide; the
latter is specified also by the 13S transcript (4) (see Figure 1). However the E1 gene products actually observed in a variety of in vivo and
in vitro studies (7,17,29,30) differ to varying degrees from these predicted values. E1A proteins, in particular, seem to be far more complex
than the pattern shown in Figure 1 and may consist of up to 6 related
polypeptides ranging in apparent molecular weight from 35 to 53 kd. In
the case of E1B on the other hand, there is only a minor discrepancy in
the molecular weight of the observed and predicted products. Thus the
protein corresponding to the larger of the two species encoded by the
22S message migrates on sodium dodecyl sulfate-polyacrylamide gels as
58 kd and that corresponding to the species transcribed from both 22S and
12S mRNAs migrates as 19 kd (21,22).
    In our studies on the role of E1 proteins in cell transformation, we
have isolated several host range mutants of Ad5 on the basis of their
ability to replicate efficiently in the Ad5-transformed human cell line
293 (which contains and expresses only the E1 region of the viral genome
(1,16). These mutants, which fall into two complementation groups, are
defective in one or more E1 functions and are also defective in transformation of rodent cells (14,18). Group I hr mutants fail to transform
rat embryo or rat embryo brain cells, but can induce an abnormal or semi-

abortive transformation of baby rat kidney (BRK) cells; in contrast, group II hr mutants fail to transform any of the rodent cells tested (14). Group I mutants, which map in E1A (9,12), are DNA negative, do not express other regions of the viral genome efficiently (2) and in particular fail to synthesize late proteins (20,22); in addition, at least one mutant of this group (hr 1) is defective in the synthesis of the product of the 13S message (25). The group II mutants, which map in E1B (9,12), are DNA positive and able to synthesize at least some late gene products (20,27), but are defective in the synthesis of the 58-kd protein transcribed from the 22S E1B message (21,26).

Since mutants of both complementation groups are altered in their ability to transform rodent cells, it would appear that both E1A and E1B functions are involved in transformation. In an attempt to shed light on the specific role of these proteins, and thereby on the mechanism of transformation, we have performed studies with both classes of mutants. These studies have shown that transformation of BRK cells by several group I hr mutants frequently results in the colinear integration of the entire viral genome, in contrast to the integration of only the left end observed most often with wild-type virus (11,28). The phenotypic properties of these transformants suggest in addition that E1A functions play a role in maintenance of transformation. In the case of group II mutants, transformation of cells cannot be induced by the virus but can be induced with viral DNA. This observation, together with the phenotypes demonstrated by the DNA-mediated transformants, suggest that the 58-kd E1B protein plays a role in initiation of transformation by virions but not by viral DNA and is not required for the maintenance of the transformed phenotype.

RESULTS AND DISCUSSION

Transformation by Group I hr Mutants

Transformation of primary BRK cells by wild-type Ad5 is typically a very inefficient process. The dose-response curve usually peaks at a relatively small number of colonies (on the order of 10/60-mm dish), and then decreases with increasing multiplicities of infection. Both phenomena are very likely due to the fact that rat cells are semipermissive for Ad5 (10,28) with the result that infection leads to extensive cytopathic effect and low cell survival. In addition, the transformed lines that can be isolated typically contain only a relatively small fraction of the viral genome (always encompassing E1) and, except in unusual circumstances (6,32), never contain the entire genome. In contrast to wild-type virus, group I hr mutants do not produce cytopathic effect in BRK cells and can induce 10- to 50-fold greater numbers of transformed colonies (14). It appears, however, that these colonies are the result of an abnormal or semiabortive transformation, since we have consistently failed to isolate and to expand them into cell lines (14,28), as can routinely be done for wild-type-induced transformants. Transformed cell lines could only be established by subculturing colonies from dishes containing many colonies and growing them initially as polyclonal populations. After a few passages, one or a few cell types predominated, and each culture became essentially monoclonal. That this process was not due to selection for wild-type transformants (induced by revertants in the mutant virus stocks) was demonstrated by the distinct phenotypes of these cell lines. Unlike wild-type transformed cells, which are typically epithelioid, the mutant-induced transformants are fibroblastic;

in addition they are incapable of growing in soft agar and do not induce tumors when injected into animals.

One particularly unusual feature of group I transformants is the structure of the integrated viral DNA sequences they contain, as revealed by Southern blot analysis. In contrast to the DNA integration pattern observed in wild-type transformants and described above, many of the cells transformed by mutant virus contain the entire viral genome colinearly integrated into the host chromosome. Two other examples of colinear integration of the Ad5 genome in transformed cells have been described (6,32). Both examples have one feature in common with the hr mutant-induced transformants described here, namely the fact that the systems used (virus and cell) amounted to very stringent nonpermissive conditions for viral replication.

Since transformation of rodent cells requires the presence and expression of only the left end of the adeno genome, integration of the entire Ad5 DNA molecule in a colinear fashion suggests that both ends of the molecule particupate in the integration process. Figure 2 illustrates a possible model for integration and the subsequent events that result in the patterns of integrated viral DNA seen under various circumstances. We suggest that initially the viral DNA molecule is inserted in its entirety into the host cell chromosome. Although this process can most easily be visualized as occurring via a circular viral DNA intermediate, circularization of the Ad5 genome is not an essential feature of the model; we do wish to emphasize however that integration involves both ends of the viral DNA molecule. After integration of the entire Ad5 genome in a colinear fashion, the stability of the integrated sequences may depend on the type of cell transformed and the resulting degree of expression of viral genes. Thus in cells that are permissive or semipermissive for Ad5 replication, the expression of late genes would not be suppressed and would likely result in cell killing. This would account for the low efficiency of transformation and extensive cytopathic effect observed in semipermissive rat cells infected with wild-type virus. In order for transformed cells to survive in such a case, expression of cytotoxic genes must be blocked: deletions or rearrangements of integrated viral sequences would be one way of achieving this while retaining the left-end sequences necessary for maintenance of the transformed phenotype. In the case of cells transformed by group I mutants, which are defective in the expression of Ad5 regions other than E1, there is no selective advantage to deletions or rearrangements of viral genes; thus the structures of integrated sequences in such cells may persist unchanged and may more frequently represent the structure formed during the initial stages of transformation, i.e., immediately after integration.

If integration into the host chromosome specifically involves the termini of the viral DNA molecule, it seems likely that one or more virally coded functions are involved in the process. In the next section we present evidence that an E1B protein, the 58-kd tumor antigen, is required only for initiation of transformation by virions but not for transformation by viral DNA. In addition, expression of this protein is not required for the maintenance of transformation. Based on this evidence we also present a case for the possibility that the 58-kd protein is required for integration of viral DNA into the host chromosome in virion-mediated transformation of cells.

Transformation by Group II hr Mutants

Hr mutants of complementation group II map in E1B, probably within those DNA sequences coding for the 58-kd protein that are spliced out

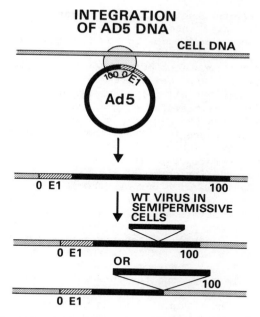

**INTEGRATION
OF AD5 DNA**

FIGURE 2. Model for the integration of the Ad5 genome into the host
chromosome. The basic assumption of the model is that integration of Ad5
DNA involves both ends of the Ad5 genome and results in colinear insertion of the entire viral moleculae into cell DNA. This could occur
through circular intermediates of viral DNA, as depicted above, but this
feature is not essential to the model. In totally nonpermissive cell
virus systems, in which cytotoxic viral functions are not expressed,
such a colinear structure might be stable and would persist, as seen with
rat cells transformed by group I hr mutants. In permissive or semipermissive systems, expression of viral functions, in addition to the transforming region E1, is assumed to result in cytopathic effect and cell
killing. Thus only transformed cells in which viral sequences to the
right of E1 have been deleted or rearranged are able to survive and give
rise to lines. This is generally what is observed in wild-type Ad2- and
Ad5-transformed rat cells.

from the region of the 13S mRNA coding for the 19-kd protein. As a
result, all of these mutants fail to synthesize the 58-kd polypeptide,
but are able to synthesize normal levels of the 19-kd species and of
most other early and late viral gene products (20,21). The role of the
58-kd protein in viral replication is still unclear; that group II mutants
are unable to transform rodent cells, however, suggests that this protein
plays a role in the transformation process. On the other hand, it is
well established that rodent cells can be fully transformed by fragments
of Ad5 DNA as small as the left 8% (<u>Hind</u>III G fragment) of the genome
which do not contain all of the coding sequences for the 58-kd antigen.
To resolve this apparent paradox, we have postulated that initiation of
transformation by viral DNA proceeds through a mechanism slightly different from that operating in the early steps of virion-mediated transformation. We suggest that this latter process requires the 58-kd function,
whereas the former is independent of it. An obvious prediction that can
be derived from this model is that DNA extracted from group II mutant

virions should be as efficient in transformation as DNA derived from wild-type virions. This proved indeed to be the case when DNA from two independent group II mutants was compared to wild-type DNA in transformation assays on both rat and hamster kidney cells: the efficiency of transformation obtained with DNA from each mutant being undistinguishable from that obtained with wild-type DNA. Cell lines established from the cultures transfected with mutant DNA all failed to synthesize the 58-kd antigen thus assuring us that the transformed foci were not induced by wild-type revertants. Morphologically these transformed lines are similar to wild-type transformants and, more important, they are able to induce tumors following infection into newborn hamsters. By these criteria, therefore, group II mutant DNA is fully capable of oncogenically transforming rodent cells in the absence of expression of the 58-kd antigen.

All of these data agree with our hypothesis that the 58-kd E1B protein is involved in initiation of transformation by virions, but has no major or obvious role in the maintenance of transformation. Exactly how this protein functions during the initiation event(s) is uncertain, but recent studies on rescue of adeno-associated virus from latently infected cells suggest that it might be involved in an integration-excision process. Ostrove and Berns (23) have in fact shown that hr 6, an Ad5 hr mutant of group II, is unable to rescue the integrated adeno-associated virus genome from latently infected Detroit 6 cells, even though it is fully capable of helping adeno-associated virus replication in mixed viral infections. Thus the group II function (58 kd) may be required for excision of the adeno-associated virus genome out of the host chromosome.

From these observations and our own studies outlined above, we suggest that, in virion-mediated transformation, the group II function might similarly be required for viral DNA integration into the host genome and subsequently plays no role, or only a minor role, in the transformed cells. In DNA-mediated transformation, on the other hand, integration of the viral genome appears to be independent of the 58-kd protein, and it is thus likely to occur through the action of cellular functions.

At present these hypotheses are based on circumstantial evidence and remain therefore quite speculative. They are, however, amenable to testing by direct studies on the mechanism of action of the 58-kd protein if this protein can be produced in larger quantities than currently available.

ACKNOWLEDGEMENT

This work was supported by the National Cancer Institute and the Medical Research Council of Canada. D.T.R. is the recipient of a NCIC Studentship and S.B. and F.L.G. are Research Associates of the NCIC.

REFERENCES

1. Aiello L, Guilfoyle R, Huebner K, Weinmann R (1979): Virology 94:460
2. Berk AJ, Lee F, Harrison T, Williams J, Sharp PA (1979): Cell 17:1935
3. Berk AJ, Sharp PA (1977): Cell 12:721
4. Bos JL, Polder LJ, Bernards R, Schrier PI, van den Elsen PJ, van der Eb AJ, van Ormondt H (1981): Cell 27:121
5. Chow LT, Broker TR, Lewis JB (1979): J Mol Biol 134:265
6. Dorsch-Hasler K, Fisher P, Weinstein B, Ginsberg H (1980): J Virol 34:305

7. Esche H, Mathews MB, Lewis JB (1980): J Mol Biol 142:399
8. Flint SJ, Sharp PA (1976): J Mol Biol 106:749
9. Frost E, Williams J (1978): Virology 91:39
10. Gallimore PH (1974): J Gen Virol 25:263
11. Gallimore PH, Sharp PA, Sambrook J (1974): J Mol Biol 89:49
12. Galos RS, Williams J, Shenk T, Jones N (1980): Virology 104:510
13. Graham FL, Abrahams PJ, Mulder C, Heyneker HL, Warnaar SJ, DeVries FAJ, Fiers W, van der Eb AJ (1974): Cold Spring Harbor Symp Quant Biol 39:637
14. Graham FL, Harrison T, Williams J (1978): Virology 86:10
15. Graham FL, Heyneker HL, van der Eb AJ (1974): Nature 251:687
16. Graham FL, Smiley J, Russell WC, Nairn R (1977): J Gen Virol 36:59
17. Halbert DN, Spector DJ, Raskas HJ (1979): J Virol 31:621
18. Harrison T, Graham F, Williams J (1977): Virology 77:319
19. Kitchingman GR, Westphal H (1980): J Mol Biol 137:23
20. Lassam NJ, Bayley ST, Graham FL (1978): Virology 87:463
21. Lassam NJ, Bayley ST, Graham FL (1979): Cell 18:781
22. Lupker JH, Davis A, Jochmesen H, van der Eb AJ (1981): J Virol 37:524
23. Ostrove JM, Berns KI (1980): Virology 104:502
24. Perricaudet M, Akusjarvi G, Virtanen A, Pettersson U (1979): Nature 281:694
25. Ricciardi RP, Jones RL, Cepko CL, Sharp PA, Roberts BE (1981): Proc Natl Acad Sci USA 78:6121
26. Ross SR, Levine AJ, Galos RS, Williams J, Shenk T (1980): Virology 103:475
27. Rowe DT, Graham FL (1981): J Virol 38:191
28. Ruben M, Bacchetti S, Graham FL (1982): J Virol 41:674
29. Smart JE, Lewis JB, Mathews MB, Harter ML, Anderson CW (1981): Virology 112:703
30. Spector DJ, Crossland LD, Halbert DN, Raskas HJ (1980): Virology 102:218
31. Spector DJ, McCrogan M, Raskas HJ (1978): J Mol Biol 126:395
32. Stabel S, Doerfler W, Friis RR (1980): J Virol 36:22
33. van der Eb AJ, Mulder C, Graham FL, Houwelling A (1977): Gene 2:115
34. van Ormondt H, Maat J, van Beveren CP (1980): Gene 11:299
35. Wilson M, Fraser N, Darnell J (1979): Virology 94:175
36. Wilson MC, Nevins JR, Blanchard JM, Ginsberg HS, Darnell JE (1979): Cold Spring Harbor Symp Quant Biol 44:447

Gene Transfer and Cancer, edited by M. L. Pearson
and N. L. Sternberg. Raven Press, New York © 1984.

Comparison of the Sequences of the Murine and Gibbon Ape Retrovirus LTR: Analysis of Elements Involved in Transcriptional Control and Provirus Integration

Stephen P. Clark and Tak W. Mak

*Department of Medical Biophysics, University of Toronto,
Toronto, Ontario, M4X 1K9 Canada*

ABSTRACT. The complete sequences of the long-terminal-repeats (LTR) of Friend spleen focus-forming virus (SFFV), two strains of Moloney murine leukemia virus (MoMuLV), three strains of Moloney murine sarcoma virus (MoMuSV), AKR murine leukemia virus (AKRMuLV), as well as the partial sequence from the LTR of Rauscher murine leukemia virus (RMuLV) and two strains of gibbon ape leukemia virus (GALV) were collected and compared. Examination of these sequences indicated that within the LTR there are highly conserved regions and highly variable regions. The former includes the terminal inverted repeats of about 11 bp and the transcriptional control elements: the CAAT box, the TATA box, the cap site and the polyadenlyation signal. In addition, a region of about 15 bp at the overlapping KpnI and SmaI restriction endonuclease sites is found to be constant, although no known function is associated with this region. The highly variable regions include the sequences immediately flanking the inverted repeats and the transcriptional control elements. An extended region of 70 to 100 bases in the U3 segment centered about 150 bases 5' of the TATA box is also found to be highly variable. This stretch of sequences encompasses the 72-bp repeat of the Moloney viruses and the 99-bp repeat of the AKRMuLV. It is within this region that a structure with extensive dyad symmetry was previously observed in the SFFV LTR. Dot matrix analysis indicated that, like the SFFV LTR, secondary structures with relatively high stabilities can be found in the Moloney and AKRMuLV. In addition, the stabilities of these proposed hairpin structures are considerably higher in LTR with duplications than the corresponding ones without these repeats. Such secondary sturctures may play an important role in the regulation of gene expression.

INTRODUCTION

The most unusual feature of retroviruses is that the genetic material of the infectious particle is single-stranded RNA, whereas the viral genome within an infected cell is double-stranded DNA (the provirus) integrated into the host nuclear DNA (see (4,7) for reviews). The RNA genome resembles a typical eucaryotic messenger RNA with a cap at the 5' end and a polyadenylic acid tail at the 3' end. Its overall length is

TABLE 1. Properties of retroviruses and their LTR

Virus	Disease	Helper virus required	Length of LTR	Length of repeat within U3 (first/second)	Source of sequence data
SFFV	Rapid erythro-leukemia and polycythemia	yes	514 bp	no repeat	(6)
MoMuLV (M3)	T-cell leukemia	no	515 bp	no repeat	(44)
MoMuLV (M6)	T-cell leukemia	no	590 bp	74/74 bp	(45)
MoMuSV (M1)	Sarcoma	yes	585 bp	70/75 bp	(35)
MoMuSV (M2)	Sarcoma	yes	588 bp	72/73 bp	(8)
MoMuSV (M5)	Sarcoma	yes	587 bp	70/75 bp	(46)
AKRMuLV	T-cell leukemia	no	622 bp	99/99 bp	(38)
RMuLV[a]	Erythroleukemia	no	-	-	(28)
GALVhi[a]	T-cell leukemia	no	-	-	(28)
GALVsf[a]	T-cell leukemia	no	-	-	(36)

[a]For these viruses, the sequences of only the R-U5 region (minus strong-stop DNA) have been reported.

approximately 6-8 kb, depending on the particular virus species. The integrated provirus is colinear with the RNA, but it is slightly longer because of the presence of a duplication of several hundred bp, the LTR, at each end. Each LTR is composed of regions that were originally present at the opposite ends of the RNA genome.

At both extremities of the RNA is a short, perfect repeat sequence called R. Adjacent to R at the 5' and 3' ends are unique sequences called U5 and U3, respectively. Immediately 3' to U5 is the primer binding site (PBS), a region approximately 20 bases long that is complementary to a specific cellular tRNA that is bound to the RNA genome and that is used as the initiation site for viral RNA-dependent DNA polymerase (reverse transcriptase) during the copying of the RNA genome into the double-stranded DNA form. Reverse transcription produces a linear provirus with the structure U3-R-U5-PBS.......U3-R-U5, where U3-R-U5 comprises the LTR that surround the viral structural genes. The provirus is then integrated into the host nuclear DNA, possibly via a circular intermediate containing either one or two LTR.

Analysis of the DNA sequences of the LTR of integrated proviruses indicates that they have structures similar to those of bacterial and eucaryotic transposons (6,37). For example, the LTR on each end of the provirus are identical in nucleotide sequence. Each of the LTR in turn are terminated by inverted repeats of 3-11 bp, and upon integration of the provirus, a few bases of cellular sequences are duplicated (29). These observations have led to the suggestion that transposition may be the mechanism of provirus integration (37). Also within the LTR are elements necessary for the control of transcription of the viral genome, including the CAAT box, the TATA box and the polyadenlyation signal.

In additon to the structural studies, much effort has been devoted to the investigation of the functional properties of LTR and their role in the activation of cellular oncogenes through downstream promotion, also known as promoter insertion (13,20). The self-contained nature of these retrovirus LTR with well-defined boundaries makes them particularly attractive for studies of eucaryotic promoters.

We have recently analyzed the sequences of the SFFV LTR and have identified a structure with extensive dyad symmetry 5' to the TATA box that may be an important control element (6). With the objective of identifying structures that are involved in the LTR regulatory processes, we have extended these analyses to six other murine retrovirus LTR and two GALV LTR.

RESULTS

The LTR of the polycythemia strain of the SFFV, three strains of the MoMuSV called M1, M2, and M5 in this paper, two strains of MoMuLV called M3 and M6, the AKRMuLV, as well as partial sequences of the RMuLV and two strains of the GALV, GALVsf and GALVhi, were compared. Some of the properties of these viruses and their LTR are listed in Table 1.

To analyze the different features of these LTR, we assembled the sequences and compared them with each other. Figure 1 shows the nucleotide positions of all the LTR aligned to give maximum homology. Spaces were introduced where necessary and represent deletions in the sequence or insertions in the other LTR. The most prevalent nucleotide at each position is represented by an open character; less common nucleotides, presumed to be mutations, are represented by closed characters. Above the sequence is a histogram (closed squares) that shows the number of different bases found at each position (five possibilities were considered: C, T, A, G and deletion). The open squares on top represent the variability index, an arbitrary number that attempts to quantitate the sequence variability at each position. This is primarily determined by the number of different bases at the position, but also takes into account the frequency of occurrence of the second most common base (for example, a position with 6 Cs and one T would have a lower variability than a position with 4 Cs and 3 Ts). An overview of the conserved and variable regions can be obtained by looking at the variability index; the individual sequences show which LTR are changed with respect to the others.

Regions within the LTR that are generally thought to be important in integration and control of transcription are marked in Figure 1. At the extreme ends are the inverted terminal repeats which confer on the LTR and proviruses a structure similar to that of transposons. This sequence is 11 bp long and does not vary among these murine viruses. Viruses from other species have inverted repeats of different lengths, but they all end with the dinucleotide TG....CA (22). This is a common feature of transposons. The GALV inverted repeats are different from the murine viruses, but because the sequence for the U3 region is not available, it is not known whether this reflects an inverted repeat with a different length from these murine viruses, a different sequence for an 11 bp inversion, or a combination of both.

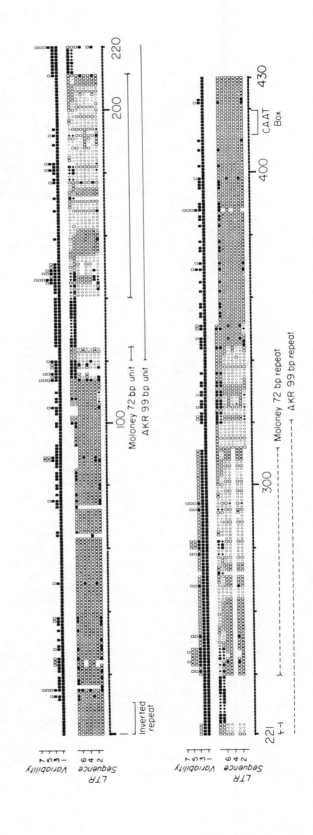

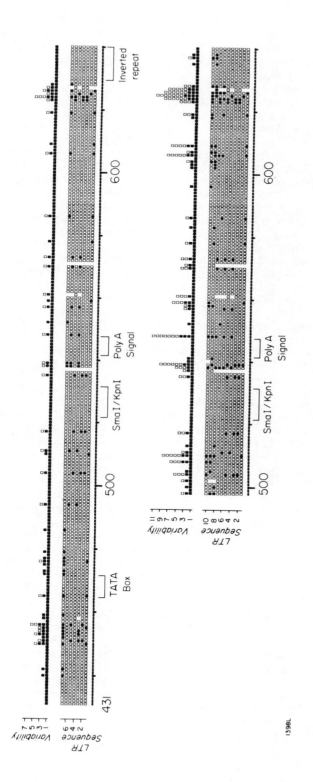

FIGURE 1. Comparison of the LTR sequences to identify the conserved and variable positions. LTR sequences are: 1) SFFV; 2) M1; 3) M2; 4) M3; 5) M5; 6) M6; 7) AKRMuLV; and from positions 488 to 640 in the bottom-most block, 8) RMuLV; 9) GALVhi; 10) GALVsf. The extra sequence from 100 to 351 is the same as that of AKRMuLV (sequence 7) and is included to show the base-pairing regions of both AKR hairpin structures. Open symbols represent the most common base at each position, closed symbols represent changes from the most common base, and spaces indicate deletions. Diamonds represent bases that are involved in base-pairing within hairpin loops; squares are positions where bases-pairing is not present. The variability histogram above each set of sequences shows the number of different bases at each position (closed squares), and the "variability index" (discussed in the text) in open squares.

The region with the highest variability occurs between positions 114 and 311, where there may or may not be a tandem duplicaiton of about 72 bp (M1, M2, M5, M6) or 99 bp (AKRMuLV). This region primarily accounts for the different lengths of the LTR (Table 1). The other regions have scattered point mutations and deletions/insertions.

The point of transcriptional initiation (cap site) has been mapped to within one or two bases of position 496 of Figure 1 (3,12). Upstream, 31 bases from the cap site, is the Goldberg-Hogness (TATA) box (15). All the Moloney strains have the sequence AATAAAA at this position, while SFFV and AKRMuLV have replaced the first A with T. Many genes have a second region of homology 40-50 bases upstream from the TATA box, known as the CAAT box (2). The consenus sequence is GGPyCAATCT (5) and is slightly different from that found in these retroviruses: AACCAATCA. The only other transcriptional control element that has been identified on the basis of its sequence is the polyadenylation signal (34) (AATAAA) at position 542, 14 bases from the last nucleotide of the RNA genome. As noted in Figure 1, regions at which these control elements occur are highly conserved. Having identified the transcriptional start and stop positions, U3, R, and U5 can be defined as occupying positions 1 to 496, 497 to 556 and 557 to 640, respectively. The sizes of these elements will vary from virus to virus depending on the number and length of any deletions. Another conserved region that has a surprisingly constant nucleotide sequence is found at the overlapping SmaI/KpnI restriction endonuclease sites at position 522, although its biological importance, if any, is not known.

As mentioned above, the most striking difference among these LTR is the presence or absence of a 70- to 99-bp direct tandem duplication. Examination of the sequence at the boundaries of this region shows that M3, the Moloney strain that lacks the duplication and therefore must be more closely related to the ancestral virus, has a nearly perfect shorter repeat sequence of 20 nucleotides approximately 70 bp apart: 5'-(99)TCA-aGGtCAgGAACAGATGGA/A.........(192)TCAgGGcCAaGAACAGATGG/T-3', where the numbers within parentheses indicate the position in Figure 1, the slashes indicate the boundaries of the region that is duplicated in M1, M2, M5, and M6 and the lower case characters represent mismatches, all of which are transitions, within the 20 bp redundancy. It is not known whether the ancestor had more or less homology between these 20 base sequences.

When the sequence of the SFFV LTR was determined, it was examined for poossible repeats and inversions (6). The region of greatest interest was that between the 5' end and the CAAT box, because of the duplication found in the Moloney viruses, and because this region was implicated in other systems as being important in controlling the efficiency of transcription. No long direct repeats were found, but an extensive imperfect dyad symmetry was identified which may be involved in DNA secondary structure in the form of a hairpin loop. Since there is evidence that the DNA upstream from the cap site in many systems is different from the bulk DNA (see discussion), other LTR were examined for similar structures.

The method used to find sequence inversions that can form hairpins involves constructing a diagonal plot and has been previously described (6). An example of such a plot is shown in Figure 2, where the (+) and (-) strands of the AKRMuLV LTR are compared. The region corresponding to the 99-bp duplication, enclosed by the dashed lines, is represented 4 times in the plot and is shown to a larger scale in Figure 3. Two possible hairpin structures were found in this LTR; the points that represent them are circled in these two figures. These hairpins and their

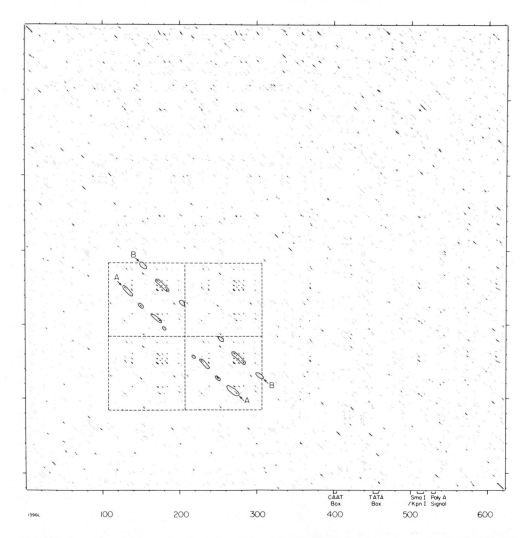

FIGURE 2. The diagonal plot used to identify the hairpins of the AKRMuLV DNA. The (+) strand LTR sequence (horizontal axis) is compared to the (−) strand sequence (vertical axis). The regions which are specified by the two copies of the 99-bp repeat are enclosed with dashed lines. The points which suggest the presence of DNA hairpins are circled. Figure 2A corresponds to Figure 1, sequence line 8, and Figure 4E, whereas Figure 2B corresponds to Figure 1, sequence line 7, and Figure 4D.

stabilities (determined as previously described (6)) are shown in Figure 4, as well as the possible structures from SFFV, M3, and M2. In the case of SFFV and M3, which do not have any duplication, the region that corresponds to the duplication is contained entirely within the hairpin, as shown by the arrows in Figure 4. The duplicated region in the Moloney LTR is entirely within the hairpin, and the AKRMuLV LTR hairpin almost completely contains the longer AKRMuLV duplication. It can be seen that

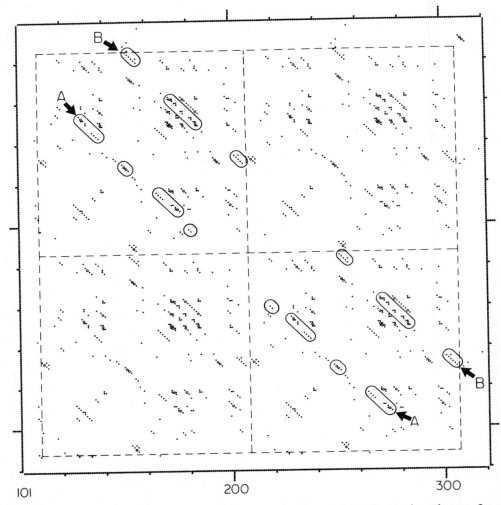

FIGURE 3. An enlargement of the 99-bp repeat region shown in Figure 2. Open circles and closed circles represent 100% and 80% homology respectively, over 5 successive bases, between the AKRMuLV LTR (+) and (-) strand sequences. See Figure 2 legend for other details.

the duplications greatly extend the size of these possible hairpins and increase their thermodynamic stability.

The hairpins that were constructed for all the LTR were compared to each other and to the changes in the DNA sequence (shown in Figure 1). The diamonds represent positions that are involved in Watson-Crick base-pairing to form the hairpin. The region from position 100 to 351 has an extra line on top of the normal seven sequences; it is a duplicate of the AKRMuLV sequence necessary to accommodate the second AKRMuLV hairpin.

All of the LTR that contain duplications have an axis of symmetry along the hairpin (Figure 4 and data not shown). In the case of the Moloney LTR, this axis (positions 190 and 290, Figure 1) corresponds to the terminal loop of the hairpin in the M3 LTR that lacks the duplication.

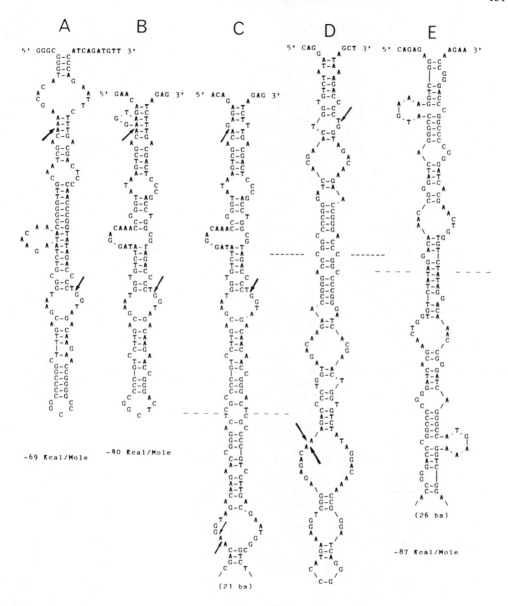

FIGURE 4. DNA hairpin structures that can be found within the LTR, and their stabilities, determined as described (6). A) SFFV; B) MoMuLV (M3); C) MoMuSV (M2); D) AKRMuLV (sequence line 7 in Figure 1; B in Figures 2 and 3); E) AKRMuLV (sequence line 8 in Figure 1, A in Figures 2 and 3). The horizontal dashed lines show the axis of symmetry; upward pointing arrows indicate the beginning of the duplicated region and downward pointing arrows indicate its end. In D, the beginning of the first copy of the duplication starts before the beginning of the hairpin. In E, the first copy starts just before the hairpin, and ends in the loop at the bottom, which is not drawn in. The second copy ends just after the end of the hairpin. bs: bases.

Identical hairpins can be drawn for M1 and M6 LTR; the other Moloney LTR loops are very similar (data not shown) but they differ slightly at the axis of symmetry. The hairpin in the AKRMuLV LTR (Figure 4D) also has an axis of symmetry that corresponds to the same region as that found in the Moloney LTR although the hairpin does not resemble the Moloney hairpins very much. The other AKRMuLV LTR hairpin has a completely different axis of symmetry (positions 160 and 260, Figure 1), but it is much more stable. The hairpin in the SFFV LTR is very similar to the hairpin in the M3 LTR overall, but has fewer bulges and loops, resulting in an increased stability. There have been several single base changes that allow it to base-pair in regions that Moloney LTR do not (black diamonds, Figure 1, line 1).

DISCUSSION

The LTR provide two functions for the provirus. They allow it to become integrated into cellular DNA and then enable it to be accurately transcribed without having to rely on cellular control elements. For these reasons it is to be expected that regions which are involved in either of these processes would be highly conserved in related viruses, even though retroviruses mutate at a very high rate (38). DNA sequences that interact with other macromolecules are expected to be highly conserved so that the correct interactions are maintained.

Examination of Figure 1 shows that some regions are identical among all the LTR and others are highly variable. The 11-bp terminal inverted repeats are identical for the AKRMuLV, SFFV, the Moloney strains and perhaps the RMuLV. If it is assumed that these inversions are important for proviral integration, this conservation probably means that they are part, if not all, of the sequence that is recognized by the integration protein, whether it is cellular or viral. In contrast to the 11-bp terminal inverted repeats, sequences adjacent to these structures within the LTR are highly variable (positions 12 to 38, 618 to 627 in Figure 1), indicating that they may be functionally unimportant.

Further evidence of the importance of the terminal inversion is obtained by comparing the LTR of endogenous virus-1 (EV-1) (22) and Rous-associated virus-2 (RAV-2) (24), two chicken retroviruses. Here the inversions are identical at both ends, despite the fact that diagonal plot analysis shows that the U3 regions of the two viruses have almost no other homology (data not shown).

The elements involved in the control of transcription are also highly conserved and often flanked by regions of variability, including point deletions/insertions, as though they indicate boundaries. The polyadenylation signal (AATAAA, position 542, Figure 1), which is usually found about 20 bases from the polyadenylation site (2), and has been found to be necessary for correct polyadenylation of the SV40 late mRNA (11), is identical in the 10 LTR. The Goldberg-Hogness box, which appears to direct transcription to start at a position about 30 nucleotides downstream (17), is the only transcriptional control region that has been identified in these LTR that is not identical in all the sequences. While the AKRMuLV and SFFV have the canonical sequence TATAAAA, all the Moloney strains have the less common sequence AATAAAA. Whether or not this represents a real biological difference among the viruses is not known. The CAAT box, like the polyadenylation signal, is completely conserved among the seven viruses. The function of this region in the promoter is unknown, but it has been found for some eucaryotic genes that deletions in this area result in a drastic reduction of transcription in

vivo (16,17,31). As with the TATA box and polyadenylation signal, this
area is flanked by variable regions.

The region containing the overlapping SmaI/KpnI restriction enzyme
sites (CCCGGGTACC) is also bounded by variable regions, although no function has been determined for it. A search of the LTR of avian sarcoma
virus (ASV) (41), RAV-2, and EV-1, (which are very similar in the R-U5
regions), baboon endogenous virus (BaEV) (42), and spleen necrosis virus
(SNV) (37) shows that a sequence closely related to CCCGGGT-C was found
approximately 60 bp 3' to the TATA box (approximately 80 bp from the
TATA box in mouse mammary tumor virus (MMTV) (10)) (data not shown). Its
position in the murine viruses, BaEV and SNV suggests that it may have
some role in transcriptional termination since it is located just 5' to
the polyadenylation signal. However, this is not supported in MMTV, EV-1,
ASV and RAV-2, where this sequence is located 3' to the polyadenylation
signal because these viruses possess shorter R regions.

As was mentioned above, the region which contributes most to the differences between the LTR is the duplicated region from positions 114 to
311 in Figure 1. The duplication is about 72 bases long when present
in the Moloney strains, 99 bases in the AKRMuLV strain analyzed in this
paper, and 26 bases in another AKRMuLV strain, which also contains substantial deletions in the region (P. Jolicoeur, personal communication).
The duplication probably arises because of the almost perfect 20 bp redundancy that flanks the larger duplication. The mechanism of generation of the normal provirus involves the jumping of reverse transcriptase
from R at the 5' end to the 3' R region (14), therefore it is easy to
envision a duplication arising in U3 by the polymerase jumping from the
5'-most repeat (starting at position 99 in Figure 1) to the 3' repeat
at position 192, thus duplicating the region between them. Although
this repeat is shorter than the murine R region by a factor of three, it
is the same length as the R region of avian retroviruses, indiccating
that such an event may well have occurred. The origin of the extra sequences present in the AKRMuLV LTR which make the duplication 99 bp long
rather than 72 is a mystery, since the extra 25 bases have no obvious
homology to the rest of the LTR (data not shown). Clearly the insertion
occurred before the duplication.

The 72- and 99-bp duplications occur in a region upstream from the
TATA box that has been found to influence the transcription of other
eucaryotic genes, even though no regions of sequence homology have been
found among them. For example, the transcription of the sea urchin
histone H2A gene is at least tripled if a 340-bp restriction fragment 80
bp upstream from the TATA box is inverted, and decreased to less than
10% of normal if the same fragment is deleted (16). In addition, this
general region has been found to be hypersensitive to digestion by DNAse
I in the chromatin of some genes (30,40), including both LTR of EV-3 (18).
In the Moloney and AKRMuLV LTR, it is likely that the duplications provide
an advantage to the viruses, or they would be lost through the same type
of error during reverse transcription which generated them. Since there
are significant differences between the SFFV, AKRMuLV and Moloney sequences in this region, it may not be the primary sturcture that is important. Despite these differences, they all have the potential to form extensive hairpins. The question of the stability of such structures in
chromatin has already been discussed (6). One additional feature of the
hairpins of LTR that have the duplication is that they possess an axis of
symmetry. If such structures exist in the chromatin, they would be very
special structures indeed.

Recently, much interest has been focused on the duplication in the LTR. There is considerable evidence to suggest the 72-bp repeat of MoMuSV may be functionally equivalent to the 72-bp repeat located approximately 120 bases upstream from the point of early gene transcriptional initiation of the DNA virus SV40, and to the corresponding region of the closely related polyoma virus (region "A" (43)), despite the fact that none of these regions shows homology to the others. SV40 requires at least one copy of its repeat for T-antigen expression and for viability. The early gene (T-antigen) is expressed regardless of the orientation of the 72-bp repeat in its natural site, or its distance from the normal site up to several kb (32). This repeat, isolated from other SV40 sequences, is also able to enhance expression approximately 100 times of cloned rabbit β-globin gene when transfected into HeLa cells, again regardless of orientation or position in the plasmid (1). In addition, region A of polyoma is required for early gene expression (43) and is able to enhance the expression of cloned rabbit β-globin gene, irrespective of orientation from as far away as 1.4 kb, when transfected into mammalian cells (9). Similarly, retrovirus LTR can induce transcription of normal cellular genes when they are integrated 5' to them not only in the orientation that would lead to downstream promotion (13,20,33), but also when they are in the opposite orientation, or even 3' to the cellular gene which is activated (33).

Deletion of the 72-bp repeat from SV40 results in loss of viability of the virus (19), which can be restored by replacing it with the Moloney 72-bp repeat (27). Apparently the Moloney repeat can mimic the action of the SV40 repeat, even though they have no sequence homology. The natural SV40-72 bp repeat region can be arranged into an extensive hairpin with a stability of -79 Kcals/mole. Replacing the SV40 repeat with that from MoMuSV would result in a hybrid structure whose base is composed of SV40 sequences, whereas most of the repeat is identical to the hairpin shown in Figure 4C, and has a stability of -44 Kcals/mole. The experiments that showed the enhancer effect of the SV40 72-bp repeat were interpreted to mean that this repeat is a cis-acting element that can drastically increase transcription (1), even at a distance, by acting as a site that enables RNA polymerase to bind to the DNA, then migrate in either direction until the point of transcription initiation is reached (32).

The observation that a region 5' to the transcribed region in many genes is hypersensitive to digestion by DNAse I in the chromatin indicates that there is discontinuity in the chromatin structure. Hairpins could well be involved in such perturbations. Consistent with this hypothesis is the mapping of the DNAse I hypersensitive site of polyoma to the A region (21) and the observation that there is the potential for secondary structure (a cloverleaf) within this region (39). In addition, the DNAse I hypersensitive region in the EV-3 LTR has been found to be also sensitive to digestion by S1 nuclease (A. Larsen and M. Groudine, personal communication). The hairpins that are found in murine LTR (shown in Figure 4) contain several single-stranded regions. However, it was found that the DNAse I hypersensitive site upstream from the chicken β-globin gene was not single-strand nuclease-sensitive (30). This might reflect an intrinsic difference between retrovirus LTR promoters and those of normal cellular genes, because, for example, the latter are closely regulated by the cell to produce the correct amount of transcript, whereas the former probably are not usually regulated to such an extent.

There are at least two (possibly nonindependent) mechanisms through which DNA secondary structure could be involved in the promotion of transcription. First, at the base of the hairpin, where the normal duplex

DNA converts to hairpin DNA, there would be a region of non-base-paired DNA to which RNA polymerase might bind. Alternatively, it could attach to one of the single-stranded loops or bulges within the hairpin itself. This effect does not necessarily have to be a direct one because accessory proteins required for transcription initiation could bind to the single-stranded regions, and then bind RNA polymerase. Extending the size of the hairpin through sequence duplication, generating an axis of symmetry at the same time, could allow twice as many accessory proteins to bind, thereby increasing the likelihood that RNA polymerase would bind and subsequently initiate transcription. Inducer or repressor proteins could conceivably bind particular hairpin structures to modulate the transcriptional rate as a mechanism of cell-specific control of gene expression. Evidence to support this comes from analyses of the A region of polyoma variants that are able to grow on mouse embryonal carcinaoma cells (wild-type strains are restricted on these cell lines). Some mutants have base substitutions (25) within the postulated (39) A region cloverleaf, whereas others have deletions and duplications (26), which can result in substantially different secondary structure. One such structure has a stem consisting of 25 bp with only one mismatch. The alterations in secondary structure may destroy a regulatory molecule binding site (25).

Another mechanism may involve phasing the nucleosomes so that some regulatory DNA signals are in the proper orientation to be recognized by nuclear proteins (reviewed in (23)). Secondary structure such as hairpins would not be expected to be packaged properly into nucleosomes, and thus could act as seeds for correct phasing, with the hairpin situated between two nucleosomes. In this role, the hairpin need not be permanent, but appearing frequently enough to maintain proper phasing.

In conclusion, comparison of the sequences of the LTR of several strains of murine retroviruses, when examined in conjunction with other LTR and various genetic elements, has formed the basis of a model that explains several observations in molecular biology: DNA secondary structure in the form of hairpins could be responsible for DNAse I hypersensitivity and S1 nuclease sensitivity within the 5' nontranscribed regions of genes; the SV40 and MoMuSV 72-bp repeats, even though they have no homology at the primary level, are functionally equivalent as shown both by replacing the natural SV40 sequence with the repeat from MoMuSV, and by the ability of both the SV40 repeat and LTR to activate genes at a distance and in either orientation - such a functional equivalence could be the result of similar secondary structure.

ACKNOWLEDGEMENTS

We wish to thank C. Shaughnessy for help with preparing this manuscript. This work was supported by grants from the National Cancer Institute of Canada and the Medical Research Council of Canada. S. Clark is a recipient of a studentship from the Medical Research Council of Canada.

REFERENCES

1. Banerji J, Rusconi S, Schaffner W (1981): Cell 27:299
2. Benoist C, O'Hare K, Breathnach R, Chambon P (1980): Nucleic Acids Res 8:127
3. Benz EW Jr, Wydro RM, Nadal-Ginard B, Dina D (1980): Nature 288:665
4. Bishop JM (1978): Annu Rev Biochem 47:35

5. Chambon P, Breathnach R (1981): Annu Rev Biochem 50:349
6. Clark SP, Mak TW (1982): Nucleic Acids Res 10:3315
7. Coffin JM (1979): J Gen Virol 42:1
8. Dahr R, McClements WL, Enquist LW, Vande Woude GF (1980): Proc Natl Acad Sci USA 77:3937
9. de Villiers J, Schaffner W (1981): Nucleic Acids Res 9:6251
10. Donehower LA, Huang AL, Hager GL (1981) J Virol 37:226
11. Fitzgerald M, Shenk T (1981): Cell 24:251
12. Fuhrman SA, Van Beveren C, Verma IM (1981): Proc Natl Acad Sci USA 78:5411
13. Fung Y-KT, Fadly AM, Crittenden LB, Kung H-J (1981): Proc Natl Acad Sci USA 78:3418
14. Gilboa E, Mitra SW, Goff S, Baltimore D (1979): Cell 18:93
15. Goldberg ML (1979): Ph.D. Thesis, Stanford University, Stanford
16. Grosschedl R, Birnstiel ML (1980): Proc Natl Acad Sci USA 77:7102
17. Grosveld GC, de Boer E, Shewmaker CK, Flavell RA (1982): Nature 295:120
18. Groudine M, Eisenman R, Weintraub H (1981): Nature 292:311
19. Gruss P, Dhar R, Khoury G (1981): Proc Natl Acad Sci USA 78:943
20. Hayward WS, Neel BG, Astrin SM (1981): Nature 290:475
21. Herbomel P, Saragosti S, Blangy D, Yaniv M (1981): Cell 25:651
22. Hishinuma F, DeBona PJ, Astrin S, Skalka AM (1981): Cell 23:155
23. Igo-Kemenes T, Zachau HG (1981): Cell 24:597
24. Ju G, Skalka AM (1980): Cell 22:379
25. Katinka M, Vasseur M, Montreau N, Yaniv M, Blangy D (1981): Nature 290:720
26. Katinka M, Yaniv M, Vasseur M, Blangy D (1980): Cell 20:393
27. Levinson B, Khoury G, Vande Woude G, Gruss P (1982): Nature 295:568
28. Lovinger GG, Schochetman G (1979): J Virol 32:803
29. Majors JE, Varmus HE (1981): Nature 289:253
30. McGhee JD, Wood WI, Dolan M, Engel JD, Felsenfeld G (1981): Cell 27:45
31. Mellon P, Parker V, Gluzman Y, Maniatis T (1981): Cell 27:279
32. Moreau P, Hen R, Wasylyk B, Everett R, Gaub MP, Chambon P (1981): Nucleic Acids Res 9:6047
33. Payne GS, Bishop JM, Varmus HE (1982): Nature 295:209
34. Proudfoot NJ, Brownlee GG (1974): Nature 252:359
35. Reddy EP, Smith MJ, Aaronson SA (1981): Science 214:445
36. Scott ML, McKereghan K, Kaplan HS, Fry KE (1981): Proc Natl Acad Sci USA 78:4213
37. Shimotohno K, Mizutani S, Temin HM (1980): Nature 285:550
38. Shimotohno K, Temin HM (1982): J Virol 41:163
39. Soeda E, Arrand JR, Smolar N, Walsh JE, Griffin BE (1980): Nature 283:445
40. Stalder J, Larsen A, Engel JD, Dolan M, Groudine M, Weintraub H (1980): Cell 20:451
41. Swanstrom R, DeLorbe WJ, Bishop JM, Varmus HE (1981): Proc Natl Acad Sci USA 78:124
42. Tamura T-A, Noda M, Takano T (1981): Nucleic Acids Res 9:6615
43. Tyndall C, La Mantia G, Thacker CM, Favaloro J, Kamen R (1981): Nucleic Acids Res 9:6231
44. Van Beveren C, Goddard JC, Berns A, Verma IM (1980): Proc Natl Acad Sci USA 77:3307
45. Van Beveren C, Rands E, Chattopadhyay SK, Lowy DR, Verma IM (1982): J Virol 41:542
46. Van Beveren C, van Straaten F, Galleshaw JA, Verma IM (1981): Cell 27:97

Gene Transfer and Cancer, edited by M. L. Pearson and N. L. Sternberg. Raven Press, New York © 1984.

DNA Transfection Studies of Endogenous Ecotropic MuLV

R. Risser, J. McCubrey, P. Green, J. Horowitz, and C. Sinaiko

McArdle Laboratory for Cancer Research, University of Wisconsin, Madison, Wisconsin 53706

ABSTRACT. We have examined the infectivity of cellular DNAs containing but not expressing endogenous murine leukemia virus (MuLV). When nonproducer genomic DNA of AKR-2B mouse cells was transfected onto NIH/3T3 mouse cells, it was not infectious, a result previously described by Lowy (8). However, when nonproducer AKR-2B DNA was transfected onto chicken cells, which were then cocultivated with Sc-1 mouse cells, infectious MuLV was recovered. The transfected chicken cell cultures produced ecotropic XC-positive MuLV that was N-tropic. Virus-producing cultures were observed approximately 25-fold less frequently when BALB/c mouse DNA was used to transfect chicken cells, but no virus-producing cultures were observed when nonproducer B6 mouse DNA was used to transfect chicken cells. Nonproducer AKR-2B DNA was also infectious for some mouse embryo fibroblast cultures. Our studies indicate that nonexpressed MuLV proviruses from several sources are activated on transfection into chicken cells. Such studies suggest that the factors governing the expression of MuLV after transfection into established cell lines (NIH/3T3) and nonestablished secondary embryo cultures (chicken and mouse) are different.

INTRODUCTION

Studies of the expression of endogenous retroviruses in inbred strains of mice have revealed diverse patterns of expression ranging from early and persistent viremia to little virus expression throughout life. The elegant genetic experiments of Rowe (12,13) demonstrated that genes identical with or adjacent to virus structural sequences are major determinants of the virological phenotype of AKR mice which are highly susceptible to leukemia. Work from the same laboratory has also shown that expression of endogenous ecotropic MuLV can be induced in cell cultures derived from AKR mice by treatment of cells with the halogenated pyrimidines iododeoxyuridine (IUdR) or bromodeoxyuridine (9). More recent studies have demonstrated that expression of ecotropic MuLV can also be induced by IUdR treatment of cells such as BALB/c, C57BL/6 and C3H (11) which have low susceptibility to leukemia. The level of virus expression induced in cultures of low leukemic strains is only 0.1% of that induced in cultures of highly leukemic strains, however (11). Genetic and molecular experiments have shown that genes that control the ecotropic virus induction phenotype in strains with low susceptibility are identical with or linked to virus structural sequences (7,

6,10,5). Thus, the proviral genomes found in mice provide amenable systems for the study of gene regulation and induction of expression in
higher eucaryotes.

Study of endogenous retroviral genome expression in DNA transfection
experiments have demonstrated another aspect of virus genome expression -
namely that changes in virus expression in cells are accompanied by
changes in DNA infectivity in transfection experiments (1). Studies by
Lowy (8) and Copeland and Cooper (2) demonstrated that cellular DNA from
AKR cells carrying but not producing ecotropic MuLV, i.e. nonproducers,
was not infectious in transfection of mouse NIH/3T3 cells, whereas cellular DNA from cells producing MuLV was infectious. The conclusion drawn
from these experiments is that a change in DNA is necessary for nonexpressed proviruses to be infectious. The results presented here demonstrate that nonproducer DNA is infectious for chicken cells and some
mouse embryo cells; thus if a change in DNA is necessary, it is one that
takes place in chicken and mouse embryo cells, but not established lines.

RESULTS

The sensitivity of a variety of cells to transfection by DNA from
AKR-2B cells producing ecotropic MuLV was tested. In all cases xeno-
geneic cells were cocultivated with SC-1 cells, and virus production was
scored in the UV-XC plaque asay (14). The results of that survey, documented below in Table 1, indicated that chick embryo fibroblasts (CEF),
mouse embryo fibroblasts (MEF) and NIH/3T3 cells were sensitive to
transfection by producer DNA.

To examine the sensitivity of these cells to transfection by DNA from
AKR-2B nonproducer cells, we transfected recipient cells with 15-25 μg
DNA/10^6 recipient cells, cocultivated with SC-1 cells, and scored for
virus production. Unexpectedly, CEF cells proved sensitive to transfection with DNA from AKR-2B nonproducer cells (Table 2). Occasional (30%)
MEF cultures also proved to be sensitive to transfection with high concentrations of AKR-2B nonproducer DNA. In addition we observed essentially no effect of treatment with IUdR on recipient cell sensitivity,
in contrast to Lowy's (8) findings.

TABLE 1. Infectivity of AKR producer DNA for various cell lines

Recipient cell	No. of virus-positive cultures[a]/ Total No. Cultures
Mouse	
NIH/3T3	17/76
SC-1	0/15
MEF	28/42
Rat (REF, Rat 1)	1/10
Monkey (Cv-1, BSC)	0/33
Human	0/6
Rabbit (SIRC)	0/12
Mink	2/20
Chicken (CEF)	27/69

[a] 15-25 μg DNA was added to each plate

TABLE 2. Infectivity of AKR nonproducer DNA for various cells

Cell type	No. positive cultures/ No. total cultures	
	+ IUdR[a]	− IUdR
NIH/3T3	1/30	0/31
MEF[b]	2/4	6/11
CEF	12/24	21/41

[a] Recipient cells were pretreated with 20 µg/ml IUdR for 24 hr.
[b] Results of four of eleven experiments; in seven experiments no infectivity was observed even with control DNA (infectious plasmid DNA).

The infectivity of genomic AKR producer DNA, genomic AKR nonproducer DNA, and cloned AKR virus DNA was compared in titration experiments on CEF cells. The results of that experiment, documented below in Table 3, demonstrate that all three DNAs are approximately equally infectious for CEF cells.

We have also examined the infectivity of DNAs from other cell types for CEF cells (Table 4). We found that four different preparations of AKR-2B nonproducer DNA were infectious when transfected into CEF. Genomic DNA containing the BALB/c ecotropic proviral genome was infectious in 10% of the experiments, whereas genomic DNA containing the C57BL/6 ecotropic provirus was not infectious.

Virus recovered from virus-positive CEF + SC-1 cell cultures proved to be an N-tropic, ecotropic, XC-positive MuLV, typical of the endogenous viruses of mice.

TABLE 3. Infectivity of genomic and cloned DNAs for CEF cells

Type of DNA[a]	µg DNA/culture	No. of virus-positive cultures/ Total no. cultures (%)	
AKR-2B cells	15	16/22	(73%)
not producing	10	21/39	(54%)
MuLV	5	2/20	(10%)
	2.5	2/25	(8%)
	1	0/18	(0%)
AKR cells	15	18/29	(62%)
producing	5	2/12	(17%)
MuLV	2.5	1/5	20%)
	1	2/16	(12%)
Cloned AKR	3×19^{-4}	7/9	(78%)
virus p623	10^{-4}	5/9	(56%)
	19^{-5}	1/6	(16%)

[a] Carrier DNA to bring the level to 15 µg/culture was added to all test DNAs below that level.

TABLE 4.   Infectivity of various DNAs for CEF cells

DNA source	No. positive cultures/ No. total cultures
AKR-2B nonproducer	
Sample 1	32/45
2	3/5
3	6/17
4	16/45
Total	57/112
AKR-2B producer	25/43
BALB/c provirus-containing	4/45
C57BL/6 provirus-containing	0/76
Ecotropic virus-negative	0/25

DISCUSSION

The results presented here demonstrate that DNA from cells that encode but do not produce ecotropic MuLV yields infectious virus on transfection to chicken and occasionally mouse embryo cells but not NIH/3T3 cells. Thus, these results confirm the earlier observations of Cooper and coworkers (1,2) and Lowy (8) and further indicate that the response of NIH/3T3 cells to nonproducer DNA may be the exception rather than the rule. That is, nonproducer DNA is indeed infectious on transfection to appropriate cells or put more generally, nonexpressed genes can be activated by the process of DNA transformation if the appropriate recipient cell is used.

In this context it is interesting to note that Jaenish and coworkers (4) have recently reported a similar change in infectivity of an endogenous Moloney MuLV genome following molecular cloning and have attributed this change in infectivity to changes in the methylation of proviral sequences. It is unknown if changes in methylation accompany changes in the expression of endogenous AKR proviruses. Clearly examples of such changes exist in endogenous avian retroviruses (3). One possibility is that enzymes in CEF cells fail to methylate or demethylate sequences in endogenous murine viruses and thereby induce virus expression.

We have also occasionally observed infectious virus production in experiments with mouse embryo cells, a result in apparent conflict with the original Cooper and Temin studies (1) on the infectivity of endogenous RAV-0 genomes from nonproducer chicken cells. In those experiments DNA from nonproducer cells was 400-fold less infectious than DNA from producer cells for CEF recipient cells (1). Our results, if substantiated in further tritration experiments, would indicate either that the regulation of infectivity of RAV-0 proviruses is different from that of AKR proviruses, or that MEF cells differ from CEF cells in their recognition and perpetuation of regulatory signals associated with endogenous proviruses. In either case this system may provide important insights into the regulation of viral gene expression in eucaryotes.

ACKNOWLEDGEMENTS

This work was supported by NCI grants CA 07175 and CA 22443. R.R. is a Scholar of the Leukemia Society of America, Inc.

REFERENCES

1. Cooper GM, Temin HM (1976): J Virol 17:422
2. Copeland N, Cooper G (1979): Cell 16:347
3. Groudine M, Eisenmen R, Weintraub H (1981): Nature 292:311
4. Habers K, Schnieke A, Stuhlmann H, Jahner D, Jaenisch R (1981): Proc Natl Acad Sci USA 78:7609
5. Horowitz J, Risser R (1982): J Virol 44:950
6. Ihle JN, Joseph DR, Domotor Jr JJ (1979): Science 204:71
7. Kozak CA, Rowe WP (1979): Science 204:69
8. Lowy D (1978): Proc Natl Acad Sci USA 75:5539
9. Lowy DR, Rowe WP, Teich N, Hartley JW (1971): Science 174:155
10. McCubrey J, Risser R (1982): J Exp Med 155:1233
11. McCubrey J, Risser R (1982): Cell 28:881
12. Rowe WP (1973): Cancer Res 33:3061
13. Rowe WP (1979): Harvey Lect 71:173
14. Rowe WP, Pugh WE, Hartley JW (1970): Virology 42:1136

Gene Transfer and Cancer, edited by M. L. Pearson
and N. L. Sternberg. Raven Press, New York © 1984.

Origins of the Structural and Transforming (rel) Genes of Reticuloendotheliosis Virus

Raymond V. Gilden, Nancy R. Rice, Robert M. Stephens,
Ronald R. Hiebsch, and Stephen Oroszlan

*Biological Carcinogenesis Program, National Cancer Institute, Frederick Cancer
Research Facility, Frederick, Maryland 21701*

ABSTRACT. Reticuloendotheliosis virus (REV) is an acute transforming
virus, horizintally transmitted in avian species and the prototype of a
serologic group that includes spleen necrosis virus (SNV), duck infectious anemia virus (DIAV), and chicken syncytial virus (CSV). REV is
distinct from the Rous group of avian retroviruses but does resemble, in
certain properties, mammalian viruses. We have demonstrated by immunological, protein sequencing, and nucleic acid hybridization techniques
that the REV structural genes are most closely related to viruses of
primate origin, namely the macaque-colobus subgroup. The rel gene, however, is clearly of avian origin, consistent with its original isolation
in turkey virus. Like many other acute transforming viruses, REV is a
complex of helper and replication-defective components. The defective
component carries the rel gene which has now been partially sequenced.
The rel insert lies between a region homologous to the 3' end of the
MoLV pol gene and carboxyl one-half of the p20(E) component of the env
gene. The rel gene product has not been characterized, and we are
attempting to identify this via synthetic peptides as immunogens. The
significance of interspecies transmission of retroviruses in the context
of cellular oncogene activation and generation of acute transforming
viruses is discussed.

INTRODUCTION

Reticuloendotheliosis is both a generic term for a small group of
highly related horizontally transmitted viruses of avian species and the
type name for an acute-acting oncogenic member of the group. In the
group are SNV, DIAV, and CSV in addition to the prototype REV. As the
names indicate, these viruses are pathogenic and thus of some consequence
to domestic flocks. REV itself was originally isolated from turkeys,
whereas SNV and DIAV probably originated in malarial plasma from a fire-
backed Borneo pheasant at the New York Zoo (18). Both of these viruses
were isolated from ducks. The REV group is clearly distinct from the
avian leukosis sarcoma virus group (AL-SV) based on serological and molecular hybridization studies, and nucleic acid sequences related to
viral structural genes are not found in normal avian DNA (9,11,22). In
fact, many early studies indicated that these viruses most closely re-

163

semble mammalian type C viruses. These observations prompted us to perform detailed studies of the relationship of REV to other viruses and to
characterize the transforming gene of REV.

RESULTS AND DISCUSSION

Early results on REV suggesting affinity to mammalian type C viruses
were based mainly on morphological criteria and also on the cation preference of the virion reverse transcriptase (8,12). Such data are, by
themselves, not indicative of genetic relationships except to suggest
differences from the AL-SV group. However, initial sequencing studies
by Hunter et al. (7) showed homology between a core protein of REV and
previously determined sequences of murine leukemia virus and feline leukemia virus (for detailed sequence data, see ref. 14), thus putting the
putative relationship to mammalian viruses on firm ground. Dr. Howard
Charman, a former colleague, then obtained REV from Dr. Ray Franklin,
University of Texas, and began immunological studies on REV p30 (the
major core protein) using antisera broadly reactive with mammalian type
C p30s. These core proteins have been extensively studied by several
laboratories and considerable protein sequence information as well as a
great deal of immunological data exist. In our assays, we found evidence of shared interspecies determinants between REV and other mammalian viruses (1). In putting together sequence information with immunological characterization (14,15), we found that REV most closely resembled the endogenous viruses of macaques, designated MAC-1 and MMC-1.
Included in this group is a third virus from colobus monkeys, designated
CPC-1 (16). The immunological and sequence data have been augmented by
molecular hybridization experiments (19) showing positive results with
REV cDNA and cloned CPC-1 proviral DNA. In addition, more recent analyses
using a variety of viral cDNAs indicate the generic affinity of REV to
mammalian viruses. This affinity is not limited to the core protein,
p30, but extends to other structural proteins, including the pol gene
(N. R. Rice, unpublished data), and by DNA sequence analysis, to the
long terminal repeats of proviral DNA (10). Thus the available evidence
strongly suggests that the structural and polymerase genes of REV originate
from mammalian DNA, i.e., REV is an escaped virus, most likely from a
primate ancestor. The obvious questions are when did this occur and
what is its observed and potential significance.

If the proposed primate to avian transmission was a recent event, REV
would be expected to show a relationship to the macaque viruses resembling that seen between types within a species. The relationship observed was much more distant, resembling that seen between retroviruses
of different species. We do not yet know the relative rates of evolution of horizontally transmitted genomes and of genomes transmitted in
the germ line. We would expect that the horizontally transmitted
viruses evolve at a much faster rate because they are continuously replicating and because of the inherent mutation rates associated with
this process. However, without clear answers to these issues, we can
only state that the evidence suggests interspecies transfer has occurred, and that the consequences (discussed below) are significant. It
therefore seems logical not to limit consideration to a remote period
(millions of years ago), but to accept the possibility that the transfer
can occur at any time.

The significance of interspecies transfer in the REV group is obvious
from the pathogenicity of these viruses. Interspecies DNA transfer may
also play an important role in oncogenesis. The observation that CSV

can induce lymphoid leukosis in chickens is interesting in this regard; the mechanism of action of CSV is similar to conventional avian leukosis virus (ALV) in that the c-myc gene is activated (5,13). Thus we can propose that horizontally transmitted retroviruses with their promotor/activator/enhancer sequences are inherently potential agents of oncogenic induction, even if they do not directly transform. A brief survey of naturally occurring cancers associated with horizontally transmitted retroviruses includes bovine leukemia, feline leukemia, gibbon ape leukemia, and most significantly, a subtype of human leukemia (17). None of these appear to be acute transforming agents.

Another role of horizontally transmitted viruses in oncogenesis is illustrated by our studies on REV itself. This is an acute transforming virus capable of inducing tumors in vivo and transforming hematopoietic cells in vitro (2,6). We established that transforming preparations contained two major species of virus-specific RNA, one associated with replication functions (helper virus) and a smaller one associated with transformation (4). Detailed restriction mapping supported by heteroduplex analysis indicated that the transforming genome had lost the reverse transcriptase gene (pol), a major portion of the envelope gene (env), and had acquired a new sequence of cellular origin (20). This new sequence is the putative transforming gene which is now designated rel. We have now determined, by sequence analysis, the points of insertion of rel within the helper virus genome (23). As expected from the restriction enzyme map, this occurs directly after a region that shows homology to the 3' terminus of the pol gene of murine retroviruses (the only other pol DNA sequences currently available for comparison) and continues for 1,500 bases to termination signals that immediately precede coding sequences for the C-terminal half of the transmembrane protein (designated p20(E) in REV, the homolog of p15(E) in murine retroviruses). P20(E) sequences are encoded in the 3'-terminal one-third of the env gene, thus ca. one-sixth of env gene sequences are retained in the recombinant genome carrying rel sequences. Cells transformed by rel do not express virion structural proteins in the absence of helper virus, which suggests that the gag gene is also not functional, although at least half of the coding sequences are present in the recombinant genome.

The nature of the rel gene product has not been established. Based on the DNA sequence, we have synthesized a dodecapeptide which has been coupled to hemocyanin for immunization purposes. Antibody to the peptide has been obtained and is currently being used to identify the rel product in nonproducer transformed cells.

Returning to the significance of horizontally transmitted retroviruses, we can emphasize another major role in oncogenesis, namely the rescue of cellular genes of presumed normal function and thus the creation of an acute transforming virus. REV thus is the end result of extraneous infection, probably by a virus with origins in primate ancestors that has captured a cellular gene of birds and has become a highly oncogenic virus. Similar creations in the laboratory account for the Harvey and Kirsten sarcoma viruses (mouse, rat 30S, and rat onc recombinants), the Rasheed rat sarcoma virus (in vitro rescue of rat onc by a rat retrovirus) (for review see ref. 3), and possibly in nature for the Woolly monkey sarcoma virus, since the helper sequences are highly related to viruses of the gibbon ape (also horizontally transmitted) (24) and the onc gene is of Woolly monkey origin (21,25).

We are now in a new era where viral onc genes have been shown to have cellular homologs which in turn appear to be activated in certain cases without known intervention of viruses. Thus, any or all of the known viral <u>onc</u> gene homologs may be involved in human cancer. Whether a <u>rel</u> homolog is relevant to human cancer we cannot yet say. The approach via nucleic acid and immunological reagents is clear. The model of REV creation by interspecies virus (gene) transfer and rescue and other consequences of interspecies transmission clearly deserves attention.

ACKNOWLEDGEMENTS

Research sponsored by the National Cancer Institute, DHHS, under Contract No. NO1-CO-75380 with Litton Bionetics, Inc. The contents of this publication do not necessarily reflect the views or policies of the Department of Health and Human Services, nor does mention of trade names, commercial products, or organizations imply endorsement by the U.S. Government.

REFERENCES

1. Charman HP, Gilden RV, Oroszlan S (1979): J Virol 29:1221
2. Franklin RB, Maldonado RL, Bose Jr HR (1974): Intervirology 3:342
3. Gilden RV, Oroszlan S, Young HA, Rice NR, Gonda MA, Cohen M, Rein A (1981): In: Frontiers in Immunogenetics (Hildemann W, ed), Elsevier/North Holland, Inc., pp 191-223
4. Gonda MA, Rice NR, Gilden RV (1980): J Virol 34:743
5. Hayward WS, Neel BL, Astrin SM (1981): Nature 209:475
6. Hoelzer JD, Lewis RB, Wasmuth CR, Bose Jr HR (1980): Virology 100: 462
7. Hunter E, Bhown AS, Bennett JC (1978): Proc Natl Acad Sci USA 75: 2708
8. Kang C-Y (1975): J Virol 16:880
9. Kang C-Y, Temin HM (1973): J Virol 12:1314
10. Lovinger GG, Mark G, Todaro GJ, Schochetman G (1981): J Virol 39: 238
11. Maldonado RL, Bose Jr HR (1976): J Virol 17:983
12. Moelling K, Gelderblum H, Pauli G, Friis R, Bauer H (1975): Virology 65:546
13. Noori-Daloii MR, Swift RA, Kung HJ, Crittenden LB, Witter RL (1981): Nature 294:574
14. Oroszlan S, Gilden RV (1980): In: Molecular Biology of RNA Tumor Viruses (Stephenson JR, ed), New York: Academic Press, pp 299-344
15. Oroszlan S, Barbacid M, Copeland TD, Aaronson SA, Gilden RV (1981): J Virol 39:845
16. Oroszlan S, Copeland TD, Gilden RV, Todaro GJ (1981): Virology 115:262
17. Poiesz BJ, Ruscetti RW, Gazdar AF, Bunn PA, Minna JD, Gallo RC (1980): Proc Natl Acad Sci USA 77:7415
18. Purchase HG, Witter RL (1975): In: Current Topics in Microbiology and Immunology (Vogt PK, ed), New York: Springer-Verlag, pp 103-124
19. Rice NR, Bonner TI, Gilden RV (1981): Virology 114:286
20. Rice NR, Hiebsch RR, Gonda MA, Bose Jr HR, Gilden RV (1982): J Virol 42:237
21. Robbins KC, Hill RL, Aaronson SA (1982): J Virol 41:721
22. Simek S, Rice NR (1980): J Virol 33:320
23. Stephens RM, Rice NR, Hiebsch RR, Bose Jr HR, Gilden RV: Proc Natl Acad Sci USA, in press

24. Todaro GJ, Lieber MM, Benveniste RE, Sherr CJ (1975): Virology 67: 335

25. Wong-Staal F, Favera RD, Gelmann EP, Manzari V, Szala S, Josephs SF, Gallo RC (1981): Nature 294:273

Gene Transfer and Cancer, edited by M. L. Pearson
and N. L. Sternberg. Raven Press, New York © 1984.

Isolation of New Mammalian Type C Transforming Viruses

*Ulf R. Rapp, **Fred H. Reynolds, Jr., and *John R. Stephenson

*Laboratory of Viral Carcinogenesis and **Carcinogenesis Intramural Research
Program, National Cancer Institute, Frederick Cancer Research Facility,
Frederick, Maryland 21701*

ABSTRACT. An acute transforming virus, designated 3611-MSV, was isolated from mice inoculated with a virus obtained by iododeoxyuridine
(IdUrd) induction of methylcholanthrene-transformed C3H/10T1/2 cells.
This virus transforms embryo fibroblasts and epithelial cells in culture.
Mice inoculated with 3611-MSV at birth develop tumors within 4 weeks;
these tumors contain several distinct mesenchymal cell types with fibroblasts as the predominant component. This new virus isolate resembles
previously described mammalian acute transforming viruses in that it is
replication-defective, requiring a type C helper virus for successful
propagation both in vitro and in vivo. Several nonproductively transformed clones have been isolated by endpoint transmission of 3611-MSV to
mouse or rat cells. Pseudotype virus stocks obtained from such clones
transform cells in vitro, are highly oncogenic in vivo, and exhibit host
range and serologic properties characteristic of the helper virus. The
major 3611-MSV translational product has been identified as a 90,000
(P90) MW polyprotein with amino terminal murine leukemia virus (MuLV)
gag gene proteins, p15 and p12, linked to an acquired sequence encoded
nonstructural component. In contrast to the gene products of many previously described mammalian transforming viruses, the 3611-MSV-encoded
polyproteins lack detectable protein kinase activity. Additionally,
3611-MSV-transformed cells resemble those of the chemically transformed
cell line, C3H/MCA-5, from which 3611-MSV was originally derived, in
that they do not exhibit overall elevated levels of phosphotyrosine. By
Southern blot hybridization analysis of the cellular DNA of 3611-MSV
nonproductively transformed rat cells, an EcoRI restriction fragment was
identified containing the entire 3611-MSV genome. This DNA fragment
hybridized strongly to MuLV gag gene specific probes but lacked detectable homology with molecular probes corresponding to the mos, ras, abl or
fes mammalian oncogenes. These findings suggest that the transformation-
specific sequences represented within the 3611-MSV genome may represent
a new as yet unidentified mammalian cellular oncogene corresponding to
sequences originally involved in transformation of C3H/MCA-5 cells by
methylcholanthrene.

Experiments were designed to generate new acute transforming retroviruses by growth of endogenous type C virus in chemically transformed
cells. These experiments were done in the hope of developing a general-
ized procedure for the isolation of recombinant virus isolates that have
picked up cellular oncogene(s) expressed in the chemically transformed
cells. The system that we chose for these studies utilized an established mouse cell line, C3H/10T1/2, characterized by sensitivity to
quantitative chemical transformation (25,26). The mouse is a suitable
model for such experiments in view of increasing evidence that cellular
homologs of viral oncogenes are highly conserved throughout evolution;
consequently genes isolated from the mouse can be used for the identification and subsequent molecular cloning of their human homologs from gene
libraries.

RESULTS

A general scheme followed for the selection of transforming viruses
from a mixed population produced by chemically transformed C3H/10T1/2
cells after induction with IdUrd (15) is shown in Figure 1 (19). Virus
from chronically producing cultures was used for infection of highly
permissive cells, such as Sc-1, a feral mouse fibroblast cell line, or
certain other transformed mouse cells. The progeny of such acute infections were sorted out by plating them on nontransformed test cells,
including C3H/10T1/2 fibroblasts as well as mink epithelial lung cells.
Infected test cells were seeded in soft agar or grown in monolayers, and
agar colonies as well as foci of criss-crossing cells were selected.
Virus produced by these cells was recovered and used to infect NIH/3T3
cells before injection into syngeneic, newborn swiss mice. Tumors that
developed were transplanted and established as cell lines in culture
providing a reservoir of tissue and cells for future work. Although
most tumors and cell lines obtained did not produce directly rescuable
transforming virus, a few did. Acutely transforming virus was cloned in
cell culture and nonproductively transformed cells were isolated.
Viruses obtained included lung carcinoma- (16), fibrosarcoma- (8) and
various lymphosarcoma-inducing isolates from which nonproductively transformed rat, mouse and mink cell lines containing rescuable transforming
virus genomes have been derived. Two representative virus isolates obtained by this approach are described in the present study.

The first virus isolate studied (CI-3) is associated with alveologen-
ic lung carcinomas and has the structure of a mink cell focus-inducing
(MCF) recombinant (4,5,18) with a substitution encompassing the gp70
coding portion of the env gene. As shown in the general isolation
scheme (Figure 1), there are several steps at which genetic variation
of the induced endogenous C3H/MuLV could have occurred so as to yield
this pathogenic derivative. We established for the MCF class virus
associated with lung carcinomas that this recombinant viral genome was
preexistent in the population of IdUrd-induced virus as a minor component.
This was accomplished by molecular cloning in the EcoRI site of λgtWES.λ B
of EcoRI-sensitive viral DNA present in a Hirt extract of cells acutely
infected with IdUrd-induced C3H/virus. Although most viral DNAs in
this preparation were resistant to EcoRI digestion, three colonies were
obtained that contained full-length viral genomes identical to the
recombinant viral genome isolated from nonproductively transformed
mink cells (20).

Virus from IdUrd-Induced C3H/MCA5 Cells

↓

Acute Infection of Permissive Cells

↓

Transfer of Progeny Virus to Test Cells:C3H/Mv-1Lu

↓

Selection of Transformed Test Cells
(Soft Agar Colonies or Foci of Crisscrossing Cells)

↓

Transfer of Virus From Test Cells to NIH/3T3

↓

Inoculate Newborn NIH Swiss Mice

↓

Reestablish Tumors in Cell Culture and Transplant Tumors

FIGURE 1. Derivation of tumor-inducing viruses from chemically transformed C3H/10T1/2 cells after induction with IdUrd.

In vitro transformed epithelial mink lung cells harboring this virus have a strongly enhanced transformed phenotype in the presence of 10 ng/ml of epidermal growth factor (EGF) which by itself does not alter the phenotype of uninfected mink lung cells. Thus the mechanism of transmation by this pathogenic recombinant virus may involve sensitization of target cells to EGF (21).

A second group of acute transforming retroviruses isolated by this procedure were replication defective, representing probable recombinants between viral and host cellular sequences. One such isolate, 3611-MSV, was found to encode a polyprotein with amino terminal gag-gene-encoded structural components. Several nonproductively transformed clonal cell lines have been derived by endpoint transmission of 3611-MSV to MMCE Cl 7 mouse (17) and FRE Cl 3 rat cells (34). Pseudotype virus stocks from such clones have been generated and shown to transform cells in vitro and in vivo (Table 1). Tumor induction occurred with a 100% incidence after a latency period of 3 weeks. Interestingly, this highly transforming virus induced tumors when injected into newborn mice, but not in weanling age mice of the same strain, NFS/N, (Table 1) or any of five other inbred mouse strains tested including AKR/N, DBA-2N, C3H/Hen, BALB/cAnN and C57BL/6N (data not shown). This resistance in weanling age mice may reflect, not the immunocompetence of these older animals but, rather the specificity for a distinct target cell in vivo that is more abundant in newborn than adult mice. Such a model is supported by the fact that weanling nude NIH swiss mice were also resistant.

Virus structural proteins expressed in mouse and rat cells nonproductively transformed by 3611-MSV included p15 and p12 (Table 2). Heterologous radioimmunoassays for the p30, p10 reverse transcriptase and gp70 were all negative with extracts of 3611-MSV nonproducer rat and mouse cells but positive for cells chronically infected with the Moloney strain of MuLV (22). Another recently isolated acute transforming virus, 2207-MSV, resembles 3611-MSV in that it is replication defective but in contrast, cells transformed by 2207-MSV do not express any viral structural proteins to any detectable extent (Table 2). Immunoprecipi-

TABLE 1. Biological Properties of 3611-MSV[a]

| Cell line | Type C helper virus | Virus titer (log $_{10}$/ml) | | Fibrosarcoma induction in vivo | | | |
| | | | | newborn | | weanlings | |
		PIU	FFU	incidence	latency (weeks)	incidence	latency (weeks)
FRE Cl 3	4070-A	6.0	< 0.5	0.4	> 36	0/20	> 36
3611-FRE Ac1	-	< 0.5	< 0.5	NT[b]	-	0/18	-
	4070-A	6.0	4.8	16/16	4	0/21	> 36
3611-FRE Ac12	4070-A	5.0	3.7	NT	-	0/20	-
MMCE Cl 7	4070-A	< 0.5	0.5	0.20	> 36	0/19	> 36
3611-MMCE Ac2	-	< 0.5	< 0.5	NT	-	NT	-
	4070-A	6.0	4.7	12/12	3	NT	> 36
3611-MMCE Ac8	4070-A	5.0	3.1	6/6	4	NT	> 36

a Cell lines were infected with 4070-A helper virus at high multiplicity and 2 weeks later culture fluids filtered and assayed for transmission to FRE Cl 3 rat cells as measured by polymerase inducing units (PIU)/ml, focus forming units (FFU)/ml, and tumorigenicity in newborn NFS/N mice according to previously described procedures (19).
b NT = not tested.

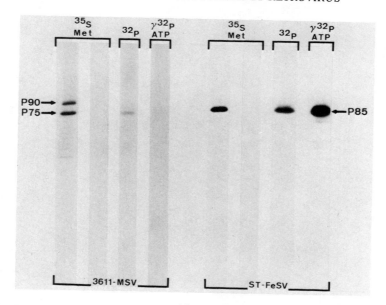

FIGURE 2. Immunoprecipitation of [^{35}S]methionine-labeled cell extracts of 3611-MSV-transformed rat cells with anti M-MuLV p12 sera.

tation of [^{35}S]methionine labeled cell extracts of 3611-MSV-transformed rat cells with anti M-MuLV p12 sera revealed 90,000 (P90) and 75,000 MW (P75) polypeptides. One of these, P75, was found to be weakly phosphorylated as was shown by immunoprecipitation of extracts from cells labeled with [^{32}P]orthophosphoric acid (Figure 2, lane 3), whereas under similar conditions no detectable phosphorylation of P90 was observed.

Acquired cellular oncogenic sequences of numerous acutely transforming retroviruses have been shown to encode polyproteins (1,2,6,11,13,22, 31,34,35,37,39) with tyrosine-specific protein kinase activity (6,11,13, 22,23,24,34,38). To test for such activity, we incubated immunoprecipitates of 3611-MSV P90 and P75 with [γ^{32}P]ATP under standard protein kinase reaction conditions (Figure 2, lane 4). These experiments showed no evidence for intrinsic or associated protein kinase activity of P90 or P75. The assays were performed with Mn^{2+} and also Mg^{2+} as the divalent metal ion under conditions by which an 85,000 MW polyprotein gene product of the Snyder-Theilen strain of feline sarcoma virus (FeSV) was efficiently phosphorylated. Phosphoamino acid analysis was performed to determine whether in vivo phosphorylation of 3611-MSV P75 involved tyrosine residues. These experiments showed that most of the labeled phosphate was on phosphoserine and a minor fraction was on phosphothreonine, whereas no ^{32}P-label was detected on tyrosine.

Cells transformed by oncogenic retroviruses with protein kinase activity generally have significantly (8- to 10-fold) elevated overall levels of phosphotyrosine (21,23,27). In contrast, when analyzed under similar conditions, none of six independently derived chemically transformed clones of C3H/10T1/2 cells, including C3H/MCA-5 (Table 3), exhibited elevated phosphotyrosine. Similarly phosphotyrosine levels in cells transformed by 3611-MSV were not significantly greater than in nontransformed control cells. In contrast both Gardner-FeSV-transformed FRE cells (23) and cells transformed in vivo by another newly isolated acute transforming retrovirus, MB65, included as positive controls, showed the expected

TABLE 2. Expression of type C virus structural proteins in cells nonproductively transformed by 3611-MSV

Cell line	Designation	Viral protein expression (ng viral protein/mg total cellular protein)[a]					
		p15	p12	p30	p10	rt	gp70
Fisher rat embryo: control	FRE Cl3	< 10	< 2	< 2	< 10	< 20	< 50
3611-transformed	3611-FRE Ac1	560	620	< 2	< 10	< 20	< 50
	3611-FRE Ac3	620	670	< 2	< 10	< 20	< 50
	3611-FRE Ac12	490	580	< 2	< 10	< 20	< 50
2207-transformed	2207-FRE Ac2-7	< 10	< 2	< 2	< 10	< 20	< 50
Wild mouse: control	MMCE Cl7	< 20	< 10	< 10	< 20	< 50	< 50
3611-transformed	3611-MMCE Ac8	1860	1670	< 10	< 20	< 50	< 50
	3611-MMCE Ac2	1910	1812	< 10	< 20	< 50	< 50
M-MuLV-infected	MMCE Cl7 (M-MuLV)	3620	4920	5620	2900	350	6200

a Cellular extracts were tested at serial 2-fold dilutions in heterologous immunoassays utilizing goat antisera against ditergene-disrupted Moloney MuLV for precipitation of 125I-labeled Rauscher MuLV p15, p12, p30, p10, reverse transcriptase (rt) and gp70 (22). The results are based on the extent of displacement relative to known protein standards and represent mean values from three separate determinations.

8- to 10-fold elevation of phosphotyrosine (Table 3). These findings are consistent with the possibility that 3611-MSV contains oncogenic sequences similar to, or even derived from, those that are active in methylcholanthrene-transformed C3H/10T1/2 cells.

In preliminary experiments we have screened C3H/MCA-5 cells (15) for elevated levels of RNA expression with a variety of molecularly cloned retrovirus-derived oncogene probes including Harvey sarcoma virus (Ha-ras), Moloney-MSV (v-mos), Abelson-MuLV (v-abl), Snyder Theilen Feline sarcoma virus (v-fes), Rouse sarcoma virus (v-src) and MC29 (v-myc) with negative results. Similarly 3611-MSV proviral DNA in non-producer transformed rat cells did not hybridize with Ha-ras, v-mos, v-abl or v-fes but hybridized strongly to MuLV gag gene-specific probes. These findings suggest that the transformation-specific sequences repre-

TABLE 3. Phosphotyrosine levels in 3611-MSV-transformed cells and C3H/MCA-5, the cell line from which 3611-MSV was derived

Cell line	Transforming agent	Growth in soft agar (%)	Phosphotyrosine (% of total phosphoamino acids)
FRE Cl 3	–	< 0.01	< 0.2
Gardner-FeSV FRE Cl 4	Gardner-FeSV	16	1.8
3611-FRE Ac1	3611-MSV	21	< 0.2
3611-FRE Ac8	3611-MSV	19	< 0.2
C3H/10T1/2	–	< 0.01	< 0.2
C3H/MCA-5	–	21	< 0.2
MB65	MB65-MSV	NT	1.3
NIH/3T3	–	–	< 0.2

[a] Growth of colonies in soft agar (16) and phosphotyrosine, expressed as a percentage of total cellular phosphoamino acids (24), were determined as previously described.

sented within the 3611-MSV genome may represent a new as-yet-unidentified mammalian cellular oncogene corresponding to sequences originally involved in transformation of C3H/MCA-5 cells. Studies are currently in progress to define the transforming sequences represented within the recombinant 2207-MSV genome and to determine whether they are related to the 3611-MSV sequences.

DISCUSSION

We have presented here the isolation in cell culture of two structurally distinct classes of transforming retroviruses. One, represented by

CI-3, is a recombinant between endogenous ecotropic and xenotropic related MuLV and belongs to the MCF class (6-9) of pathogenic MuLV. The other class, of which 3611-MSV represents a prototype isolate, exhibits all the characteristics of a recombinant that has acquired a cellular oncogene that may be active in the chemically transformed cells from which it originated. The mechanism by which these recombinants are generated is not clear at present and may involve two steps, the first of which would be the formation of a readthrough transcript between MuLV and a cellular oncogene located 3' to the integrated virus. The transcript in this model would initiate from the 5' long-terminal repeat (LTR) of the virus which may have deleted a 3' portion of its genome including the 3' LTR with its transcription stop signal (32). The joint transcript, which contains viral sequences required for RNA packaging, in addition to the cellular oncogenic sequences, could subsequently become incorporated into pseudotype virus particles. Upon transfer and reverse transcription in another cell which also received intact infectious MuLV, the 3' end of the infectious virus might be transferred to the virus-oncogene mosaic transcript by a copy-choice mechanism (7). Alternatively, incorporation of a cellular gene might require packaging of an oncogene mRNA in one step and incorporation into the viral genome during reverse transcription, again by a copy-choice mechanism, during a subsequent cycle of infection. While these two models appear most compatible with the few facts currently known about this process, other mechanisms are still possible.

So far we have described biological approaches for the use of MuLV as a transducing agent. It might also be possible to incrase this activity by altering the genome of molecularly cloned virus. The usefulness of retroviral genomes as vectors for eucaryotic genes has been explored in several laboratories (10,29,36) but we are not aware of attempts to increase its transduction frequency. This might be achieved in several ways. Transcription of RNA from proviral DNA terminates at the 3' end, presumably because of the presence of a short termination sequence which is part of RNA in the LTR (32). It might be possible to remove this sequence without hampering the ability of the virus to be replicated into DNA. Lack of this transcription stop signal might then increase the frequency of readthrough into genes adjacent to the integration site, a possible first step in the formation of a transductant.

Another approach would be to increase the number of integration events that take place in an infected cell. Reverse transcription of genomic RNA transcribed from an integrated provirus into DNA within the same infected cell does not seem to occur, probably because there is little or no active reverse transcriptase produced from proviral transcripts. It might be possible to delete the gag gene in molecularly cloned MuLV in such a way that large amounts of reverse transcriptase would be produced from proviral transcripts. Such a construct, if it leads to intracellular reverse transcription and reintegration, presumably would be highly toxic to cells, and it is therefore important that reintegration events should be controlled possibly by use of a conditional polymerase mutant or by use of mouse mammary tumor virus (MMTV) for the construct since its transcription is under hormonal control (9,33).

Transduction by retrovirus is one of several available techniques for the isolation of eucaryotic genes; others include cDNA cloning (12) and DNA transfection (3,14,28,30). cDNA cloning is limited to more abundant mRNA species and requires expression of a gene before it can be cloned. The isolation of genes selected by DNA transfection has the disadvantage of the frequent presence of introns within cloned genes and the occurrence of so-called poison sequences. The construction of a retrovirus which can be used for biological cloning of expressed or unexpressed genes would therefore be an important tool to develop.

ACKNOWLEDGEMENT

Research sponsored in part by the National Cancer Institute, DHHS, under contract No. NO1-CO-75380 with Litton Bionetics, Inc. The contents of this publication do not necessarily reflect the fiews or policies of the Department of Health and Human Services, nor does mention of trade names, commercial products, or organizations imply endorsement by the U.S. Government.

REFERENCES

1. Barbacid M, Lauver AV, Devare SG (1980): J Virol 33:196
2. Bister K, Hayman MJ, Vogt PK (1977): Virology 82:431
3. Cooper GM, Okenquist S, Silverman L (1980): Nature 284:418
4. Devare SG, Rapp UR, Todaro GJ, Stephenson JR (1978): J Virol 28:457
5. Elder JH, Gautsch JW, Jensen FC, Lerner RA, Hartley JW, Rowe WP (1977): Proc Natl Acad Sci USA 74:4676
6. Feldman RA, Hanafusa T, Hanafusa H (1980): Cell 22:757
7. Goldfarb MP, Weinberg RA (1981): J Virol 38:136
8. Hartley JW, Wolford HK, Old LJ, Rowe WP (1977): Proc Natl Acad Sci USA 74:789
9. Huang AL, Ostrowski MC, Berard D, Hager GL (1981): Cell 27:245
10. Joyner A, Yamamoto Y, Bernstein A (1981): In: ICN-UCLA Symp. on Molecular and Cellular Biology (Brown DD, Fox CF, eds), Vol. XXIII, New York: Academic Press, p 535
11. Neil JC, Delamarter JF, Vogt PK (1981): Proc Natl Acad Sci USA 78:1906
12. Okayama H, Berg P (1981): Mol Cell Biol 2:161
13. Pawson T, Guyden J, Kung T-H, Radke K, Gilmore T, Martin GS (1980): Cell 22:767
14. Pulciani S, Santos E, Lauver AV, Long LK, Robbins KC, Barbacid M (1982): Proc Natl Acad Sci USA 79:2845
15. Rapp UR, Nowinski RC, Reznikoff A, Heidelberger C (1975): Virology 65:392
16. Rapp UR, Todaro GJ (1978): Science 201:821
17. Rapp UR, Keski-Oja J, Heine UI (1979): Cancer Res 39:4111
18. Rapp UR, Todaro GJ (1979): Proc Natl Acad Sci USA 75:2468
19. Rapp UR, Todaro GJ (1980): Proc Natl Acad Sci USA 77:624
20. Rapp UR, Birkenmeier E, Bonner TI, Gonda MA, Gunnell M (1983): J Virol 45:740
21. Rapp UR, Reynolds F.J. Jr, Stephenson JR (1983): J Virol 45:914
22. Reynolds FJ Jr, Sacks TL, Deobagkar DN, Stephenson JR (1979): Proc Natl Acad Sci USA 75:3974
23. Reynolds FH Jr, Van de Ven WJM, Stephenson JR (1980): J Biol Chem 255:11040
24. Reynolds FH Jr, Van de Ven WJM, Blomberg J, Stephenson JR (1981): J Virol 38:1084
25. Reznikoff CA, Bertram JS, Brankow DW, Heidelberger C (1973): Cancer Res 33:3239
26. Reznikoff CA, Brankow DW, Heidelberger C (1973): Cancer Res 33:3231
27. Sefton BM, Hunter T, Beemon K, Eckhart W (1980): Cell 20:807

28. Shih C, Shilo B-Z, Goldfarb MP, Dannenberg A, Weinberg RA (1979): Proc Natl Acad Sci USA 76:5714
29. Shimotohno K, Temin HM 91981): Cell 26:67
30. Shilo B-Z, Weinberg RA (1981): Nature 289:607
31. Stephenson JR, Khan AS, Sliski AH, Essex M (1977): Proc Natl Acad Sci USA 74:5608
32. Temin HM (1981): Cell 27:1
33. Ucker DS, Ross SR, Yamamoto KR (1981): Cell 27:257
34. Van de Ven WJM, Reynolds FH Jr, Stephenson JR (1980): Virology 101:185
35. Van de Ven WJM, Reynolds FH Jr, Nalewaik RP, Stephenson JR (1980): J Virol 35:165
36. Wei C-M, Gibson M, Spear P, Scolnick E (1981): J Virol 39:935
37. Witte ON, Rosenberg N, Paskind M, Shields A, Baltimore D (1978): Proc Natl Acad Sci USA 75:2488
38. Witte ON, Dasgupta A, Baltimore D (1980): Nature 283:826
39. Young HA, Rasheed S, Sowder R, Benton CV, Henderson LE (1981): J Virol 38:286

Gene Transfer and Cancer, edited by M. L. Pearson and N. L. Sternberg. Raven Press, New York © 1984.

Isolation of v-*fes*/v-*fps* Homologous Sequences from a Human Lung Carcinoma Cosmid Library

John Groffen, Nora Heisterkamp, and John R. Stephenson

Laboratory of Viral Carcinogenesis, National Cancer Institute, Frederick Cancer Research Facility, Frederick, Maryland 21701

ABSTRACT. The Gardner and Snyder-Theilen isolates of feline sarcoma virus (FeSV) represent genetic recombinants between feline leukemia virus (FeLV) and transformation-specific sequences of cat cellular origin (v-fes gene). A related transforming gene (v-fps) common to the Fujinami and PRC II strains of avian sarcoma virus (ASV) has also been described. Polyprotein gene products of each of these virus isolates exhibit tyrosine-specific protein kinase activity. By restriction endonuclease and molecular hybridization analysis, the v-fes and v-fps genes have been found to contain highly related sequences. Moreover, molecular probes corresponding to each hybridize to a single well-resolved 12-kb EcoRI restriction fragment of human cellular DNA. DNA clones containing v-fes and v-fps homologous sequences were isolated from a representative cosmid library of human lung carcinoma DNA. Cellular inserts within these cosmids, ranging from 32 to 42 kb in length, represent overlapping regions corresponding to 56 kb of contiguous human DNA sequences. Sequences both homologous to, and colinear with the Gardner/Snyder-Theilen FeSV v-fes and Fujinami ASV v-fps genes are distributed discontinuously over a region of up to 9.5 kb and contain a minimum of 3 distinct noncoding regions (introns). A 12-kb EcoRI restriction fragment representing the entire v-fes/v-fps human homolog has been subcloned in pBR328 and subjected to fine structure mapping. By this means the arrangement of human DNA sequences homologous to acquired sequences of each virus isolate were accurately defined. Upon transfection to RAT 2 cells, using the thymidine kinase gene as a selective marker, the human v-fes/v-fps homolog lacked transforming activity. These findings strongly argue that transforming sequences independently acquired by avian and mammalian retroviruses correspond to a common cellular gene that has been highly conserved throughout vertebrate evolution.

INTRODUCTION

Acute transforming retroviruses represent rare spontaneously arising genetic recombinants between type C viruses and cellular oncogenes (7,19). Several virus isolates of this nature have been shown to encode as their major translation products, tyrosine-specific protein kinases that are closely associated with their transforming function. Such viruses can be separated into classes on the basis of their cellular oncogenic sequences

TABLE 1:   Transforming Retroviruses Encoding Tyrosine-Specific Protein
           Kinases

Gene[a]	Virus Isolate	Transforming Protein	gag Gene Structural Components
Mammalian			
abl	Abelson MuLV	P120	+
fes	Gardner FeSV	P110	+
	Snyder Theilen FeSV	P85	+
Avian			
fps	Fujinami ASV, UR1	P140, P150	+
	PRCII, PRCIV	P105, P170	+,+
yes	Y73, Esh	P90, P80	+,+
ros	UR2	P68	+
src	RSV	pp60	−

[a]Designation of viral transforming (onc) sequences and their translational products is according to convention (4).

(Table 1). Acquired cellular oncogenes and representative virus isolates
of each group include: v-src (RSV), v-fes (ST- and GA-FeSV), v-fps (FSV,
PRCII, UR1), v-yes (Y73, Esh), v-ros (UR2) and v-abl (A MuLV) (4). Two
of these genes (v-fes and v-abl) are of mammalian cellular origin while
the remaining four (v-src, v-fps, v-yes and v-ros) were derived from
naturally occurring avian tumors. Earlier studies indicating low levels
of sequence homology between the v-fes and v-fps genes, raised the possibility that these either represent distantly related genes or correspond
to a common cellular locus that has remained highly conserved throughout
vertebrate evolution (17). Such a model was supported by the demonstra-
tion of immunologic cross-reactive (2) and structural relatedness (3) of
their major translational products. The present study was undertaken to
molecularly clone human cellular v-fes and v-fps homologous sequences in
an effort to resolve these alternative possibilities and provide information regarding the number of potentially oncogenic sequences within the
human genome encoding tyrosine specific protein kinases.

RESULTS AND DISCUSSION

As an initial measure of the relatedness of the avian Fujinami sarcoma
virus (FSV)-v-fps gene to the Gardner (GA) and Snyder-Theilen (ST) FeSV
v-fes genes, molecular probes corresponding to the complete GA-FeSV and
ST-FeSV genomes, designated GA-v-fes and ST-v-fes, respectively, and to
0.5 kbp PstI subgenomic fragments of ST-FeSV, designated v-fes S_L and
v-fes S_R (Figure 1), were prepared (8,9). Each was tested for hybridization by Southern blot analysis to a series of restriction fragments of a
previously described molecular clone of FSV in λgtWES-λB (10,18).
As shown in Figure 1, the extent of v-fps homology with the individual
v-fes probes varied in a manner colinear with their arrangement in the
ST-FeSV and GA-FeSV genomes. For instance, homology to v-fes S_R was
restricted to the PstI-SmaI fragment at 3' region of FSV-v-fps, whereas
v-fes-S_L lacked homology with the 3' terminal BamHI-SmaI fragment and

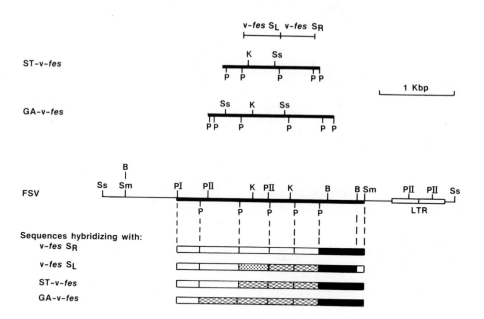

FIGURE 1. Homology between FSV-v-<u>fps</u> and acquired cellular sequences
(v-<u>fes</u>) of the Gardner and Snyder-Theilen strains of FeSV. An <u>Sst</u>I
restriction fragment, representing the entire molecularly cloned FSV
genome was purified from recombinant phage FSV-1 by gel electrophoresis
(9). After digestion with the indicated restriction enzymes, hybridization was performed using previously described [^{32}P]-labeled v-<u>fes</u>-
specific probes including GA-v-<u>fes</u>, ST-v-<u>fes</u>, v-<u>fes</u>-S$_L$, and v-<u>fes</u>-S$_R$ (8,
9). Extents of hybridization of FSV-v-<u>fps</u> with each of the four probes
is shown as negative (☐); weak (▨); intermediate (▨); and strong
(■). Restriction endonucleases include <u>Bam</u>HI (B), <u>Kpn</u>I (K), <u>Pst</u>I (P),
<u>Pvu</u>I (PI), <u>Pvu</u>II (PII), <u>Sma</u>I (Sm), and <u>Sst</u>I (Ss).

v-<u>fes</u> S$_L$ homology extended much further into the 5' region of FSV-v-<u>fps</u>.
The most extensive homology was observed with GA-v-<u>fes</u> which included
all but the extreme 5' region of v-<u>fps</u>.

These results demonstrate extensive homology between v-<u>fes</u> and v-<u>fps</u>
and establish colinearity in their structural organization. To resolve
whether these viral transforming sequences correspond to the same, or
alternatively, to related but genetically distinct cellular genes, high-
molecular-weight DNAs of several mammalian species were analyzed for
sequence homology to v-<u>fes</u> and v-<u>fps</u> specific probes. In each case
single 7.0- to 12.0-kb <u>Eco</u>RI DNA restriction fragments hybridized to
probes specific for both viral transforming genes (data not shown). The
lack of identifiable DNA restriction fragments exhibiting exclusive or
preferential hybridization with either v-<u>fes</u> or v-<u>fps</u> specific probes
strongly argues for the involvement of a common cellular genetic locus
in derivation of viruses containing these genes.

To further define human v-<u>fes</u>/v-<u>fps</u> homologous sequences, a cosmid
library of <u>Mbo</u>I partially digested human DNA was constructed and screened
for hybridization to v-<u>fes</u> specific probes (Figure 2). The cosmid system
was chosen for this purpose because of its capacity for cloning large

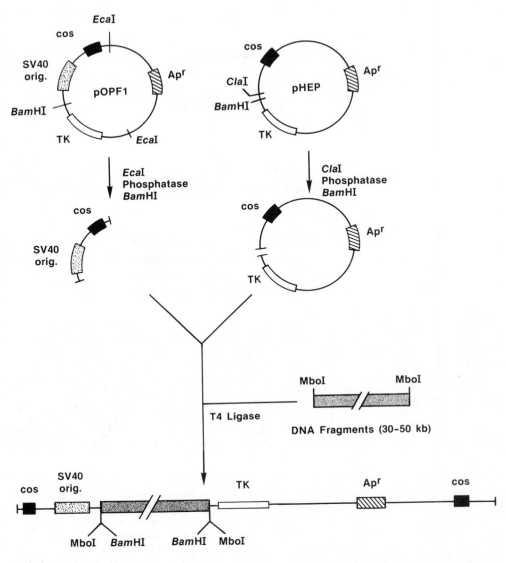

FIGURE 2. Schematic representation of the construction of a human lung carcinoma DNA library in a cosmid vector system. High-molecular-weight cellular DNA was purified from human lung carcinoma tissue, partially digested with MboI and size fractionated over a 5–20% sucrose gradient. DNAs of plasmids pOPF1 and pHEP were digested with EcaI and ClaI, respectively, treated with calf intestine phosphatase, and redigested with BamHI. 1.0 μg of a 1:1 molar ratio of the restricted plasmid DNAs and 2.0 μg of restricted cellular DNA fragments (30–50 kb) were ligated, in vitro packaged, and transduced into Escherichia coli ED8767 according to previously described procedures (9). A total of approximately 250,000 ampicillin-resistant colonies were obtained representing three to four times that required for representation of the entire human genome.

inserts representing extensive contiguous regions of human cellular DNA
(9). A total of three clones were initially selected and subjected to
further analysis. Two of the clones contained a 12.0-kb EcoRI restriction fragment with homology to both v-fes S_L and v-fes S_R, whereas only
the 9.8-kb 5' region of this fragment was represented in the third clone.
Further restriction enzyme analysis indicated that sequences within
these clones were overlapping and represented a 58-kb contiguous region
of the human genome. The orientation and positioning of the cellular
inserts within these clones, both relative to each other and to the
cosmid vector, are summarized in Figure 3.

For purposes of fine structure mapping, the above described 12.0-kb
EcoRI v-fes homologous restriction fragment was subcloned in pBR328.
The regions of hybridization shown in Figure 3 are based on identification of restriction fragments hybridizing with each of the four indicated
probes. These encompass a total of 4.5 kb of homology distributed discontinuously over a 9.5 kb region. No additional homology with either
GA or ST FeSV were observed within the entire 58 kb of human DNA represented within the three cosmid clones. The similarity in arrangement
of homologous sequences within the viral and cellular DNAs establishes
colinearity between v-fes and its human homolog (9).

To accurately define regions of sequence homology of the v-fps gene
with the human cellular homolog of v-fes, the same series of three cosmid clones were examined (Figure 3). Hybridization with FSV-v-fps was
restricted to the 12.0-kb EcoRI restriction fragment containing v-fes
homologous sequences. Although FSV-v-fps homology to human DNA most
closely resembled that of GA-FeSV v-fes, the 3' terminal v-fes homologous region of human DNA common to ST-v-fes and GA-v-fes did not hybridize to detectable extent with the FSV-v-fps probe. ST-v-fes
homologous sequences differed from those of both GA-v-fes and FSV-v-fps
in that they are not represented within the 5' terminal region hybridizing to the other two. Finally, two regions of human DNA homology
unique to FSV-v-fps were identified in the 5' half of the 12.0-kbp human
EcoRI DNA fragment. Thus although all three viral oncogenes appear to
be entirely represented by homologous sequences within a single c-fes/
c-fps human genetic locus, the exact positions at which regions of
homology map differ among the individual viral transforming genes. The
lack of detectable hybridization of v-fps with the 3' region of the
c-fes/c-fps locus could reflect evolutionary divergence. Alternatively,
a comparison of the 5' terminal position of ST-v-fes, and 3' position of
FSV-v-fps homologous sequences within the human c-fes/c-fps locus, indicated by the dotted lines, may provide a maximum estimate of human DNA
sequences required for transformation.

The larger size of the FSV-v-fps gene (18) as compared to that of GA-
v-fes (5,9) may be accounted for by regions of the human c-fes/c-fps
locus which are uniquely homologous with FSV-v-fes. These FSV-v-fps
unique sequences can be explained by one of several alternative possibilities. For instance such sequences may have been initially represented
within GA-v-fes but deleted during passage of GA-FeSV subsequent to its
initial derivation. Alternatively, the differences in sequences in these
viruses may reflect differences in the positions of coding and noncoding
regions of the c-fes/c-fps RNA transcripts of the divergent host species
from which they were isolated. Finally, mechanisms of incorporation of
cellular oncogenic sequences in retroviral genomes may be imprecise and
the resulting insert within the viral genomic RNA may not necessarily
correspond exactly to the cellular mRNA from which it was derived. Either
the first or third possibilities appear most probable in that one of

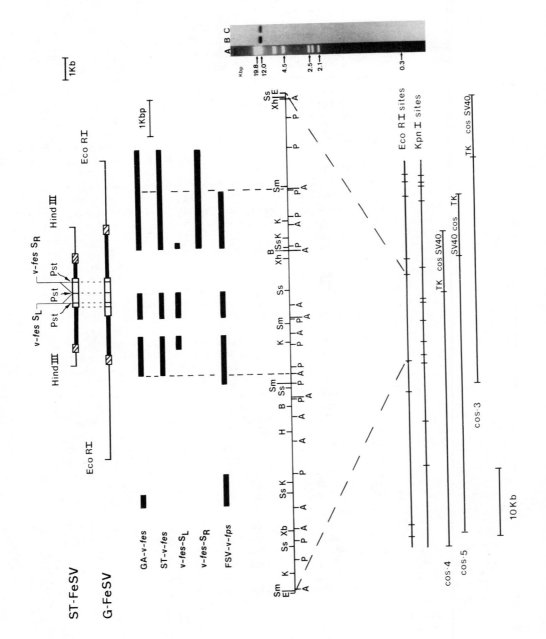

these must be evoked to explain the differences between the acquired cellular sequences of GA-v-fes and ST-v-fes. Resolution of these alternative models may provide insight into mechanisms by which cellular oncogenes become stably associated with the genomes of retroviruses.

The present findings strongly favor the possibility that the v-fes and v-fps sequences correspond to a common cellular genetic locus which has been highly conserved throughout vertebrate evolution (10). Thus tyrosine-specific protein kinase activities associated with the translational product of such sequences (1,6,12-16,20) have probable functional significance to their host. Although the mammalian homologs of other avian retrovirus encoding tyrosine specific protein kinases have not been characterized, the human homolog of the mouse v-abl has been identified, molecularly cloned, and shown to be independent of the v-fes/v-fps locus (unpublished observations).

To date, the human c-fes/c-fps sequence has lacked detectable transforming activity upon transfection to cultured fibroblast cells. It seems highly probable, however, that this sequence has oncogenic potential considering the frequent representation of analogous sequences in transforming retroviruses isolated from species as widely divergent as the chicken and cat. The inability to demonstrate transforming activity by transfection could reflect either a block to c-fes/c-fps expression at the level of transcription, or the requirement for secondary mutations for the generation of sequences with transforming function. The recent development of hybridomas producing monoclonal antibody specific for the fes gene product should be of value in resolving these alternative possibilities (21).

The human carcinoma DNA cosmid library generated in the present study provides a unique reagent for the molecular cloning of cellular homologs of viral transforming genes. In particular, this library should be valuable for the isolation of those human transforming genes with extensive

FIGURE 3. Comparison of v-fes and v-fps homologous sequences within the c-fes/c-fps human genetic locus. Open boxes (▢) within the viral genomes represent the relative positions of acquired cellular sequences, whereas FeLV cross reactive sequences are shown as solid lines (▬). The position of long terminal repeats (▨) and cellular flanking sequences (——) are also indicated. The 12.0-kb EcoRI restriction fragment shown in the center of the figure contains all detectable v-fes and v-fps homologous human DNA sequences. Restriction fragments hybridizing to GA-v-fes; ST-v-fes; v-fes S_L; v-fes S_R; and FSV-v-fps are indicated as solid bars in the upper portion of the figure. The position of the 12.0-kb EcoRI fragment within a 58-kb contiguous sequence of human cellular DNA is indicated by the dotted diagonal lines. The restriction map of this latter sequence was deduced as a composite of individually mapped overlapping cellular sequences represented within the cosmids shown at the bottom of the figure. The relative positions of the tk gene, cos site, and SV40 restriction fragment within the 9-kb vector is shown for purposes of orientation. Hybridization of EcoRI restriction fragments within the inserted cellular sequence of one such cosmid clone (cos-5) with GA-v-fes (B) and FSV-v-fps (C) (^{32}P)-labeled probes are shown on the right side of the figure. Restriction enzymes include: AvaI (A); BamHI (B); EcoRI (E); HindIII (H); KpnI (K); PstI (P); SmaI (Sm); Sst (Ss); Xba (Xb); and XhoI (Xh).

intervening sequences such as c-abl. An important feature of this system is the presence of a functionally active thymidine kinase gene allowing for selection of minority populations of eukaryotic cells containing such cosmids following transfection. In addition, SV40 DNA sequences situated in one of the cosmid arms have been shown to exert a positive influence on transcription in the globin system (11). If this sequence similarly influences expression of cellular homologs of viral transforming genes, its presence may be an important factor for identification of the translational products of these sequences and a determination of their transforming potential.

ACKNOWLEDGEMENT

We thank G. T. Blennerhassett and P. Hansen for excellent technical assistance. This work was supported under Public Health Service Contract No. NOI-CO-75380 and by Grant No. CA-14935 from the National Cancer Institute.

REFERENCES

1. Barbacid M, Beemon K, Devare SG (1980): Proc Natl Acad Sci USA 77: 5158
2. Barbacid M, Breitman ML, Lauver AV, Long LK, Vogt PK (1981): Virology 110:411
3. Beemon K (1981): Cell 24:145
4. Coffin JM, Varmus HE, Bishop JM, Essex M, Hardy WD Jr., Martin GS, Rosenberg NE, Scolnick EM, Weinberg RA, Vogt PK (1981): J Virol 40:953
5. Fedele LA, Even J, Garon CF, Donner L, Sherr CJ (1981): Proc Natl Acad Sci USA 78:4036
6. Feldman RA, Hanafusa T, Hanafusa H (1980): Cell 22:757
7. Fischinger PJ (1980): In: Molecular Biology of RNA Tumor Viruses (Stephenson JR, ed), New York: Academic Press, pp 163-198
8. Franchini G, Even J, Sherr CJ, Wong-Staal F (1981): Nature 290:154
9. Groffen J, Heisterkamp N, Grosveld F, Van de Ven WJM, Stephenson JR (1982): Science 216:1136
10. Groffen J, Heisterkamp N, Shibuya M, Hanafusa H, Stephenson JR (1983): Virology 125:480
11. Grosveld F, Lund T, Murray EJ, Mellor AL, Dahl HHM, Flavell RA (1982): Nucleic Acids Res 10:6715
12. Kawai S, Yoshida M, Segawa K, Sugiyama H, Ishizaki R, Toyoshima K (1980): Proc Natl Acad Sci USA 77:6199
13. Neil JC, Ghysdael J, Vogt PK (1981): Virology 109:223
14. Pawson T, Guyden J, Kung T-H, Radke K, Gilmore T, Martin GS (1980): Cell 22:767
15. Reynolds FH Jr, Van de Ven WJM, Blomberg J, Stephenson JR (1981): J Virol 37:643
16. Reynolds FH Jr, Van de Ven WJM, Stephenson JR (1980): J Biol Chem 255:11040
17. Shibuya M, Hanafusa T, Hanafusa H, Stephenson JR (1980): Proc Natl Acad Sci USA 77:6536
18. Shibuya M, Wang L-W, Hanafusa H (1982): J Virol 42:1007

19. Stephenson JR, Todaro GJ (1982): In: Advances in Viral Oncology (Klein G, ed), New York: Raven Press, pp 59-81
20. Van de V3n WJM, Reynolds FH Jr, Stephenson JR (1980): Virology 101:185
21. Veronese F, Kelloff GJ, Reynolds, FH Jr, Hill RW, Stephenson JR (1982): J Virol 43:896

Gene Transfer and Cancer, edited by M. L. Pearson and N. L. Sternberg. Raven Press, New York © 1984.

Characterization of Four Members of the P21 Gene Family Isolated from Normal Human Genomic DNA and Demonstration of Their Oncogenic Potential

*,†Esther H. Chang, ‡Mathew A. Gonda, **Mark E. Furth, †Jerome L. Goodwin, §Shirley S. Yu, **Ronald W. Ellis, **Edward M. Scolnick, and *Douglas R. Lowy

*Dermatology Branch and **Laboratory of Tumor Virus Genetics, National Cancer Institute, Bethesda, Maryland 20205; †Department of Pathology, Uniformed Services University of the Health Sciences, Bethesda, Maryland 20014; ‡NCI-Frederick Cancer Research Facility, Frederick, Maryland 21701; and §Meloy Laboratory, Springfield, Virginia 22151*

ABSTRACT. We have studied the structure and function of the p21 gene family in human cells. Using probes derived from the v-onc genes of Harvey murine sarcoma virus (Ha-MuSV) and Kirsten murine sarcoma virus (Ki-MuSV), called v-Ha-ras and v-Ki-ras, respectively, we molecularly cloned from normal human genomic DNA four distinct restriction endonuclease fragments. Two (called c-Ha-ras1 and c-Ha-ras2) preferentially hybridized to v-Ha-ras; two (called c-Ki-ras1 and c-Ki-ras2) hybridized to v-Ki-ras. These ras clones contain all the sequences in human DNA that hybridize to these probes under our hybridization conditions.

Human c-Ha-ras1, with three intervening sequences, contained 0.9-kb homology with v-Ha-ras; c-Ha-ras1 contained even more homology with the previously isolated rat c-Ha-ras gene with 3 intervening sequences. Human c-Ha-ras2 diverged from v-Ha-ras more than c-Ha-ras1 and did not appear to contain intervening sequences. c-Ki-ras1, with a single intervening sequence, contained 0.9-kb homology with v-Ki-ras, whereas c-Ki-ras2 had only 0.3 kb homology with v-Ki-ras or c-Ki-ras1.

After ligation of a long terminal repeat, derived from either Ha-MuSV or Gardner feline sarcoma virus, 0.5 kb upstream from the 5' end of the region homologous to v-Ha-ras, foci of transformed NIH/3T3 cells were induced by transfection. The DNA in the transformants contained the LTR ligated to c-Ha-ras1. Using a monoclonal antibody that reacts specifically with v-Ha-ras or rat c-Ha-ras, high levels p21 were precipitated. This p21 was similar to that induced by the rat c-Ha-ras gene with intervening sequences and was distinguishable from the viral p21 both in its migration rate in one-dimensional gel electrophoresis and in its lack of

phosphorylation at a threonine residue. The transformed cells formed
tumors in nude mice.

We conclude that human cells contain several p21 genes and that high
levels of the p21 encoded by at least one of these genes can induce oncogenic transformation.

INTRODUCTION

The transforming genes (v-onc) of RNA tumor viruses have recently been
found to be derived from a group of normal cellular homologs (c-onc) of
avian, rodent, and nonprimate origin. These c-onc genes are evolutionarily highly conserved (15). The gene products encoded by the v-onc
genes of several viruses have been identified. Low levels of immunologically related proteins have been detected in normal cells of many vertebrate species. The relationship between the viral transforming genes and
their cellular homologs is an interesting and important area to study. In
this report, we will concentrate on the v-onc genes of two of these transforming viruses, Ha-MuSV (13) and Ki-MuSV (14) and on their c-onc genes
(8,10).

RESULTS AND DISCUSSION

p21-coding (ras) Gene Family

Ha-MuSV and Ki-MuSV belong to a subgroup of viruses encoding a transforming protein of 21 kd (p21) (24). The viral genes which specify p21
are called v-ras (7). Four p21 coding sarcoma viruses have been identified. Ha-MuSV was isolated from the plasma of a Chester-Beatty rat following inoculation of Moloney murine leukemia virus. Ki-MuSV was isolated
after repeated passages of Kirsten murine leukemia virus, a helper independent virus also of mouse origin, through Wistar-Furth rats. The two
other members of p21 coding viruses are BALB murine sarcoma virus (B-MuSV)
(1,20) which was isolated from a BALB mouse, and the rat murine sarcoma
virus (R-MuSV) (21,29). The latter virus was isolated from cultured
Sprague-Dawley rat cells cocultivated with any of several chemically
transformed rat cell lines. Both B-MuSV and R-MuSV have transduced a
Harvey-type c-onc gene (1,29). Although Ha-MuSV, Ki-MuSV and R-MuSV were
isolated from different strains of rats and B-MuSV was isolated from mice,
the viruses encode proteins that cross-react immunologically and are
functionally related (19,22-24). All the viral p21s bind guanine nucleoside phosphates (GDP and GTP) noncovalently, but do not bind adenine
nucleoside phosphates (22).

These four viruses are highly tumorigenic in vivo and transform many
kinds of human and rodent cells, including primary and epithelial cells.
The transformed cells express high levels of p21. Like other transforming
retroviruses, these four viruses have been found to have acquired a fragment of their host cell sequences.

Results obtained from peptide mapping of Ha-MuSV and Ki-MuSV p21 demonstrated that these viral p21s are homologous in only 2/3 of their tryptic
peptides (10). DNA sequencing of the p21 coding region of the viral genomes has confirmed these findings and has localized most of their amino
acid divergence to the C-terminus of the protein (9,26). The v-ras sequences of both Ha-MuSV and Ki-MuSV were found to be composed of about
1 kb of evolutionarily conserved host cellular sequences (called c-ras)
(10). These rat-derived sequences were located in the 5' half of the

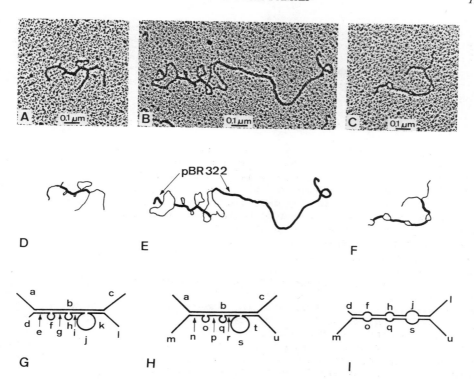

FIGURE 1. Heteroduplex analyses of v-Ha-<u>ras</u> (<u>BamHI-EcoRI</u>, 2.3-kb insert),
rat c-Ha-<u>ras</u>1 (<u>EcoRI-XbaI</u>, 2.3-kb insert), and human c-Ha-<u>ras</u>1 (<u>Sac</u>1, 2.9-
kb insert) pBR322 clones (5). Heteroduplexes v-Ha-<u>ras</u> x rat c-Ha-<u>ras</u>1 and
rat c-Ha-<u>ras</u>1 x human c-Ha-<u>ras</u>1 were prepared from the insert. The v-Ha-
<u>ras</u> x human c-Ha-<u>ras</u>1 heteroduplex was formed from the intact clones
after <u>Sal</u>I cleavage. Electron micrograph, interpretive tracing and schematic drawing of v-Ha-<u>ras</u> x rat c-Ha-<u>ras</u>1 are shown in A, D, and E respectively. B, E, and H represent v-Ha-<u>ras</u> x human c-Ha-<u>ras</u>1 and C, F, and
I represent rat c-Ha-<u>ras</u>1 x human c-Ha-<u>ras</u>1. The methods for preparing
heteroduplex molecules were as described previously (8,28). The heteroduplex molecules were spread from a hyperphase containing 60% formamide,
0.1 M Tris, pH 8.5, and 0.01 M EDTA onto a hypophase of 18% formamide.
The contour lengths in kb, based on measurements of 15 molecules were
as follows: a = 0.56 ± 0.07, b = 1.00 ± 0.07, c = 0.68 ± 0.04, d = 0.05
± 0.1, e = 0.24 ± 0.03, f = 0.22 ± 0.03, g = 0.19 ± 0.03, h = 0.21 ±
0.20, i = 0.18 ± 0.02, j = 0.89 ± 0.04, k = 0.35 ± 0.05, l = 3.4 ± 0.30,
m = 1.00 ± 0.09, n = 0.14 ± 0.01, o = 0.31 ± 0.03, p = 0.18 ± 0.02, q =
0.21 ± 0.02, r = 0.19 ± 0.02, s = 0.76 ± 0.07, t = 0.27 ± 0.04, u =
1.01 ± 0.09. Contour lengths for v-Ha-<u>ras</u> (a-c) and rat c-Ha-<u>ras</u>1 (d-i)
are from values previously published (8). Human c-Ha-<u>ras</u>1 clone = m-u
and human c-Ha-<u>ras</u>1 = n-t. The values of the four duplexes in I are
0.21, 0.30, 0.39 and 0.33 kb. The letter designations are merely to
show the location of the various flanking and intervening sequences. The
duplexed regions between the lettered features in I represent the homologous portions of the Ha-<u>ras</u> gene but also include some regions of homology between the intervening sequences.

Ha and Ki genomes (6,27,28). The sequence divergence between v-Ha-ras and
v-Ki-ras was such that ras probes derived from v-Ha-ras or v-Ki-ras detected different restriction endonuclease fragments in various normal
vertebrate DNAs. These results suggested that the c-ras genes are a
multigene family of divergent genes that are conserved throughout evolution (5,10).

Structure of Rat and Human c-ras Genes

In order to study the c-ras genes in more detail, and to demonstrate
directly the existence of several ras genes, we used the v-Ha-ras or v-Ki-
ras probes to molecularly clone some of these c-ras sequences from genomic
rat (8) and human DNA libraries (5). Two c-Ha-ras genes have been isolated from each species, and two c-Ki-ras genes have been isolated from human
DNA. Both rat c-Ha-ras clones contained 0.9-kb sequences homologous to
in v-Ha-ras. The 0.9-kb region of homology in one clone (designated rat
c-Ha-ras1) was interspersed with 3 sets of intervening sequences. In the
second rat clone (rat-c-Ha-ras2) the region of homology was colinear with
v-Ha-ras (8).

One human Ha clone (human c-Ha-ras1), isolated from a HaeIII-limit
digest library (18) contained an 18-kb insert. In this insert of human
DNA, the sequences that hybridize to v-Ha-ras are contained in 8.5-kb
BglII, 6.6-kb BamHI, or 3-kb SacI fragments. The 3-kb SacI fragment
subcloned in pBR322 HLTR clone 5, has been studied in greatest detail.
Heteroduplexes formed between this clone of human c-Ha-ras1 and v-Ha-ras
have homologous 0.9-kb sequences (Figure 1). As was also true of rat
c-Ha-ras1, human c-Ha-ras1 was interrupted by 3 sets of intervening
sequences. The structure of this human gene therefore resembles that of
rat c-Ha-ras1, since both genes contain four exons of similar size.
Heteroduplexes formed between these two clones revealed 1.2 kb of homology,
0.3-0.4 kb longer than the homologous sequences in v-Ha-ras and either
c-Ha-ras1 gene. Since length of each substitution loop was shorter than
that for the corresponding intervening sequence in the heteroduplex with
the viral DNA, the homology between these two genes apparently extends
beyond the exons and includes portions of each intervening sequence.
Conservation within the same intervening sequences has also been found
between other human rodent genes, such as globin (16).

The second human c-Ha-ras clone contained a 15-kb EcoRI insert; it was
isolated from an EcoRI-limit digest library (25). This clone was designated human c-Ha-ras2. A 2.7-kb BamHI/EcoRI fragment contained all the
sequences homologous with v-Ha-ras (Figure 2). Analysis of heteroduplex-
ing under usual spreading conditions (60% formamide and 0.1 M Tris pH 8.5)
has shown a duplex of 0.4 kb with v-Ha-ras. When lowering the hybridization stringency (30% formamide and 0.1 M Tris pH 8.5), a longer homologous sequence of 0.6-0.7 kb was observed.

Both human c-Ki-ras fragments were isolated from the HaeIII-limit
digest library (18). A 3.8-kb HindIII fragment from one recombinant and
a 3-kb EcoRI fragment from the other contained all the sequences of each
clone homologous to v-Ki-ras (Figure 3). These clones were designated
c-Ki-ras1 and c-Ki-ras2, respectively.

The structure of both c-Ki-ras genes was analyzed by forming heteroduplexes between v-Ki-ras and each human c-Ki-ras gene. 0.9 kb of homology was detected between v-Ki-ras and c-Ki-ras1. There was a 0.2-kb
intervening sequence in c-Ki-ras1 located 0.6 kb downstream from the 5'
end of the homologous region. By contrast, only 0.3 kb of homology was
found between v-Ki-ras1 and c-Ki-ras2. Lowering the hybridization strin-

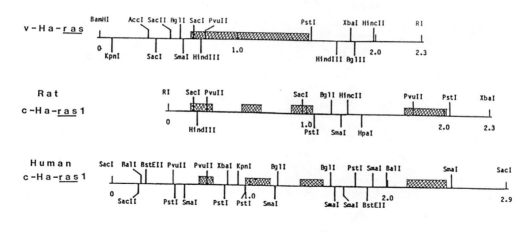

FIGURE 2. Restriction endonuclease maps in kbp of v-Ha-<u>ras</u> and c-Ha-<u>ras</u> sequences. As compiled from Southern blot hybridization, heteroduplex analysis and partial sequence analysis (Chang et al., unpublished data). The homologous v-Ha-<u>ras</u> and c-Ha-<u>ras</u> sequences in the four fragments are highlighted by crosshatches.

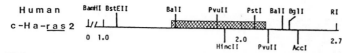

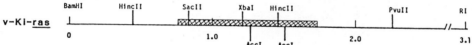

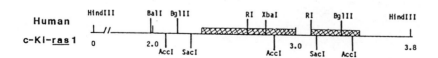

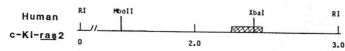

FIGURE 3. Restriction endonuclease maps in kbp of v-Ki-<u>ras</u> and c-Ki-<u>ras</u> sequences based on Southern blot hybridization and heteroduplex analysis. The homologous v-Ki-<u>ras</u> and c-Ki-<u>ras</u> sequences in the three fragments are highlighted by crosshatches.

gency did not increase the length of the duplexed DNA. Since almost 600 nucleotides are required to encode p21, this 0.3 kb homology presumably represents only a portion of the p21 coding sequences.

Transforming Activity of Human c-Ha-ras1

It has been shown that two previously cloned c-<u>onc</u> retroviral homologs, mouse c-<u>mos</u> (2) and rat c-Ha-<u>ras</u>1 (8) when ligated to a viral LTR (the retroviral control element which contains sequences for activation, pro- motion, and transcription of RNA) upstream from the 5' end of the gene,

can transform NIH/3T3 cells. Given the conservation of c-Ha-ras1 in rat
and human genomes, we have first concentrated our effort in the human ras
genes on exploring the biological activity of c-Ha-ras1. The 18-kb recombinant, as well as the BamHI 6.6-kb fragment and the SacI 3.0-kb fragment
did not induce transformation in NIH/3T3 cells. This human gene can, however, induce oncogenic transformation of NIH/3T3 cells when an LTR is
present upstream (Figure 4). The transformants induce tumors in nude
mice and contain high levels of p21 (4). Analysis of genomic DNA from
transformants has revealed that both viral LTR and human c-Ha-ras1 sequences are present. These data suggest that normal cellular sequences
can transform upon upstream addition of an LTR leading to enhanced expression of downstream sequences. These results provide experimental evidence
that increased expression of a normal human gene product is one way by
which malignant transformation of cells can occur.

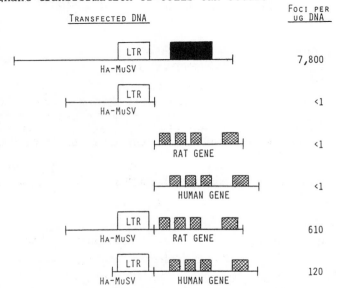

TRANSFECTED DNA

FOCI PER
ug DNA

7,800

<1

<1

<1

610

120

FIGURE 4. DNAs were precipitated with calcium chloride (11) and 0.2 ml
was added to 35-mm dishes seeded on the previous day with 2.25×10^5 NIH/
3T3 cells. Calf thymus DNA (25 µg/ml) was used as carrier. Each DNA
insert shown in the Table was cloned in pBR322; 0.1 or 0.2 µg of insert DNA was used per dish. The DNAs were added without digestion by a
restriction endonuclease. The cells were treated as described (17) except that dimethylsulfoxide was not used. Foci were counted 16 days
later. The viral LTR is represented by the open rectangle, v-Ha-ras by
the black rectangle, and the exons of c-Ha-ras1 (defined by their homology to v-Ha-ras) by the cross-hatched rectangles. Ha-MuSV DNA was genomic clone H-1, which is a 5.4-kb circularly permuted copy of the viral DNA
genome (3,8,12); Ha-MuSV LTR DNA was clone P-14 (4,10). Human c-Ha-ras1
DNA contained the 2.9-kb SacI fragment described in Figure 2; Ha-MuSV
LTR-human c-Ha-ras1 DNA was clone 6-2 (4). Ha-MuSV LTR rat c-Ha-ras1 DNA
was clone P-14 into which a 2.3-kb fragment of rat c-Ha-ras1 had been
inserted (by M. Haiken, R. Ellis, and E. Chang) at the BamHI site. This
2.3-kb fragment of rat c-Ha-ras1 extends from EcoRI to XbaI in clone
LHBE (8); these sites were converted (by R. Ellis) to BamHI by the addition of oligonucleotide linkers and cloned at the BamHI site in pBR322
(this latter clone is called LXBE).

ACKNOWLEDGEMENT

This work was supported in part by a NCI research support contract to Meloy Laboratories, Springfield, Virginia.

REFERENCES

1. Andersen P, Ellis RW, Tronick SR, Devare SG, Aaronson SA, Scolnick EM (1981): Cell 26:129
2. Blair DG, Oskarsson MK, Wood TG, McClements WL, Fischinger PJ, Vande Woude GF (1981): Science 212:941
3. Chang EH, Ellis RW, Scolnick EM, Lowy DR (1980): Science 210:1249
4. Chang EH, Furth ME, Scolnick EM, Lowy DR (1982): Nature 297:497
5. Chang EH, Gonda MA, Ellis RW, Scolnick EM, Lowy DR (1982): Proc Natl Acad Sci USA 79:4848
6. Chang EH, Maryak JM, Wei C-M, Shih TY, Shober R, Cheung HL, Ellis RW, Hager GL, Scolnick EM, Lowy DR (1980): J Virol 35:76
7. Coffin JM, Varmus HE, Bishop JM, Essex M, Hardy WD, Martin GS, Rosenberg NE, Scolnick EM, Weinberg RA, Vogt PK (1981): J Virol 40:953
8. DeFeo D, Gonda MA, Young HA, Chang Eh, Lowy DR, Scolnick EM, Ellis RW (1981): Proc Natl Acad Sci USA 78:3328
9. Dhar R, Ellis RW, Shih TY, Oroszlan S, Shapiro B, Maizel J, Lowy DR, Scolnick E (1982): Science 217:934
10. Ellis RW, DeFeo D, Shih TY, Gonda MA, Young HA, Tsuchida N, Lowy DR, Scolnick EM (1981): Nature 292:506
11. Graham FLM, Van der Eb, AJ (1973): Virology 52:456
12. Hager GL, Chang EH, Chan HW, Garon CF, Israel MA, Martin MA, Scolnick EM, Lowy DR (1979): J Virol 31:795
13. Harvey JJ (1964): Nature 204:1104
14. Kirsten WH, Mayer LA (1967): J Natl Cancer Inst 39:311
15. Klein G (ed) (1981): Advances in Viral Oncology: Cell-Derived Oncogenes (Volume 1). New York: Raven Press
16. Konkel DA, Majel JV Jr, Leder P (1975): Cell 18:865
17. Lowy DR, Rands E, Scolnick EMJ (1978): J Virol 26:291
18. Maniatis T, Hardison RC, Lacy E, Lauer U, O'Connell C, Quon D, Sim GK, Efstratiadis (1978): Cell 15:687
19. Papageorge AG, Lowy DR, Scolnick EM (1982) J Virol 44:509
20. Peters RL, Rabstein LS, Louise S, Van Vleck R, Kelloff GJ, Heubner RJ (1974): J Natl Cancer Inst 53:1725
21. Rasheed S, Gardner MB, Heubner RJ (1978): Proc Natl Acad Sci USA 75:2972
22. Scolnick EM, Papageorge AG, Shih TY (1979): Proc Natl Acad Sci USA 76:5355
23. Shih TY, Papageorge AG, Stokes PE, Weeks MO, Scolnick EM (1980): Nature 287:686
24. Shih TY, Weeks MO, Young HA, Scolnick EM (1979): Virology 96:64
25. Slightom JL, Blechl AE, Smithies O (1980): Cell 21:627
26. Tsuchida N, Ryder T, Ohtsubo E (1982): Science 217:937
27. Wei C-M, Lowy D, Scolnick EM (1980): Proc Natl Acad Sci USA 77:4674
28. Young HA, Gonda MA, DeFeo D, Ellis RW, Nagashima K, Scolnick, EM (1980): Virology 107:89
29. Young HA, Rasheed S, Sowder R, Benton CV, Henderson LE (1981): J Virol 38:286

Gene Transfer and Cancer, edited by M. L. Pearson
and N. L. Sternberg. Raven Press, New York © 1984.

Chromosomal Mapping of Tumor Virus Transforming Gene Analogs in Human Cells

*O. W. McBride, **D. C. Swan, **K. C. Robbins, **K. Prakash,
and **S. A. Aaronson

*Laboratories of *Biochemistry and **Cellular and Molecular Biology, National Cancer
Institute, National Institutes of Health, Bethesda, Maryland 20205*

ABSTRACT. A series of human/rodent hybrid somatic cell lines containing a reduced complement of human chromosomes has been analyzed to determine the chromosomal location of cellular onc genes in human cells. The
transforming gene (v-sis) of simian sarcoma virus (SSV) was subcloned in
pBR322 and the human homolog (c-mos) of the transforming gene (v-mos) of
Moloney murine sarcoma virus (MoMSV) was cloned from a human recombinant
phage library. Both v-sis and c-mos (human) were then used as molecular
probes for detection of the corresponding cellular genes in EcoRI-digested,
size-fractionated DNAs. By testing for the presence of v-sis and c-mos
(human) in somatic cell hybrids possessing varying numbers of human chromosomes, it was possible to assign c-sis and c-mos (human) to human chromosomes 22 and 8, respectively. The location of these cellular onc genes
is intriguing since very specific reciprocal translocations involving
each of these chromosomes have previously been associated with specific
human neoplasms. Neither the regional location of the onc genes relative
to the specific chromosomal break points in the neoplastic cells nor the
level of expression of these onc genes in the transformed cells has been
determined yet. We are currently using cloned probes for additional
human onc gene analogs (c-myb, c-myc, c-abl, and c-bas) to assign these
onc genes to specific human chromosomes.

INTRODUCTION

Transforming retroviruses have arisen by recombination of replication-
competent type C RNA viruses with evolutionarily well-conserved cellular
genes, termed onc genes (2). It is now well established that these genes
are required both for induction and maintenance of viral transformation in
vitro and in vivo. Among more than two dozen independent transforming
retrovirus isolates, some have been shown to possess highly related onc
sequences. These findings have indicated that the number of cellular genes
that can acquire transforming activity when incorporated within the retroviral genome may be limited. The protein products of some onc genes have
been identified (6), but their mechanism of action are not as yet well
understood.

Accumulating evidence suggests that neoplastic transformation may result
directly from the activation of onc genes within the cell. Highly efficient transformation by the cellular analogs of acute virus transforming

genes has been demonstrated after ligation of these cellular genes to a
viral long terminal repeat (LTR) (3-5). Hayward et al. (14) have shown
that in avian leukosis virus-induced B cell lymphomas, transcription of a
cellular analog (c-myc) of the transforming gene of an acute leukemia virus
(MC 29) is activated by integration of viral promoter sequences adjacent
to this cellular gene. They proposed a promoter insertion model for oncogenesis and suggested that activation of a c-onc gene may be the common
initiation event in neoplastic transformation by both viral and nonviral
agents. It has been suggested that specific chromosome translocations
associated with certain tumors may also provide a mechanism for activating
a cellular onc gene (17,34).

   The importance of cellular oncogenes also has been demonstrated by an
entirely different approach. Several groups have transformed normal mouse
cells with DNA isolated from human tumors and various tumor cell lines (8,
12,18-21,26,29,31,36,37). The results currently indicate that common
transforming genes may be activated in neoplasms of the same cell type
and that different transforming genes are activated in neoplasms of cells
at different stages of development (20,21,26,29). Moreover, some of
these transforming genes have been shown to have sequences homologous to
sequences in the onc genes found in acute transforming viruses (8,12,24,
31). Hence, it appears that the cellular onc genes found in these viruses
may be similar, or identical, to transforming genes in nonvirally induced
human tumors.

   Thus, acute transforming RNA tumor viruses provide a potentially valuable approach to elucidate the mechanisms involved in human malignancies.
We have used somatic cell hybrids to determine the chromosomal location
of several cellular onc genes. This information should facilitate an
evaluation of possible interactions of these genes with other genetic
elements.

                              RESULTS

   Analysis of somatic cell hybrids segregating human chromosomes allows
the localization of human genes to specific chromosomes. A chromosomal
assignment is dependent on concordant segregation of a gene with a single
chromosome, and discordant segregation of the gene with all other chromosomes in a large group of hybrid cell lines. Concordancy refers to
either retention or loss of both a chromosome and the gene from each
line, whereas independent segregation of a chromosome and the gene represents discordancy. Several large series of independent hybrid cell
lines were isolated in selective medium containing HAT (100 μM hypoxanthine, 1 μM amethopterin, and 16 μM thymidine) and 100 μM ouabain
after polyethylene glycol 1000-induced fusion of human cells with hprt⁻
or tk⁻ mutant rodent fibroblasts. Cloned hybrid lines were usually subcloned at least once to obtain segregant hybrid cell populations containing a reduced, and relatively homogeneous, content of specific human
chromosomes. Since at least one enzyme marker has been assigned to each
human chromosome, the specific human chromosome content of each hybrid
cell line or subclone was determined by standard isoenzyme analyses (13,
27) and sometimes confirmed by karyotyping (35,40). DNA was simultaneously
isolated from these same hybrid cell populations, and DNA fragments were
transferred to nitrocellulose after restriction endonuclease digestions
and agarose gel electrophoresis. Hybridization of the transferred DNA
with isotopically labeled, cloned DNA probes thereby permitted assignments
of genes to specific human chromosomes. It was possible to distinguish human
onc sequences from corresponding sequences present in rodent DNAs by dif-

ferences in DNA fragment sizes after digestion with appropriate restriction enzymes.

The primate cell-derived transforming gene v-sis of SSV has been assigned to a specific human chromosome by this procedure (38). The full length linear 5.2-bp SSV genome (Figure 1A) contains a 1.0-bp segment of helper virus-unrelated information (v-sis) localized toward the 3' end with respect to SSV RNA (11,32). A 970-bp subgenomic SacI/DbaI fragment composed entirely of v-sis sequences was subcloned in pBR322, labeled with ^{32}P by nick translation, and used as a molecular probe for the detection of c-sis (human). Unlabeled hybrid DNA samples were digested with a restriction enzyme (EcoRI) which made it possible to distinguish c-sis (human) from corresponding sequences present in rodent DNAs. A single (20-bp) human DNA fragment hybridiz ing with the v-sis probe was readily distinguished from smaller sis-related fragments present in Chinese hamster and mouse DNA (Figure 1B).

Using hybridization of a v-sis probe to EcoRI-digested DNAs from 24 human/rodent somatic cell hybrids, we were able to detect the homologous human sequence in only 6 of these lines, and the results (Figure 2) indicate that c-sis is located on human chromosome 22. There were no discordancies between the segregation of c-sis (human) and chromosome

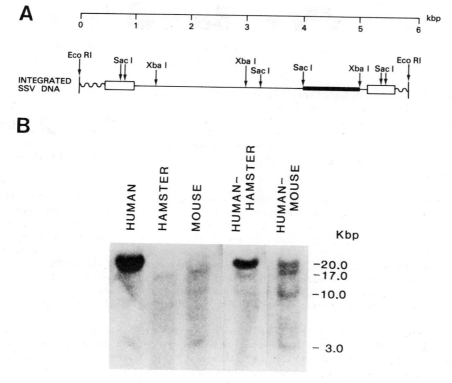

FIGURE 1. (A) Map of the cloned SSV genome. ☐ denotes the LTR sequences; ■ denotes the v-sis transforming region. (B) Hybridization of v-sis to EcoRI-digested DNAs. Human placenta, Chines hamster kidney, and mouse liver DNAs were digested with EcoRI, size-fractionated by 1% agarose gel elecrophoresis, transferred to nitrocellulose, and hybridized with a ^{32}P-labeled v-sis probe. Individual DNA digests were run in the first three lanes; 1:1 mixtures of human: Chinese hamster and human: mouse DNA digests were run in the remaining lanes (from ref. 38).

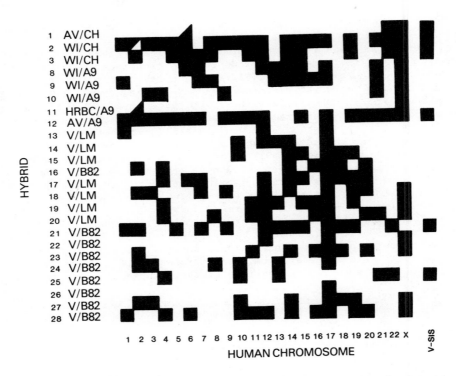

FIGURE 2. Human chromosome and c-<u>sis</u> (human) distribution in somatic cell hybrids. Individual hybrid cell lines are represented on the ordinate and specific human chromosomes on the abscissa. Solid squares indicate the presence of a particular chromosome in a hybrid line; symbols ◣ and ◢ indicate the presence of only the short arm or long arm, respectively. Solid squares in the last column indicate the presence of c-<u>sis</u> (human) (from ref 38).

22, whereas this sequence segregated discordantly ($\geq$ 21%) with all other human chromosomes except chromosome 5 (8% discordancy). The assignment of c-<u>sis</u> (human) to chromosome 22 was confirmed by two additional procedures. Four of the hybrid cell lines containing human chromosome 22 were subcloned (i.e., 8 to 12 subclones from each line) thereby permitting analysis after additional human chromsome segregation. An additional panel of 16 different human/Chinese hamster hybrid lines was also analyzed. Detection of c-<u>sis</u> (human) by molecular hybridization was concordant with chromosome 22 in all these lines and discordant with all other human chromosomes.

The human analog of the transforming gene (v-<u>mos</u>) from the MoMSV has been molecularly cloned and used as a probe to detect c-<u>mos</u> (human) sequences in human/rodent hybrid cell lines (30). <u>Eco</u>RI-restricted human placental DNA was fractionated by RPC-5 column chromatography and agarose gel electrophoresis. Fractions hybridizing to a labeled v-<u>mos</u> probe were ligated to <u>Eco</u>RI-cut λ Charon 16A DNA, packaged in vitro, plated onto <u>Escherichia coli</u> LE392, and a recombinant phage was detected by plaque hybridization. The purified recombinant contained a 2.5-kbp insert that hybridized with a v-<u>mos</u> probe under relaxed conditions. The extent of homology between c-<u>mos</u> (human) and v-<u>mos</u> was determined by

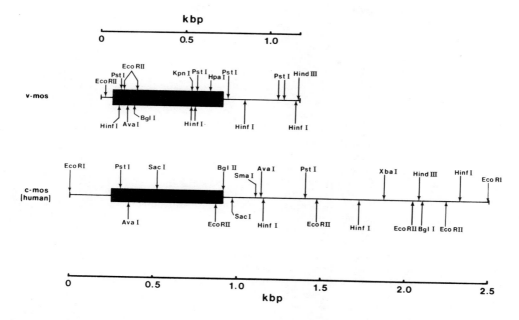

FIGURE 3. Comparison of the restriction enzyme maps of c-mos (human) and v-mos. The region of homology (0.65-kbp) between the two DNAs is indicated by a solid bar on each molecule; homology was determined by heteroduplex analysis and by analysis of restriction digests of each DNA with a labeled probe prepared from the alternate DNA mos-related sequence (from ref 30).

heteroduplex analysis and by reciprocal restriction analyses of MoMSV DNA with a c-mos (human) probe and c-mos (human) with a v-mos probe (Figure 3). Based upon the combined results from heteroduplex and restriction analyses, it was concluded that these two sequences contain 0.65-kbp uninterrupted region of homology commencing about 100 bp from the 5' terminus of the 1.15-kbp v-mos sequence.

Hybridization of the c-mos (human) DNA probe to size fractionated, Eco-RI-digested DNAs from a panel of 24 human/rodent somatic cell hybrids detected this human sequence in 7 of these lines. Rodent mos-related sequences were not detected under the stringent hybridization conditions used. Analysis of the human chromosome content of these 24 hybrid cell lines revealed discordant segregation ($\geq$ 21%) of c-mos with all human chromosomes except chromosome 8. This chromosome was present in the two human/Chinese hamster hybrids containing c-mos, but chromosome 8 could not be identified unambiguously in human/mouse hybrid cell lines. Sub-clones of two human/Chinese hamster hybrids containing c-mos were then analyzed and concordant segregation of chromosome 8 and c-mos was found in these 22 subclones. Two additional panels of human/Chinese hamster hybrids were also analyzed (Figure 4) and concordancy (11 positive/20 total) of c-mos with chromosome 8 was observed. Discordant segregation ($\geq$ 20%) of c-mos with all other chromosomes except chromsome 19 (5% dis-cordancy) was found in this series. However, chromosome 19 segregated discordantly (46%) with c-mos in the original series of 24 hybrid cell lines and in human/Chinese hamster subclones. The combination of these results provides an unambiguous assignment of c-mos to human chromosome

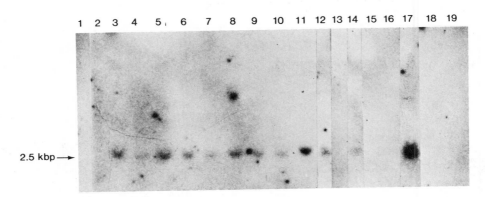

FIGURE 4: Chromosomal mapping of c-<u>mos</u> (human). DNAs isolated from human/
hamster somatic cell hybrids and controls were digested with <u>Eco</u>RI, size
fractionated by 0.7% agarose gel electrophoresis, transferred to nitrocellulose, and hybridized with a ^{32}P-labeled c-<u>mos</u> (human) probe. Lanes 1
through 16 represent hybrid cell DNAs; lanes 17, 18, and 19 represent
human placenta, Chinese hamster, and λ (<u>Hin</u>dIII cut) DNAs, respectively.
A 2.5-kbp <u>Eco</u>RI fragment hybridizing with c-<u>mos</u> human is present in all
lanes except 1, 2, 13, 15, 16, 18, and 19 (from ref. 30).

8. The human analogs of several other viral <u>onc</u> genes (c-<u>myb</u>, c-<u>myc</u>, c-
<u>abl</u>, c-<u>bas</u>) have been cloned and are presently being used as probes to
localize these genes to specific human chromosomes.

DISCUSSION

    As an approach toward examining the interactions of <u>onc</u> genes with
other cellular genetic elements, we have undertaken chromosomal mapping
of these genes. The procedures utilized molecular hybridization of
cloned c-<u>onc</u> (human) DNA probes to DNAs of human/rodent somatic cell
hybrids that segregate human chromosomes. By analysis of a large number
of hybrid cell lines containing different numbers of human chromosomes,
as well as segregant subclones, it was possible to assign c-<u>sis</u> (human)
and c-<u>mos</u> (human) to human chromosomes 22 and 8, respectively.
    Consistent and relatively specific chromosome translocations have
been reported in some human leukemias and lymphomas (33,34). The involvement of chromosome 8 in chromosomal rearrangements in Burkitt's lymphoma
and other B cell neoplasms has been documented (1,17,33,34,41). The
most frequent rearrangement in Burkitt's lymphoma is a reciprocal translocation between chromosome 14 and 8 (1,41), but two alternate reciprocal
translocations between 8 and chromosomes 2 and 22 have been described
(1). The break point on chromosome 8 (8q24) is consistent in all three
translocations (1). It is interesting that the human immunoglobulin
(Ig) genes for K (23,25) and λ (9, 25) light chains and the heavy chains
(7) are located on chromosomes 2, 22, and 14, respectively. It is also
relevant that the human heavy chain Ig genes have been localized to that
region of chromosome 14 (14q32) exhibiting the break site in Burkitt's
lymphomas both by in situ hybridization with a γ4 constant region
probe (16) and by analysis of somatic cell hybrids containing a human
14q32 translocation using hybridization with V_H, D_H, J_H, and C_E probes

(W. McBride, J. Battey, G. Hollis, D. Swan and P. Leder, unpublished results). The kappa light chain genes have also been mapped to the same chromosome region ($2p_{12-13}$) as the break point in those Burkitt's lymphomas exhibiting the 2:8 translocation (23). Since Ig genes undergo both productive and aberrant rearrangements in lymphocytes (15), these events could include the activation of a cellular onc gene by the rare translocation of a portion of an Ig locus to the vicinity of an onc gene as proposed by Klein (17) and Rowley (34). The report by Lenoir et al. (22) of complete concordance between the class of secreted Ig light chains in lymphomas and the specific chromosome translocation (i.e., 2:8 or 8:22 translocations are associated with K or λ light chain secretion, respectively) is consistent with this hypothesis, although it makes some potentially simple mechanisms for onc gene activation unlikely. Analogous translocations involving chromosome 15 and chromosomes bearing kappa (chromosome 6) and heavy chain (chromosome 12) genes also have been reported in mouse plasmacytomas (28).

The location of the analog of v-mos to human chromosome 8 indicates that c-mos (human) is a possible candidate for activation in human B cell lymphomas. Blair et al. (3,4) have shown highly efficient transformation with c-mos (mouse) ligated to a viral LTR. There is still uncertainty whether c-mos (human) can be similarly activated. It is possible that other human onc gene analog(s) may also be located on chromosome 8. Another nonrandom reciprocal translocation involving chromosome 8 has been reported (34) in acute myeloblastic leukemia but the localization (8q22) and reciprocal chromosme (21q22) differ from those involved in B cell neoplasms.

The localization of c-sis (human) on chromosome 22 is interesting. Chronic myelogenous leukemia (CML) was the first human neoplastic disease to be associated with a specific chromosome rearrangement, the Philadelphia (Ph') chromosome, and this most frequently represents a reciprocal 9:22 translocation (34). The constant break point (22q11) is similar to that reported in B cell neoplasms involving an 8:22 translocation, but chromosomal banding is not sufficiently sensitive to preclude a difference as large as 5,000 to 10,000 kbp in the actual break point sites in these two neoplasms. The failure to detect sis-related transcripts (39) in one cell line derived from a patient with CML and in fresh cells from a patient in CML blast crisis currently argues against activation of c-sis by this translocation involving chromosome 22. In situ hybridization has shown sis to be located at 22q13 (I. Kirsch, personal communication) which may also argue against its possible activation by such chromosomal translocations.

Evaluation of the possibility that human neoplasms arise by activation of cellular onc genes (14,17,34) will be facilitated by the assignment of human onc gene analogs to specific chromosomes, and regional chromosomal assignments will also be important. Those neoplasms involving consistent chromosome translocations can be especially useful for this analysis. It should be possible to detect the activation of specific cellular onc genes by blot hybridization of fractionated RNA with cloned onc sequence probes (10,14,39). It is also important to determine whether there are DNA sequence alterations in the vicinity of specific onc genes in tumors by restriction endonuclease analyses and examination of phage or cosmid libraries prepared from tumor cell lines.

REFERENCES

1. Bernheim A, Berger R, Lenoir G (1981): Cancer Genet Cytogenet 3:307

2. Bishop JM (1978): Annu Rev Biochem 47:35.
3. Blair DG, Oskarsson M, Wood TG, McClements WL, Fischinger PJ, Vande Woude GF (1981): Science 212:941
4. Blair DG, McClements WL, Wood TG, Vande Woude GF (1983): this volume
5. Chang EH, Gonda MA, Ellis RW, Furth ME, Scolnick EM, Lowy DR (1983): this volume
6. Cold Spring Harbor Symp Quant Biol (1980) 44:721
7. Croce CM, Shander M, Martinis J, Cicurel L, D'Ancona GG, Dolby TW, Koprowski H (1979): Proc Natl Acad Sci USA 76:3416
8. Der CJ, Krontiris TG, Cooper GM (1982): Proc Natl Acad Sci USA 79: 3637
9. Erikson J, Martinis J, Croce CM (1981): Nature 294:173
10. Eva A, Robbins KC, Andersen PR, Srinivasan A, Tronick SR, Reddy EP, Ellmore NW, Galen AT, Lautenberger JA, Papas TS, Westin EH, Wong-Staal F, Gallo RC, Aaronson SA (1982): Nature 295:116
11. Gelman EP, Wong-Staal F, Kramer RA, Gallo RC (1981): Proc Natl Acad Sci USA 78:3373
12. Goldfarb M, Shimizu K, Perucho M, Wigler M (1983): This volume
13. Harris H, Hopkinson DA (1976): In: Handbook of Enzyme Electro-phoresis in Human Genetics, Amsterdam: North Holland Publishing Co.
14. Hayward WS, Neel BG, Astrin SM (1981): Nature (Lond) 290:475
15. Heiter PA, Korsmeyer SJ, Waldman TA, Leder P (1981): Nature 290:368
16. Kirsch IR, Morton CC, Nakahara K, Leder P (1982): Science 216:301
17. Klein G (1981): Naturae 294:313
18. Krontiris TG, Cooper GM (1981): Proc Natl Acad Sci USA 78:1181
19. Lane MA, Sainten AC, Cooper GM (1981): Proc Natl Acad Sci USA 78: 5185
20. Lane MA, Sainten AC, Cooper GM (1982): Cell 28:873
21. Lane MA, Sainten AC, Cooper GM (1982): this volume
22. Lenoir GM, Preud'homme JL, Bernheim A, Berger R (1982) Nature 298: 474
23. Malcolm S, Barton P, Bentley DL, Ferguson-Smith MA, Murphy CS, Rab-bits TH (in press): In Human Gene Mapping VI, Basel: Karger
24. Marx JL (1982): Science 216:724
25. McBride OW, Hieter PA, Hollis GF, Swan D, Otey MC, Leder P (1982): J Exp Med 155:1480
26. Murray MJ, Shilo BZ, Shih C, Cowing D, Hsu HW, Weinberg RA (1981): Cell 25:355
27. Nichols EA, Ruddle FH (1973): J Histochem Cytochem 21:1066
28. Ohno S, Babonits M, Weiner F, Spira J, Klein G, Potter, M (1979): Cell 18:1001
29. Perucho M, Goldfarb M, Shimizu K, Lama C, Fogh J, Wigler M (1981): Cell 27:467
30. Prakash K, McBride OW, Swan DC, Devare SG, Tronick SR, Aaronson SA (1982) Proc Natl Acad Sci USA 79:5210
31. Pulciani S, Santos E, Lauver AV, Long LK, Robbins KC, Barbacid M (1982): Proc Natl Acad Sci USA 79:2845
32. Robbins KC, Devare SG, Aaronson SA (1981): Proc Natl Acad Sci USA 78:2918.
33. Rowley JD (1980): Annu Rev Genet 14:17
34. Rowley JD (1982): Science 216:749
35. Seabright M (1971): Lancet II:971
36. Shih C, Padhy LC, Murray M, Weinberg RA (1981): Nature 290:261
37. Shih C, Weinberg RA (1982): Cell 29:161
38. Swan DC, McBride OW, Robbins KC, Keithley DA, Reddy EP, Aaronson SA (1982): Proc Natl Acad Sci USA 79:4691

39. Westin EH, Wong-Staal F, Gelmann EP, Favera RD, Papas TS, Lauten-
    berger JA, Eva A, Reddy EP, Tronick SR, Aaronson SA, Gallo RC
    (1982): Proc Natl Acad Sci USA 79:2490
40. Wyandt HE, Wysham DG, Mindern SK, Anderson RS, Hecht F (1976):
    Exp Cell Res 102:85
41. Zech L, Maglund U, Nilsson K, Klein G (1976):   Int J Cancer 17:47

Gene Transfer and Cancer, edited by M. L. Pearson and N. L. Sternberg. Raven Press, New York © 1984.

Cellular Oncogenes: Enhancement of Their Expression in Animal and Human Tumors

[1]U. G. Rovigatti and S. M. Astrin

Institute for Cancer Research, Fox Chase Cancer Center, Philadelphia, Pennsylvania 19111

ABSTRACT. The expression of the cellular oncogene chicken c-myc is enhanced several fold in bursal lymphomas induced by avian leukosis virus (ALV). Integration of the ALV provirus next to c-myc activates its transcription by providing a strong viral promoter. This mechanism of oncogenesis has been called promoter insertion and represents an interesting model for in vivo tumorigenesis by activation of a cellular oncogene. With this model in mind, we collected samples from patients with acute lymphoblastic leukemia (ALL), chronic lymphocytic leukemia (CLL), and non-Hodgkin's lymphoma (NHL) for the purpose of analyzing expression of human sequences homologous to retroviral oncogenes. An analysis of the transcripts present in peripheral blood leukocytes or lymph nodes from these patients was performed with the use of either v-myc (from MC29) or chicken c-myc as a probe. An elevated level of human c-myc transcripts was found in peripheral blood leukocytes (PBL) from some of the leukemia/lymphoma patients as compared to the level in PBL from normal donors. In addition, evidence was obtained that HL60, a human promyelocytic leukemia cell line expressing elevated myc transcripts, has an increased copy number of myc DNA sequences. The significance of these results will be discussed in relationship to possible mechanisms of oncogenesis.

INTRODUCTION

The notion that specific genes, called viral oncogenes, are present in the genome of the acutely transforming retroviruses and are responsible for in vitro transformation and in vivo tumorigenesis has been supported in the past 10 years by several pieces of evidence (70).

First of all, temperature-sensitive mutants have been isolated for several acutely transforming retroviruses. Their conditional mutation showed for the first time that a viral gene function was required not only for the establishment but also for the maintenance of transformation (33,43). Furthermore, genetic and biochemical studies have consistently shown that transformation-defective mutants lose a segment of the viral genome corresponding to a portion or the whole viral oncogene, where all

---

[1] Present address: Laboratory of Molecular Oncology, NCI-Frederick Cancer Research Facility, Frederick, Maryland 21701.

the temperature-sensitive mutants also mapped (5,19,60).

The gene products encoded by different viral oncogenes have been identified in several instances. In the best studied example, the helper-
independent (or replication nondefective) Rous sarcoma virus (RSV), a
protein of MW 60,000 is encoded by the RSV oncogene src (6,12). This
protein is phosphorylated and associated with a tyrosine-phosphorylating
activity (pp60 src). Furthermore, the presence of phosphotyrosine may
be associated with the transformed phenotype, since RSV-transformed cells
contain about 10 times as much phosphotyrosine in protein as uninfected
cells (41,57).

Finally, the development of recombinant DNA technology has led to the
isolation, cloning, and sequencing of several different viral oncogenes.
Purified oncogenes have been shown to cause in vitro transformation as
well as in vivo tumorigenesis. They have also been shown to encode the
specific transforming proteins, for example pp60 src and its tyrosine
phosphorylating activity in the case of RSV src, as previously mentioned
(1,14,21,23).

A second very important notion about oncogenes is the fact that they
are present as cellular oncogenes, a form very similar to the viral
genes, in the genomes of all the vertebrate species studied so far and
also in some invertebrate species (11,61,63). This general property has
two implications: 1) cellular oncogenes should encode for important
cellular functions, since they have been highly conserved throughout
evolution. These functions may be important in cellular physiology and
also in cellular differentiation and embryonic development, since differences in oncogene expression have been found in different cell types
and organs (10,25,58,59); 2) cellular oncogenes may be involved in in
vitro transformation or in vivo tumorigenesis. Preliminary evidence for
such a statement came from studies in which the transforming oncogene of
so-called recovered ASV was shown to be derived from the normal cellular
oncogene c-src (31,32). Other studies have shown that at least two different cellular oncogenes: c-mos and c-ras, which are normally inactive
and not capable of inducing transformation after transfection, can be
activated to a high level of expression and can transform NIH/3T3 cells
in culture after being linked to a strong viral promoter [present in the
Long Terminal Repeat (LTR)] (5,7,8).

To analyze the involvement of endogenous cellular oncogenes in tumorigenesis and transformation, we will discuss in this paper two different
systems, chicken B cell lymphomas induced by ALV and human lymphoid malignancies, such as ALL, CLL, and NHL.

RESULTS

Chicken B Cell Lymphomas

ALV causes B cell lymphomas 4 to 12 months after injection into day-
old chickens. Unlike the acutely transforming viruses, ALV does not
contain an oncogene, does not transform target cells in culture, and
induces neoplasia only after a long period of latency (70). The absence
of an oncogene in ALV and in other leukosis and leukemia viruses ruled
out the most obvious models for the mechanism of pathogenesis in ALV-
induced chicken B cell lymphomas. However, recent work from the laboratories of S.M. Astrin and W.S. Hayward has elucidated such a mechanism.

The structure of ALV suggested a mechanism of cellular activation. As
it is schematically represented in Figure 1, the ALV provirus contains
an LTR sequence that is repeated at both ends and is in direct contact

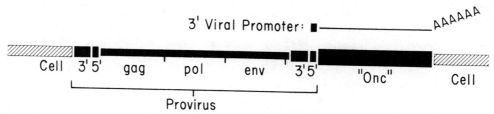

FIGURE 1. This figure briefly illustrates the promoter insertion model of viral leukemogenesis. The integrated provirus, with two viral LTRs, the cellular oncogene, and flanking cellular DNA sequences are represented. A scheme of the <u>onc</u> sequence transcript with viral sequences at the 5' end and a polyA stretch at the 3' end is presented above the DNA sequences. The <u>onc</u> sequence is in most of the lymphomas we have studied; <u>myc</u>, the cellular oncogene homologous to the MC29 virus transforming gene.

with the adjacent cellular sequences. As previously mentioned, an LTR contains a strong viral promoter that is utilized in the case of the left LTR for viral transcription (64,65). The right LTR could also promote transcription, in this case of the flanking cellular sequences. According to this model, now called the promoter insertion model, such a viral promoter would be able to integrate next to a cellular oncogene and to activate it, resulting in neoplastic transformation (Figure 1) (29,48). Predictions of the model are:

1) Assuming that ALV integrates randomly in the host genome, the integration event(s) leading to neoplastic transformation should be rare. Therefore, the outgrowing tumor and subsequent metastases should have a clonal origin.

2) Since oncogenes are probably limited in number (15 retroviral oncogenes have been identified so far) (11), it would be conceivable to find activation of the same oncogene in different tumors. Similar ALV integration sites are therefore expected.

3) Although the total provirus does not seem to be required for oncogene activation in the promoter insertion model, at least one of the two LTRs must be present in the tumors. Furthermore, transscripts containing the viral promoter covalently linked to cellular sequences should be specifically present in the tumor, but not present in infected nontumor cells.

All these predictions of the model have been tested and verified (2, 29,48,53a): 1) Clonality of the tumors and their metastases has been determined in most cases, with one possible exception. 2) At least five different clusters or classes of integration sites have been identified as present in one or more than one tumor. Furthermore, the cellular region flanking two different provirus integration classes was cloned and shown to contain the same sequence. This cellular sequence appeared to be normally present in the nontumor cell genome. In 85% of the lymphomas on the other hand, a new fragment was present beside the normal sequence. This new DNA fragment in most of the cases, comigrated with and was, therefore, adjacent to an ALV integration site. 3) Cellular transcripts covalently linked to the viral LTR were identified in the lymphomas. 4) Finally, W.S. Hayward et al. (29), utilizing retroviral oncogenes cDNA probes, showed that such cellular transcripts hybridized with a <u>myc</u> (Myelocytomatosis virus 29 oncogene) probe; in most of the chicken B cell lymphomas there was a 30- to 300-fold elevation of such c-myc RNA sequences.

Therefore, in about 85% of the ALV-induced chicken B cell lymphomas, the ALV provirus (often defective) is integrated next to a cellular oncogene (c-myc) and activates its transcription by providing a viral promoter. This event might be the initial step leading eventually to neoplastic transformation.

Human Leukemias and Lymphomas

The discovery of c-myc oncogene activation in ALV-induced chicken B cell lymphomas prompted us to investigate whether oncogene activation was also present in human leukemias and lymphomas. We analyzed total RNA extracted from peripheral blood leukocytes (PBL) obtained from different ALL, AML, and CML patients or from normal blood donors.

A typical experiment, where a difference was found between some of the patients' RNA and normal blood donors RNA, is shown in Figures 2A and 2B. Total RNA from an ALL patient, (KS), hybridized strongly with a v-myc probe (kindly provided by T. Papas). This result seemed to be consistent: different preparations from the same sample showed a similarity in the hybridization pattern [the lowest RNA concentration still hybridizing with the probe (2A:3,4,6)]. Additional patient RNA-positive samples included a NHL (Mi:2A:12) and a second ALL (JL:2B:10,11), whereas two additional patient samples (CLL: Me and F4; 2A:2,10,11) appeared to be negative for the hybridization with v-myc. Other samples were included as controls and they also appeared to be negative. Interestingly, total RNA extracted from PBL obtained from the parents and two brothers of the child with ALL (KS) showed low level of hybridization to v-myc (2B:2,3,6, 7,8) and the same ALL patient (KS) after chemotherapy and remission appeared to be negative for the hybridization with this oncogene probe (2B:4). From this and other experiments, we concluded that myc-related sequences might be expressed at higher level in some hematopoietic cells. Table I summarizes the data we have obtained with PBL from different patients and normal blood donors. Are myc sequences present only in lymphoid or hematopoietic cells? To answer this question, we have analyzed (in collaboration with P.O.P. Ts'o and R.K. Moyzis of The Johns Hopkins University) several samples obtained from normal human fibroblasts, human tumor cell lines and mouse or Syrian hamster embryos. As shown in Figure 3, total or poly-A-selected RNA extracted from such cell lines or embryos hybridized very weakly with our v-myc probe (even at high concentrations of RNA). In contrast to this result, a NHL patient showed a strong hybridization (Figure 3, lane 12), possibly even higher than our chicken B cell lymphoma control (Figure 3, lane 11) containing approximately 100 copies of c-myc RNA per cell (29). What is the cause of this differential expression of c-myc sequences? Even though it would be extremely difficult to completely answer this question, we have recently been very interested in detecting genetic differences which might explain this variation in myc sequences expression. Although we could not detect major differences by Southern blot analysis in the DNAs from patients' PBL, we found that a human promyelocytic leukemia cell line (HL60) contained a higher number of copies of myc related sequences. In Figure 4, two identical Southern blots have been hybridized with our v-myc probe at low (4A) and high (4B) stringency. A more intense hybridization band is clearly detected in the lane corresponding to HL60, particularly when high stringency conditions were used.

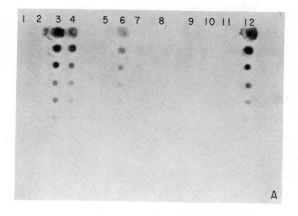

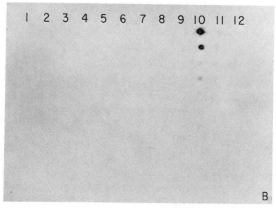

FIGURE 2. Example of c-myc sequence analysis by dot blot hybridization
with total cellular RNA extracted from normal blood donor PBL or leuke-
mia/lymphoma patient PBL. Dot blot analysis was performed as previously
described (2) and according to Thomas (66). The probe utilized in this
experiment was a chicken c-myc clone isolated from an ALV-induced lymphoma (47). In most of the other experiments, we have used a v-myc
clone kindly provided by T. Papas (39). The two probes gave essentially
identical results. An additional clone containing human c-myc sequences,
kindly provided by B.G. Neel and W.S. Hayward, gave similar results.
Samples and RNA amounts in the first dilution of dot blot experiments
are as follows: A and B) lanes 1, 5, and 9 wheat germ total RNA used as
a negative control (5 mg).
    A, lanes 3, 4, and 5) different RNA preparation from PBL of ALL pa-
tient (SK) (1.0; 0.7; and 0.5 mg, respectively; lane 7) ALL patient (SK),
bone marrow (BM) (0.5 mg); lane 8) normal blood donor (CR-2) PBL (0.5
mg); lanes 10 and 11) CL patient (Me) (PBL) (10) and BM (11) (1 mg);
lane 12) NHL patient (Mi) PBL (1 mg).
    B, lanes 2, 3, 6, 7, and 8) relatives of the ALL patient SK: total
RNA from PBL (0.5 mg); lane 10 and 11) ALL patients (JL). Fracations
enreached for lymphocytes (10) and granulocytes (12) (1 mg RNA).
    B, lane 12 and A lane 2) CLL patient (F4) PBL RNA (1 mg).

TABLE I. <u>myc</u> gene expression in PBL from normal and tumor samples.

	Number analyzed	Positive RNA hybridization with v-<u>myc</u>
Total normal blood donors	9	0
CLL	8	3
ALL	3	3
NHL	4	3
Total tumor samples	15	9

These results are particularly interesting in view of the fact that <u>myc</u> sequences are expressed at a level about 10- to 20-fold higher in the HL60 cell line (53b,71). The data are best explained by assuming that <u>myc</u>-related DNA sequences have been amplified in the HL60 cell line. The biological significance of these results is still not clear.

DISCUSSION

We have reported in this paper that the cellular oncogene c-<u>myc</u> is activated in ALV-induced chicken B cell lymphomas by the integration of the provirus next to the endogenous oncogene. We have also presented data showing that in some lymphoid and myeloid human neoplasias there is an elevated expression of c-<u>myc</u> sequences.

In the case of chicken B cell lymphomas, the mechanism of c-<u>myc</u> activation has been elucidated; in most of the tumors, the integrated provirus provides a strong viral promoter for transcription reading into the cellular oncogene. The proposed model of promoter insertion is supported by: 1) classes of ALV integration sites mapping at the left end of c-<u>myc</u>; 2) the presence of specific transcripts containing both viral and cellular (c-<u>myc</u>) sequences in most of the tumors examined; 3) cloning and sequencing of the provirus-host cell junction from two ALV-induced lymphomas. The viral LTR has been localized upstream from the c-<u>myc</u> oncogene, and its integration site identified in relation to the normal oncogene, which has been also cloned and partially sequenced (29,47,48,53a).

Results in agreement with the promoter insertion model have been reported by other groups (22). However, Payne et al. have found that in ALV-induced B cell lymphomas, proviral DNA (viral LTR) can also be integrated at the 3' end of the oncogene or at the 5' end but in the orientation opposite to transcription and still enhance the expression of c-<u>myc</u> sequences (50). These different results are difficult to be explained by a classical promoter activation hypothesis. Alternative explanations might involve the effect(s) of new regulatory elements, transcription enhancer sequences, which have been identified in the SV40 genome (72-bp repeats near the origin of SV40 replication) (28). Although similar sequences have been identified in murine leukemia viruses, there is no evidence as yet that they are also present in avian retroviruses (26,42).

What is the mechanism of neoplastic transformation induced by ALV infection? Activation of c-<u>myc</u> oncogene transcription in 85% of the B cell lymphomas or activation of other oncogenes in the remaining tumors may be the initiating event leading eventually to neoplastic transforma-

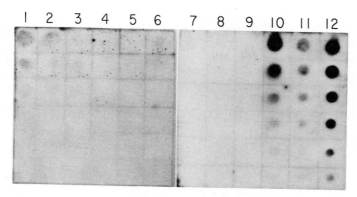

FIGURE 3. Analysis of different tumor or normal human cell lines RNA by dot blot hybridization. This analysis was performed as described in Figure 2. Total RNA or polyA selected RNA was spotted on nitrocellulose filter paper in 2-fold serial dilutions. Filters were then hybridized with ^{32}P-labeled v-myc probe. Samples and RNA amount in the first dot blot dilution were as follows:

Lane 1 and 2) JHU-2 (normal human cells) total RNA (0.6 and 0.72 mg; lane 3) IMR-90 (normal human cell lines) total RNA (0.72 mg); lanes 4 and 5) SKES, 2A and 2G Ewing sarcoma cell lines total RNA (0.3 and 0.32 mg); lanes 6 and 7) 130T B1 and D1 Rhabddomyosarcoma cell lines total RNA (1220 and 0.66 mg); lane 8) polyA selected RNA from Syrian hamster embryo (1 mg); lane 9) polyA-selected RNA from Syrian hamster brain tissue (1.1 mg); lane 10) MC29 virus-purified RNA (0.030 mg of RNA in the first dilution); lane 11) chicken B cell lymphoma (36 L) total cellular RNA. The estimated number of c-myc transcripts in this lymphoma was about 11/cell (30) (0.2 mg); lane 12) NHL patient (PE) total RNA from PBL (0.9 mg of RNA in the first dilution.

tion. As previously mentioned, viral oncogenes have been shown to be responsible for neoplastic transformation. Also in the case of avian myelocytomatosis virus 29, there is fairly good evidence that this is the case. Transformation-defective mutants and revertants that have reacquired transforming potential have been isolated by Ramsay et al., and the mutations all have been shown to map in the oncogene region (4,52). Furthermore, the v-myc oncogene has been cloned in T. Papas' and M. Bishop's laboratories and shown to induce transformation upon transfection into NIH/3T3 cells (39,68).

Despite the oncogenic potential of v-myc, when cellular DNA from ALV-induced chicken B cell lymphomas were transfected into NIH/3T3 cells, the resulting foci of transformed mouse cells completely lacked both viral (ALV) and chicken c-myc sequences. A different gene has been identified by Cooper et al. in such transfected NIH/3T3 cells and recently cloned (13). The relationship between c-myc and this new transforming gene is still unclear. Assuming that ALV integration next to c-myc is the event initiating neoplastic transformation, the c-myc gene product or another effector molecule could eventually activate the actual B cell lymphoma transforming gene, which is identified by NIH/3T3 transfection. Alternatively, NIH/3T3 cells have already reached a semi-transformed state, in which the myc gene-encoded function is no longer required, but another B cell lymphoma activated gene is still required in order to obtain neoplastic transformation.

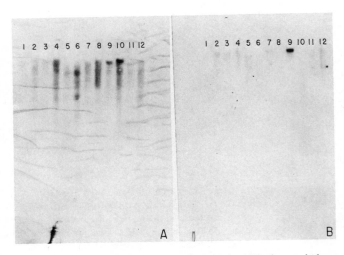

FIGURE 4. Amplification of the sequences hybridizing with v-myc in the promyelocytic leukemia cell line HL60. Southern blot analysis of different normal blood donors or leukemia/lymphoma patient PBL-DNA and of the DNA from the cell line HL60. DNA samples were processed as described (62). 5 μg (#1,3,5,7,9,11) or 10 μg (#2,4,8,10,12) of DNA were digested with BamHI restriction enzyme. (DNA sample 2B 10 was accidentally degraded). The DNA transferred to a nitrocellulose filter was hybridized with a ^{32}P-labeled v-myc probe at 37°C for 72 hr at the following conditions: A) lower stringency: 30% formamide, 5 x SSC, 1 x Denhardt, 0.1% sodium dodecyl sulfate (SDS), 10% dextran sulphate. B) Higher stringency: 50% formamide, 5 xx SSC, 1 x Denhardt, 0.1% SDS, 10% dextran sulphate.

In both cases, washings were performed at 65°C in 1 x SSC, 0.1% SDS and 0.1 SSC, 0.1% SDS. Dry filters were exposed to an X-ray film for 24 hr. Samples are as follows: lanes 1 and 2) NHL (WF): lanes 3 and 4) NHL (PE); lanes 5 and 6) BALB/c mouse DNA; lanes 7 and 8) CLL) CF; lanes 9 and 10) HL60; lanes 11 and 12) PBL from a normal blood donor.

A link between human cancer and retroviruses (or retroviral oncogene activation) has been searched for for several years (30). Only recently, the availability of recombinant DNA clones specific for retroviral oncogenes has allowed the analysis of the cellular homologous oncogenes present in human normal cells or tumor cell lines. Different human oncogenes (human c-fes, c-ras, c-sis, c-myc, c-myb (9,16,17,24,27,67,72) have recently been cloned and characterized. In some cases, the expression of such oncogenes has also been analyzed in normal and tumor cell lines of human origin (2,53a,71).

Furthermore, the development of DNA transfection techniques in the last few years has led to the analysis of several different human tumors or human tumor cell lines. Particularly in the case of bladder, lung, and colon carcinoma cell lines, human genes have been detected that transform mouse NIH/3T3 cells upon transfection (36,37,46,51,60). Independent reports from at least four different laboratories identified the transfected human genes as human bas and Ha-ras for the bladder carcinoma cell lines and human Ki-ras for the lung and colon cell lines (18,49,56).

Also in the case of lymphoid neoplasms, human genes have been identified that are transfectable into NIH/3T3 cells. Such genes appear to be specific for the differentiation state of leukemic cells (38). Human lymphoid neoplasms seem to be particularly interesting for this sort of analysis, because in several instances a form of leukemia or lymphoma has been associated with a specific chromosomal abnormality (35,54). In Burkitt's Lymphomas (BL) or BL cell lines, such aberrations involve beside chromosome 8, chromosomes 2, 14, and 22, where immunoglobulin (Ig) genes have been mapped (15,20,44). This association led Klein (35) and Rowley (54) to postulate that Ig genes might activate cellular oncogenes after being translocated or rearranged next to them. This hypothesis appears to be particularly appealing in view of the fact that chromosome breaks have been localized very close to the Ig genes and that there is a good correlation in BL between variant translocations and Ig chain produced (t 8;2 produces k and t 8;22 produces λ) (34,44).

What is the significance of the higher c-myc expression present in some of the ALL, CLL, and NHL we have studied? Very recently, Westin et al. have reported that they can find a single band of Northern blots of RNA from various human leukemic blood cells and hematopoietic cell lines with only 1- to 2-fold variation in the intensity of the hybridization. The only exception they reported was the promyelocytic leukemia cell line HL60, which expresses approximately 5- to 10-fold more MC29-related onc sequences (71). In our case, we found differences in the expression of myc-related sequences among different leukemic and normal blood donor samples. Although a constant low level of myc hybridization was detected in total RNAs from normal blood donor samples, the intensity of the hybridization was much higher in some of the leukemic blood samples or in some cell lines like HL60 (data not shown). In our experience, the higher intensity of hybridization seen in HL60 was certainly not as high as the hybridization we have detected in certain human tumor samples (for example, sample 12 in Figure 3). This difference in the results might be explained either by the fact that different samples were analyzed by the two groups or that different techniques were employed (Northern blot versus dot blot hybridization). Experiments are in progress in order to clarify these points.

A difference in the expression of c-myc sequences could be explained in different ways: 1) c-myc expression is increased in certain types of differentiated cells normally absent from peripheral blood or present as a very small fraction of the leukocyte population, but which are present as a higher percentage of cells in certain kinds of leukemias and lymphomas. In this case, higher c-myc expression would be just a marker of certain stages of differentiation; 2) the elevated expression of c-myc is abnormal and somehow related to the pathological properties of patient samples or of a cell line like HL60. In either case, the mechanism of such an increase in c-myc expression observed in several samples of human leukemias and lymphomas we have studied, is not clear. These observations cannot all be explained by the amplification phenomenon we have discovered in HL60 DNA (unpublished results). However, HL60 amplification appears to be an interesting example of genetic alteration correlated with higher gene expression. The causal links might be: 1) the increased number of available templates leads to increased transcription; 2) one or more of the amplified genes is more actively transcribed.

Gene amplification is a very well known phenomenon in the development of Drosophila melanogaster and Xenopus Laevis but it may have a broader biological relevance than originally thought. The availability of a cell line such as HL60 and of transfection and molecular cloning techniques may shed some more light on complex phenomena such as amplification and neoplastic transformation.

ACKNOWLEDGEMENTS

We acknowledge the technical assistance of R. Diehl. We are grateful to several people who provided us with some of the material used in this work: T. Papas for a v-myc recombinant plasmid bacterial strain; W.S. Hayward and B.G. Neel for 36L and MC29 virus RNA and a human DNA recombinant phage containing c-myc sequences; P.O.P. Ts'o and R.K. Moyzis for different human and Syrian hamster cell RNAs.

REFERENCES

1. Andersson P, Goldfarb MP, Weinberg RA (1979):   Cell 16:63
2. Astrin SM, Rovigatti UG: Progress in Cancer Research and Therapy. Vol. 27, Raven Press, New York (in press)
3. Bernstein A, MacCormick R, Martin GS (1976):   Virology 70:206
4. Bister K, Ramsay GM, Hayman MJ (1982):   J Virol 41:754
5. Blair DG, Oskarsson M, Wood TG, McClements WL, Fishinger PJ, Vande Woude GC (1981):   Science 212:941
6. Brugge JS, Erikson RL (1977):   Nature 269:346
7. Chang EH, Ellis RW, Scolnick RM, Lowy DR (1980):   Science 210:1249
8. Chang EH, Furth ME, Scolnick EM, Lowy DR (1982):   Nature 297:479
9. Chang EH, Gonda MA, Ellis RW, Scolnick EM, Lowy DR (1982):   Proc Natl Acad Sci USA 79:4848
10. Chen JH (1980):   J Virol 36:162
11. Coffin JM, Varmus HE, Bishop JM, Essex M, Hardy WD, Martin SG, Rosenberg NE, Scolnick EM, Weinberg RA, Vogt PK (1981):   J Virol 36:162
12. Collett MS, Erikson RL (1980):   Proc Natl Acad Sci USA 75:2021
13. Cooper GM, Neiman PE (1981):   Nature 292:857
14. Copeland NG, Zelenetz AD, Cooper GM (1979):   Cell 17:993
15. Croce CM, Shander M, Martinis J, Cicurel L, D'Ancona GG, Dolby TW, Koprowski H (1977):   Proc Natl Acad Sci USA 76:3416
16. Dalla Favera R, Gelmann EP, Gallo RC, Wong Stall F (1981):   Nature 292:31
17. Dalla Favera R, Gelmann EP, Martinotti S, Franchini G, Takis Papas S, Gallo RC, Wong-Staal F (1982):   Proc Natl Acad Sci USA 79:6497
18. Der CJ, Krontiris TG, Cooper GM (1982):   Proc Natl Acad Sci USA 79:3637
19. Duesberg PH, Vogt PK (1970):   Proc Natl Acad Sci USA 67:1673
20. Erikson J, Martinis J, Croce CM (1981):   Nature 294:173
21. Fedele LA, Even J, Garon CF, Donner L, Sherr CJ (1981):   Proc Natl Acad Sci USA 78:4036
22. Fung YT, Fadly AM, Crittenden LB, Kung HJ (1981):   Proc Natl Acad Sci USA 78:3418
23. Gilmer TM, Erikson RL (1981):   Nature 294:771
24. Goldfarb M, Shimizu K, Perucho M, Wigler M (1982):   Nature 296:404
25. Gonda TJ, Sheiness DK, Bishop MJ (1982):   Mol Cell Biol 2:617
26. Gorman CM, Merlino GT, Willinghan MC, Howard BH (1982):   Proc Natl Acad Sci USA 79:6777
27. Groffen J, Heisteerkamp N, Grosveld F, Van De Ven W, Stephenson JR (1982):   Science 216:1136
28. Gross P, Dhar R, Khoury G (1981):   Proc Natl Acad Sci USA 78:943
29. Hayward WS, Neel BG, Astrin SM (1981):   Nature 290:475.
30. Hiatt HH, Watson JD, Winsten JA, eds. "Origin of Human Cancer", Cold Spring Harbor Conferences on Cell Proliferation, Vol. 4, Book B. Cold Spring Harbor Laboratory Press, 1977.
31. Karess RE, Hanafusa H (1981):   Cell 24:155.

32. Karess RE, Hayward WS, Hanafusa H (1979): Proc Natl Acad Sci USA 76:3154
33. Kawai W, Hanafusa H (1971): Virol 46:470
34. Kirsh IR, Morton CC, Nakahara K, Leder P (1982): Science 216:301
35. Klein G (1981): Nature 294:313
36. Krontiris TG, Cooper GM (1981): Proc Natl Acad Sci USA 78:1181
37. Lane MA, Sainten A, Cooper GM (1981): Proc Natl Acad Sci USA 78:5185
38. Lane MA, Sainten A, Cooper GM (1982): Cell 28:873
39. Lautenberger JA, Schulz RA, Garon CF, Tsichlis PN, Papas TS (1981): Proc Natl Acad Sci USA 78:1518
40. Lenoir GM, Prend'Homme JL, Bernheim A, Berger R (1982): Nature 278:474
41. Levinson AD, Oppermann H, Levintow L, Varmus HE, Bishop MJ (1978): Cell 15:561
42. Levinson B, Khoury G, Vande Woude G, Gross P (1982): Nature 295:568
43. Martin GS (1970): Nature 227:1021.
44. McBride OW, Hieteer PA, Hollis GF, Swan D, Otey MC, Leder P (1982): J Exp Med 155:1480
45. Mittelman F (1981): Adv Cancer Res 34:141
46. Murray M, Shilo BZ, Shih C, Cowing D, Hsu HW, Weinberg RA (1981): Cell 25:355
47. Neel BG, Gasic GP, Rogler CE, Shalka AM, Ju G, Hishinuma F, Papas T, Astrin SM, Hayward WS (1982): J Virol 44:167
48. Neel BG, Hayward WS, Robinson HL, Fang J, Astrin SM (1981): Cell 23:323
49. Parada LF, Tabin CJ, Shih C, Weinberg R (1982): Nature 297:474
50. Payne GS, Bishop JM, Varmus HE (1982): Nature 295:209
51. Perucho M, Goldfarb M, Shimizu K, Concepcion L, Fogh J, Wigler M (1981): Cell 27:467
52. Ramsay G, Graf T, Hayman MJ (1980): Nature 288:170
53a. Rovigatti UG, Rogler CE, Neel BG, Hayward WS, Astrin SM (1982): In: Tumor Cell Heterogeneity: Origins and Implications (Owens Jr AH, Coffey DS, Baylin SB, eds), New York: Academic Press, pp 319–330
53b. Rovigatti UG, Astrin SM (1983): In: Genes and Proteins in Oncogenesis (Vogel H, Weinstein R, eds), New York: Academic Press, pp 241–251
54. Rowley J (1980): Annu Rev Gen 14:17
55. Rowley JD (1982): Science 216:749
56. Santos E, Tronick SR, Aaronson SA, Pulciani S, Barbacid M (1982): Nature 298:343
57. Sefton BM, Hunter T, Beemon K, Ekhart W (1980): Cell 20:807
58. Sheines D, Bishop JM (1979): J Virol 31:514
59. Shibuya M, Hanafusa H, Balduzzi PC (1982): J Virol 42:143
60. Shih C, Padhy LC, Murray M, Weinberg RA (1981): Nature 290:261
61. Shilo BZ, Weinberg RA (1981): Proc Natl Acad Sci USA 78:6789
62. Southern EM (1975): J Mol Biol 98:503
63. Stehelin D, Varmus HE, Bishop JM, Vogt PK (1976): Nature 260:170
64. Temin HM (1981): Cell 27:1
65. Temin HM (1982): Cell 28:3
66. Thomas PS (1980): Proc Natl Acad Sci USA 77:5201
67. Truss MD, Sodroski JG, Haseltine WA (1982): J Biol Chem 257:2730
68. Vennstrom B, Moscovici C, Goodman HM, Bishop JM (1981): J Virol 39:625
69. Vogt PK (1977): In: Comprehensive Virology (Fraenkel-Conrat H, Wagner RR, eds), Vol 9, Plenum Press, p 341

70. Weiss RA, Teich NM, Varmus H, Coffin JM, eds., (1982): RNA Tumor Viruses, New York: Cold Spring Harbor Laboratory

71. Westin EH, Wong-Staal F, Gelmann EP, Dalla-Favera R, Papas TS, Lautenberger JA, Eva A, Reddy EP, Tronick SR, Aaronson SA, Gallo RC (1982): Proc Natl Acad Sci USA 79:2490

72. Wong-Stall F, Dalla Favera R, Franchini G, Gelmann EP, Gallo RC (1981): Science 213:226

Gene Transfer and Cancer, edited by M. L. Pearson
and N. L. Sternberg. Raven Press, New York © 1984.

Cellular Transforming Genes in Cancer

*Mary-Ann Lane, *Adrienne Sainten, *Dorothy Neary,
**Dorothea Becker, and **Geoffrey M. Cooper

*Laboratory of Immunobiology and **Laboratory of Molecular Carcinogenesis,
Department of Pathology, Harvard Medical School, Sidney Farber Cancer Institute,
Boston, Massachusetts 02115

ABSTRACT. A common cellular transforming gene activated in six mouse
mammary tumors induced by mouse mammary tumor virus (MMTV) or dimethylbenzanthracene and in the human mammary tumor cell line MCF7 was identified by restriction endonuclease analysis. Transforming activity of all
seven tumor DNAs was inactivated by the enzymes SacI and PvuII, but not
by EcoRI, HindIII, XhoI, BamHI or KpnI (9). Isolation of a molecular
clone containing the human mammary tumor transforming sequence has recently been completed. The transforming efficiency of this gene in NIH/
3T3 cells is 2 x 10^4 foci per µg of cell DNA.

To determine whether one or several genes were activated in neoplasms
representative of different normal stages of a complex differentiative
lineage, we also studied a number of T- and B-lymphocyte neoplasms representative of early, intermediate, and mature stages of cellular differentiation. By analysis of the susceptibility of transforming activity
to inactivation by restriction endonuclease digestion, we have identified
three transforming genes in the B-lymphocyte lineage: one common to pre-
B lymphocyte neoplasms, one common to intermediate B neoplasms, and one
common to mature B neoplasms. Two additional genes were identified in
T-lymphocyte neoplasms: one common to intermediate T-lymphocyte neoplasms and one common to mature T neoplasms. These results indicate that
within a complex differentiative lineage common transforming genes are
activated in neoplasms representative of the same stage of differentiation but that different genes are activated in neoplasms representative
of different stages of differentiation.

INTRODUCTION

Genes that regulate growth in normal cells during differentiation
function in response to appropriate signals that allow proliferation and
maturation to proceed in an orderly manner. In the neoplastic cell,
genetic control of proliferation appears to be lost. Nonneoplastic cells
may contain a number of genes with potential transforming activity that
are normally well regulated and expressed only at a particular phase of
cell differentiation. Abnormal expression of these genes may result in
neoplastic growth. Experiments by Cooper and co-workers have addressed
the question of the potential transforming activity of genes from normal

cells (2). In this series of experiments, DNA from normal cells was prepared, sheared to a size range of 0.5 to 5.0 kb and transfected as a calcium phosphate precipitate into NIH/3T3 cells. Transforming efficiencies high-molecular-weight DNAs from these cells were approximately 3×10^{-4} transformants per μg of DNA, whereas transforming efficiencies for sheared DNAs were 10-fold greater. Transforming efficiencies of DNAs from foci isolated in primary transfection of sheared DNA when tested in secondary transfection were 100- to 1000-fold higher (0.1 to 1.0 foci per μg of DNA), comparable to transforming activities of strongly oncogenic viruses (5,12). These studies suggest that normal cell genes can transform at high efficiencies when they are expressed abnormally.

High-molecular-weight DNA from neoplastic cells, unlike that from normal cells, transforms NIH/3T3 cells in primary transfection with high efficiencies of 0.1 to 1.0 transformants per μg of DNA, suggesting that events that have already occurred at the DNA level have freed these genes from appropriate control. Activated transforming genes that can be efficiently transmitted by transfection with high-molecular-weight DNAs have been found in chemically transformed mouse fibroblasts (17), B-cell lymphomas and a nephroblastoma induced by avian lymphoid leukosis viruses (LLV) (3), human bladder carcinomas (8,16), mammary tumors of mouse and human origin (9), gliomas and neuroblastomas of rat and mouse origin (15), and human colon carcinoma and promyelocytic leukemia (14). The transforming genes detected by transfection of DNAs of tumors induced by LLV, a class of retroviruses that lack viral transforming genes, and those of mammary tumors associated with MMTV, which also lacks a viral transforming gene, are not linked to viral DNA sequences, suggesting that oncogenesis by these viruses involves indirect activation of cellular transforming genes (3,9).

Hayward and co-workers (7) have demonstrated that in LLV-induced tumors, a cellular gene (c-myc), homologous to the transforming gene of acute leukemia virus, is activated by adjacent integration of viral DNA (long terminal repeat insertion). However, analysis of NIH cells transformed by DNAs of these neoplasms indicates that transformation was not mediated by transfer of the c-myc gene to the NIH cells (4). These observations indicate that at least two different cellular genes are activated in LLV-induced neoplasms. Since carcinogenesis is a multistage process, activation of c-myc may precede or complement activation of the cellular transforming gene detected by transfection. Alternatively, LLV may act at an early preneoplastic stage to expand the population of cells in which transforming events occur, which is consistent with the mechanism proposed by McGrath and Weissman for induction of T-cell lymphomas by analogous retroviruses of the AKR mouse (13). Thus, these findings suggest that transformation by a variety of carcinogenic agents can involve dominant mutations or gene rearrangements that result in the activation of cellular transforming genes, which are then detectable by transfection.

Weinberg and co-workers have demonstrated that mouse fibroblasts transformed by several different chemical carcinogens contained related activated transforming genes as determined by restriction enzyme analysis (17). We have studied a series of mammary tumors of mouse and human origin. In these experiments, high-molecular-weight DNAs of five mouse mammary tumors, two chemical carcinogen-induced mouse mammary tumors, and one human mammary tumor cell line (MCF07) were assayed for the presence of transmissible activated transforming genes by transfection. DNAs of six mouse tumor and the human tumor cell line induced transformation with high efficiencies. The transforming activities of DNAs of all five MMTV-induced tumors, the chemical carcinogen-induced mouse tumor, and the human tumor cell line were inactivated by digestion with the restriction endonucleases PvuII and SacI but not by BamHI, EcoRI, HindIII, KpnI or XhoI. These results suggest that the same transforming gene was activated in six different mouse mammary carcinomas, induced by either MMTV or a chemical carcinogen, and in a human mammary carcinoma cell line (9). This transforming gene differs by restriction analysis from that activated in two human bladder carcinomas (8) and from the gene activated in chemically transformed fibroblasts (17). These findings suggest that within neoplasms of a particular differentiated cell type, a common transforming gene is activated. Cloning of the human mammary tumor transforming sequence has recently been completed. The transforming efficiency of this clone is 40,000 foci/µg of cell DNA insert, and as expected from our previous studies, the transforming sequence contains both SacI and PvuII sites.

Sera from mice bearing tumors induced by NIH/3T3 cells transformed by mouse or human mammary tumor DNA immunoprecipitated an 86 kd glycoprotein in extracts of NIH cells transformed by human mammary carcinoma DNA. This antigen was also immunoprecipitated by sera from mice bearing tumors induced by mouse mammary carcinoma DNAs and from mice bearing primary carcinomas. These results indicate that this protein represents an antigen that is specifically associated with expression of the transmissible transforming genes of human and mouse mammary carcinomas (1).

Molecular cloning of the transforming gene activated in chicken bursal lymphoma has been carried out by Goubin et al. (6). The use of this cloned gene as a probe in Southern blotting analysis indicates that this gene is evolutionarily well conserved in that hybridization to human DNAs is of comparable intensity to that observed in hybridization of the probe to chicken DNA. The cloned chicken bursal gene is biologically active and transforms with efficiencies 10^5 times enriched over uncloned bursal tumor cell DNA.

Several conclusions can be drawn from these studies. We may first assume that cellular transforming genes, in their normal state, are carefully regulated and may only be expressed or "turned on" at a particular phase of cellular differentiation in response to the appropriate external signals. We can speculate that, as a rare event, a dominant genetic change in the control elements of these genes can lead to unregulated growth that results in the production of a neoplasm. Clearly, one or several steps may be involved in the deregulation of such a gene. The end result, however, may be successfully scored by transfection. A second point which emerges is that these genes appear to be well conserved in evolution, based upon the results of restriction enzyme analysis, which indicate an apparent similarity between human and mouse mammary tumor transforming genes (9,1), and upon results obtained with the cloned chicken bursal transforming gene (6). This suggests that a gene cloned from a neoplasm of mice may share substantial homology with the analogous gene in humans. These studies also demonstrate that within a particular differentiated phenotype, a common transforming gene is activated that may be particular to the differentiated state of the neoplasm.

Considering these data, we have speculated that in a specific cell lineage that undergoes several differentiative steps to maturity, one or several of the genes expressed at these steps may be susceptible to rearrangements or mutations that can lead to neoplastic transformation. To examine this hypothesis more closely, we chose a cell lineage where differentiation can be described in terms of migration, surface markers, and cellular function in maturity. Cells of the immune system seemed most appropriate for these investigations.

Within the immune system, the differentiative lineages of B- and T-lymphocytes are perhaps the best characterized. Cell surface markers exist which allow classification of cell types as early, intermediate, or mature in both human and murine systems. Neoplasms that arise from T- and B-lymphocyte populations have been characterized with regard to their state of differentiation by surface markers, by function in in vitro assays, and, in B-cell neoplasms, by the degree of heavy and light chain production, assembly, and secretion. These neoplasms can be categorized as representative of early, intermediate, or mature counterparts of normal T- and B-lymphocyte differentiation. Identification, characterization, and molecular cloning of cellular transforming genes from T- and B-lymphocyte neoplasms, which are representative of early, intermediate, and mature stages of normal cellular differentiation, will provide the tools to examine genetic events that lead to neoplastic transformation. These studies will allow us to assess the number of genes at risk for neoplastic transformation within a well-described normal cell differentiative lineage. Probes generated in these experiments may provide new insights into the mechanisms by which growth is regulated in normal lymphocytes and may lead to an understanding of molecular events that signal cellular proliferation and differentiation.

RESULTS AND DISCUSSION

To determine whether transmissible transforming genes could be detected in T- and B-lymphocyte neoplasms by transfection of NIH/3T3 cells, we prepared high-molecular-weight DNA (>20 kb) from more than twenty different neoplastic cell lines or primary patient isolates from T- and B-lymphocyte neoplasms of mouse or human origin. Calcium phosphate precipitates of these DNAs were applied to NIH/3T3 cells, and primary transformation efficiencies were scored after 12 to 14 days of culture (10). Efficiencies of these DNAs in primary transfection ranged from 0.05 to 0.5 foci/µg of DNA. Four to six foci from each primary transfection were picked and grown in mass culture. DNAs were prepared from these foci and were used as donor DNAs in secondary transfection assays. Transforming efficiencies in secondary transfection also ranged from 0.05 to 0.5 foci/µg of DNA, indicating that transmissible activated transforming genes from the neoplasms were present in the transformed NIH cells. DNA from spontaneous transformants, which occasionally arise in NIH/3T3 cells, does not retransform in secondary transfection assays; thus we were assured that these assays were identifying only dominant activated transmissible transforming genes in transformants from these neoplasms. Transforming efficiencies for some of the T- and B-neoplasm DNAs tested in primary and secondary transfection assays are presented in Tables 1 and 2. Efficient transformation of NIH cells were achieved with DNAs from frozen patient cells, primary tumors, or cell lines of both mouse and human origin. From neoplasms of B-lymphocyte lineage, we have obtained transformation using DNA from tumors representataive of early, intermediate, and mature stages of normal differentiation. From neoplasms of the T-lymphocyte lineage, we have identified transformants representative of intermediate and mature stages of normal differentiation. Because of a lack of cell surface markers to characterize pre-T-lymphocyte tumors, obtaining a representative for this classification has proved difficult. At present, we have several candidate neoplasms which show no heavy chain gene rearrangement, have no theta on their surface, and are terminal transferase inducible. Assays are currently in progress to determine whether DNAs from these tumors will transform NIH/3T3 cells

TABLE 1. T-lymphocyte neoplasms possessing transmissible transforming genes

| Species | Type of Neoplasm | | |
	Pre-T	Intermediate-T	Mature-T
Human	None	T10[a]	Sezary syndrome[a]
Mouse	SJL[b,c]	S49	Clone A
		W7.1	104.6
		L691	
		WKT2	
		SL3	
		SL7	

[a]Primary tumors.

[b]Cell line from M. Schied (see ref. 10 for other cell lines or patient isolates).

[c]Transforming efficiency = 0.15 foci/μg DNA for SJL, 0.10-1.0 foci/ μg DNA for intermediate T neoplasms and 0.05-0.55 foci/μg DNA for mature T neoplasms. Control values for DNA from normal mouse thymocytes, helper clone 101.6, human embryo fibroblasts or salmon sperm were $\leq$ 0.005 foci/μg DNA.

in culture. With the completion of these studies, we will have identified transmissible transforming genes from T- and B-lymphocyte neoplasms which represent early, intermediate, and mature stages of normal differentiation, and will have completed our first goal in these studies.

Restriction enzyme analysis of transforming genes has proved useful in two ways. First, it has allowed us to demonstrate that activation of a specific transforming gene is correlated with a particular differentiated cell type in neoplasms representative of that particular stage of normal differentiation. Second, identification of restriction enzymes that do not inactivate transforming genes provides a useful cloning strategy by means of a transforming gene enrichment step.

To carry out this type of analysis, we selected four restriction endonucleases that recognize a 6-base sequence and that cleave cellular DNA statistically once every 4 kb. We chose EcoRI, HindIII, BamHI, and XhoI to cleave whole cell DNA containing transforming genes of interest. Digestions were monitored by gel electrophoresis to assure that complete digestion had occurred. Both digested DNAs and companion undigested samples were transfected onto NIH/3T3 cells and foci were enumerated. If a transforming gene possessed the 6-base sequence recognized by the restriction endonuclease, the gene would be cleaved. Cleavage within the transforming gene sequence resulted in a reduction in transformation efficiency by direct inactivation of the transforming gene. In this manner, a "fingerprint" of the transforming gene could be generated based upon enzyme inactivation patterns.

These findings are summarized in Table 3. We are currently continuing and expanding these. To date, by this method of analysis, we have identified three different B-cell transforming genes and two different T-lineage transforming genes. In these groups, a common gene appears to be activated in both mouse and human neoplasms within a differentiated cell

TABLE 2. B-lymphocyte neoplasms possessing transmissible transforming genes

Species	Type of Neoplasms		
	Pre-B	Intermediate-B	Mature-B
Human	$C^+B^+1^a$	Rajie	GM1500
	$C^+B^+2^a$	Namalwa[e]	GM2132
	$C^-B^-1^a$	BJAB[e]	
	$C^-B^-2^a$	MC116[f]	
	207	EW36[f]	
	697	CW678[f]	
	SMS-SB[b]		
	NALM-1[c]		
Mouse	B6T4E4[d]	W231	S107
	B6T1E1[d]	2PK3	M315
		BCL-1	NS2.1

[a] primary tumors.
[b] Cell line prepared by G. Smith and B. Ozan, manuscript in preparation.
[c] See J. Ritz et al., Blood 58:648 (1981).
[d] Abelson-induced pre-B tumor, C57BL/6 strain from R. Risser.
[e] African Burkitts patient cell lines from I. McGrath.
American Burkitts patient cell lines from I. McGrath.
[f] Transforming efficiencies ranged from 0.09-1.10 foci/µg DNA for pre-B neoplasms, 0.15-1.2 for intermediate-B, and 0.11-0.20 for mature B neoplasms. Controls as in Table I or EBV-immortalized B lymphocytes gave <0.005 foci/µg DNA.

type, again suggesting the presence of evolutionarily well-conserved genes. The restriction analysis of each of these genes establishes them as distinct from transforming genes of human bladder carcinoma (8), mouse and human mammary tumors (9), and chemically transformed fibroblasts (17). The transforming genes thus far identified correlate well with phenotypic expression within particular differentiated cell types. It is our hypothesis that these genes represent cell growth genes that have been freed of normal regulatory constraints. When cloning of a representative gene from each of the five groups is completed, we will use these genes as probes to determine the signals that trigger their expression during normal cellular differentiation and to determine the stage at which these genes are at risk for neoplastic changes.

TABLE 3. Restriction enzyme sensitivity of B- and T-lymphocyte neoplasm transforming sequences

Neoplasm	Restriction enzyme				
	EcoRI	BamHI	XhoI	HindIII	SacI
Pre-B neoplasms					
6 human	−	+	+	−	ND
2 mouse	−	+	+	−	ND
Intermediate B neoplasms					
2 human	−	+	−	−	ND
3 mouse	−	+	−	−	ND
Mature B neoplasms					
2 human	−	−	−	−	+
2 mouse	−	−	−	−	+
Intermediate T neoplasms					
1 human	+	−	−	−	ND
6 mouse	+	−	+/−	−	ND
Mature T neoplasms					
1 human	−	−	+	+	ND
1 mouse	−	−	+	+	ND

+ indicates that restriction enzyme treatment inactivated the focus forming activity of the DNA tested.
ND = not determined.

ACKNOWLEDGEMENTS

We would like to thank J. Ritz and E. Ritz for cell phenotyping and for providing primary patient isolates; M. McGrath, I. Weissman, S. Lanier, N. Warner, A. Ragab, J. Lenz, C. Reinisch, D. Eardley, C. Terhorst, J. Reinwald, R. Risser, The Human Genetic Mutant Cell Repository, and the Salk Institute for providing cells and cell lines used in these studies; and H. Cantor and S. Schlossman for useful discussions. This work was supported by CA26825, CA18689, CA28946, CA06721, and an American Cancer Society Faculty Research Award to G.M.C. and by Biomedical Research Support Grants from the National Cancer Institute and the American Cancer Society.

REFERENCES

1. Becker D, Lane MA, Cooper GM (1982):   Proc Natl Acad Sci USA 79:3315
2. Cooper GM, Okenquist S, Silverman L (1980):   Nature 284:418
3. Cooper GM, Nieman PE (1980):   Nature 287:656
4. Cooper GM, Nieman PE (1981):   Nature 292:857
5. Copeland NG, Zelenetz AD, Cooper GM (1979):   Cell 17:993
6. Goubin G, Luce J, Nieman P, Cooper GM (manuscript in preparation)
7. Haywood WS, Neel BG, Astrin SM (1981):   Nature 290:475
8. Krontiris TG, Cooper GM (1981):   Proc Natl Acad Sci USA 78:1181
9. Lane MA, Sainten AC, Cooper GM (1981):   Proc Natl Acad Sci USA 78:
    5185
10. Lane MA, Sainten AC, Cooper GM (1982):   Cell 28:873
11. Lanier LL, Warner NJ, Ledbetter JA, Herzenberg LA (1981):   Immunolo-
    gy 127:1691
12. Lowy DR, Rands E, Scolnick EM (1978):   J Virol 26:291
13. McGrath MS, Weissman IL (1979):   Cell 17:65
14. Murray MJ, Shilo BZ, Shih C, Cowing D, Hsu HW, Weinberg RA (1981):
    Cell 25:355
15. Shih C, Padhy LC, Murray M, Weinberg RA (1981):   Nature 290:261
16. Shih C, Shilo BZ, Goldfarb MP, Dannenberg A, Weinberg RA (1981):
    Nature 290:261
17. Shilo BZ, Weinberg RA (1981):   Nature 289:607
18. Strober S (1981):   Twentieth Midwinter Conference of Immunologists,
    Pacific Grove, Calif.

Gene Transfer and Cancer, edited by M. L. Pearson
and N. L. Sternberg. Raven Press, New York © 1984.

Genetic Analysis of the Transformed Phenotype in Mouse Cells

*Michael B. Small, *Esau Simmons, *Krishna K. Jha,
*Harvey L. Ozer, **Lawrence A. Feldman, †Jayashree Pyati,
†Stephen Hann, and †Dino Dina

*Department of Biological Sciences, Hunter College, New York, New York 10021;
**Department of Microbiology, University of Medicine and Dentistry, Newark,
New Jersey 01703; and †Department of Genetics, Albert Einstein College of Medicine,
Bronx, New York 10461*

ABSTRACT. BALB/c 3T3 clone A31 has been transformed in vitro by a
variety of virological, physical, and chemical agents. Analysis of
several transformants has demonstrated expression of the transformed
phenotype in somatic cell hybrids between viral [Simian virus 40 (SV40),
avian sarcoma virus (ASV)] or chemical carcinogen transformed and untransformed 3T3. Such dominant transformants have been used for DNA-mediated
gene transfer using the calcium-phosphate co-precipitation technique
into NIH/3T3. Primary transfectants have been isolated by growth in
agarose. Restriction enzyme sensitivity of two donor DNAs derived from
chemically transformed cells is similar to that previously reported by
Weinberg and coworkers for other transformed mouse cell lines. We have
recovered a transforming agent following infection by Moloney murine
leukemia virus in the case of one chemical transformant and its primary
transfectants. The relationship of this agent to previously identified
oncogenic retroviruses is currently under investigation.

INTRODUCTION

Several years ago, we initiated an investigation addressed toward the
question of the genetic basis of "malignant transformation" in mouse cells
in culture. Insights into the regulation of expression of the transformed
phenotype can be approached through the analysis of cell hybrids. Considerable work had been perofrmed on the tumor phenotype in vivo in cell
hybrids, but rather little had been done with the transformed cell
phenotype in vitro. A review we wrote at that time emphasized the un-
certainties in the field (17). Because we had been involved in multiple
aspects of the cellular interaction of the small DNA tumor virus SV40,
we chose initially to exploit that system. Multiple transformants were

already available by the mid-1970s for SV40-transformed mouse cells,
especially 3T3 cells (1). These included cell lines with different phenotypes obtained through direct selection or as revertants of previously
transformed cells. We developed a set of untransformed and SV40-trans-
formed cell lines which would be amenable to cell fusion analysis to
assess questions related to expression and suppression of the transformed
phenotype. Studies were designed to emphasize phenotypes relevant to
in vitro transformation because that aspect had been the subject of much
study and it was particularly amenable to the analysis of multiple
isolates. Similarly, a wide variety of transformants could be analyzed,
not merely those involving SV40 as the oncogenic agent; this was significant because we anticipated that different patterns of expression could
be operative in independent transformants and even in different hybrids
within a single cross. Finally, we considered it important to work with
a limited number of cell lineages and, as much as possible, with presumably a single cell type (fibroblasts). To accomplish these purposes,
we isolated a subline of BALB/3T3, designated THO, which was both resistant to 10^{-5}M thioguanine (TG^R) due to deficient activity of the enzyme
HPRT (unable to grow in HAT medium composed of hypoxanthine, aminopterin,
and thymidine) and also resistant to 3 mM ouabain (OUA^R), presumably due
to an altered membrane ATPase (11). This cell line retained the growth
properties of the untransformed BALB/3T3 parent (A31) with respect to
saturation density, low efficiency of colony formation in 1% calf serum,
anchorage dependence (Aga^-), and lack of tumorigenicity in nude mice. It
is aneuploid, as is A31, with changes in chromosome number but few rearrangements. Coupling of a recessive (TG^R) and a co-dominant (OUA^R)
marker made THO a "universal hybridizer" for selection of cell hybrids
(in HAT plus 1.5 to 2 mM ouabain), i.e., with cells lacking additional
selective markers (3,11). We transformed THO with SV40 (SV/THO) and
introduced $TG^R OUA^R$ into a conventional SV40-transformed 3T3 for compara-
tive purposes.

RESULTS AND DISCUSSION

   Hybrids between THO and SV40-transformed 3T3 (SV/3T3) consistently
expressed the relevant transformed phenotype in vitro (11). In one series
of experiments, over 100 colonies were assessed for density-dependent
inhibition of growth (DDIG) using an autoradiographic procedure for DNA
synthesis. Expression was not due to the inability of THO to suppress,
as shown by the fact that hybrids between SV/THO and secondary mouse
embryo fibroblasts gave identical results. Control experiments ruled
out the unlikely possibility that the selection procedure itself (HAT
plus ouabain in complete growth medium in monolayer) was responsible for
inducing or preferentially selecting rare transformed hybrids in such
crosses (11,13). These results are not in themselves startling: it has
become well-accepted that a single SV40 genome is sufficient to maintain
the transformed phenotype (5). It is also important to emphasize that
cellular genes are an integral component of the manifestation of that
expression at all levels. In its simplest sense, transformation is a
cellular phenomenon. More precisely, several laboratories have demonstrated experimentally the effect of alteration of cellular genes, as
in revertants of SV/3T3 isolated by Vogel and Pollack (26) and temperature
sensitive mutants of SV/3T3 isolated by Renger and Basilico (20). We also
concluded that the basis for the phenotype is more complex than simple
genetic models of dominance and recessiveness would imply. We analyzed
a novel revertant of SV40-transformed mouse embryo fibroblasts (SV-T2)

in which the untransformed cell growth patterns had been restored (9).
If reversion were due to a "dominant" cellular mutation resulting in
suppression, we would expect that hybrids between the revertant and SV/THO
would not express the transformed phenotype. Conversely, if reversion
were due to a "recessive" cellular mutation resulting in an inability to
express the transformed phenotype, hybrids between the revertant and
untranformed THO would restore the transformed phenotype. When such
hybrids were isolated and analyzed for multiple parameters of the transformed phenotype, neither result was observed (13). These data, not
consistent with either simple model, indicate a more complex interaction
such as that proposed in a gene dosage model.

These studies were extended to BALB/3T3 transformed either by avian
(ASV) or murine [Moloney murine sarcoma virus (MSV)] retroviruses (K.K.
Jha and H.L. Ozer, unpublished data). The most common finding was that
expression of the transformed phenotype occurred in hybrids with THO,
although only some parameters were amenable to testing. In the case of
the ASV transformant (B77/3T3), in which a single integrated copy is
reportedly present (25), most, but not all, hybrids were morphologically
transformed. B77/3T3 itself readily developed less-transformed morphological variants, even following recloning, so that the heterogeneity among
the hybrids was in part a reflection of that phenomenon. This interpretation was supported by the findings that even these "flat" hybrids were
anchorage independent (Aga+). These results are to be contrasted with
the experience with ASV-tranformed rat embryo fibroblasts (REF), in which
suppression is often observed in hybrids with REF, including suppression
of anchorage independence (M.J. Weber and J. Wycke, personal communication). Because, in all cases, the transformed phenotype is dependent
on the B77 src gene, the results argue for a cell-dependent difference
in behavior. A possible noteworthy factor is that transformation by B77
occurred in an aneuploid host in one case (3T3) and a diploid cell in
the other (REF). In several crosses with different MSV/3T3, all of
which were nonproducers for virus (as THO), expression was most commonly
observed as well. Suppression was observed in one cross in 7 of 10
hybrid colonies. The transformed phenotype reappeared on subsequent
passage in several cases, indicating that loss of the MSV genome was not
responsible for the apparent suppression. Neither this cross nor the
majority of crosses which showed expression were investigated further.

We shifted attention to chemical transformants of 3T3, anticipating
that such dominant expression in cell hybrids might be less common because a variety of mechanisms might be involved in carcinogenesis and suppression of the tumor phenotype in vivo (as reviewed in reference 17).
Multiple hybrids have been isolated between THO and two putative chemical
transformants of A31 provided by other laboratories: clone H, which was
induced by nitrosocarboryl and obtained from Quarles and Tennant (19),
and A31.DMBA 4-35, which was induced by dimethylbenzanthracene and obtained
from Todaro (21). Care was taken to include for detailed analysis many
examples of possible suppression (based on initial colonial morphology),
yet expression of the tranformed phenotype was consistently observed in
the different assays. Although differences among the hybrid clones were
apparent, none approached the untransformed THO phenotype. Results for
multiple parameters of the transformed phenotype for THO x clone H are
summarized in Table 1 and for anchorage independence (Aga+) for THO x
A31.DMBA in Table 2. Taken together, these data are strikingly uniform
(i.e., expression) in contrast to the more varied findings in other systems.
The genetics of A31 and many other established mouse cell lines offer a
plausible explanation. A31 is heteroploid with 68 to 78 chromosomes per

cell (28). Not unexpectedly, obtaining autosomal recessive mutants has
been experimentally difficult (14). One might predict, therefore, that
chemical carcinogenesis in this system might well be expected to show a
strong bias for a "dominant" (one-hit) mode of expression. Similarly,
expression of a virus-induced transformed phenotype, once established,
would tend to appear dosage independent (as subsequently assessed in a

TABLE 1. Growth properties of cell hybrids: THO x clone H[a]

Cell line	Colonial morphology[b]	Saturation density (cells x 10^{-4}/cm^2)		Colony formation (%)		
		10% serum	1% serum	Plastic	Mono-layer of A31	Agarose
clone H	round/dense	30	7.0	23	18	10.0
THO2	flat	7	3.6	8	<0.1	<0.1
hyb. clone 1	fibroblastoid	36	3.6	20	33	5.0
hyb. clone 2	round/dense	25	4.6	25	60	8.0
hyb. clone 3	intermediate	25	3.6	21	11	8.0
hyb. clone 4	round/dense	18	5.2	ND[c]	ND	18.0
hyb. clone 5	round/dense	18	4.6	ND	ND	0.8
hyb. clone 6	intermediate	21	5.3	19	33	0.8
hyb. clone 7	round/dense	18	3.2	ND	ND	9.3
hyb. clone 8	round/dense	18	4.2	ND	ND	7.0
hyb. clone 9	round/dense	21	3.2	ND	ND	11.0
hyb. clone 10	round/dense	18	3.6	ND	ND	7.0

[a]Data redrawn from Jha et al. (12).
[b]More than 90% of the hybrid colonies displayed the rounded refractile
appearance typical of clone H. The hybrid clones isolated for analysis
deliberately included a disproportionate number with atypical morphology.
[c]ND = not determined.

TABLE 2. Growth properties of cell hybrids: THO x A31.DMBA 4-35[a]

Cell line	Colonial morphology[b]	Colony formation (5)	
		Plastic	Agarose
A31.DMBA	dense/piled	36	30
THO2-2	flat	10	<0.01
hybrid clone 6	dense/piled	22	3.1
hybrid clone 8	intermediate	nd[c]	2.5
hybrid clone 10	dense/flat	nd	0.5
hybrid clone 12	intermediate	30	19.0
hybrid clone 14	dense/flat	nd	2.0
hybrid clone 16	intermediate	nd	0.4
hybrid clone 18	intermediate	nd	1.0

[a]Analyses performed as described previously (12).
[b]Additional colonies observed in this experiment had a dense/piled morphology characteristic of A31.DMBA and hybrid clone 6.
[c]ND = not determined.

cell hybrid). Such an interpretation is also supported by gene transfer experiments with these cell lines by us and others (22) in which a high proportion of carcinogen-transformed cell lines were successful donors.

We have performed DNA-mediated gene transfer into NIH/3T3 (10) with high-molecular-weight cellular DNA using the DNA co-precipitation technique of Graham and van der Eb (8) as modified by Wigler et al. (27). We have relied exclusively on anchorage independence (Aga$^+$) as a criterion of gene transfer. Our results are summarized in Table 3. These data confirm those of Shih et al. (22), and their results are included for comparison. We consider differences, as with MC5-5 and MB66MCA AC1 13, more apparent than real in view of the limited number of experiments performed. The sensitivity of DNA transfer to different restriction endonucleases has been reported as a useful criterion for similarity of the responsible donor sequence (15,16,18,23). Multiple experiments have been performed with DNA from clone H and a more limited number with A31.DMBA, as shown in Table 4. The pattern of sensitivity is quite similar to that reported for carcinogen-transformed mouse cells (23). XhoI and SalI had little or no effect. EcoRI and HindIII markedly reduced (or eliminated) activity.

TABLE 3. Transfection by DNA from chemically transformed cell lines

Cell line	Agent[a]	Source	Agarose EOC[b]	Cell fusion[c]	DNA TF[d]
BALB/3T3 clone A31					
A31S	none	Scher	$<10^{-5}$	NT	NT(−)[e]
clone H	NC	Tennant	$\geqslant 30\%$	D	++(NT)
A31.DMBA 4-35	DMBA	Todaro	$\geqslant 30\%$	D	+(NT)
3T3.DMBA	DMBA	DiPaolo	$\leqslant 1\%(v)$[f]	D(v)[f]	NT(+)[g]
BP.A31	BP	Todaro	$\geqslant 30\%$	NT	−(NT)
MC-5	3-MC	Todaro	$\geqslant 30\%$	NT	−(+)
C3H 10T 1/2					
C3H 10T 1/2	none	−−	$<10^{-5}$	NT	NT(−)
MB66 MCA ACL 13	3-MC	Todaro	$\sim .01\%$[h]	NT	+(−)
MB66 MCA C136	3-MC	Todaro	$\sim .01\%$	NT	+(+)
MCA-16	3-MC	Heidelberger	$\sim .01\%$	NT	+(+)
NIH/3T3					
NIH/3T3	none	Weinberg	$<10^{-5}$	NT	−(−)

[a]NC = nitrosocarboryl; DMBA = 7,12-dimethylbenzanthracene; BP = benzo[a]-pyrene; 3MC = 3-methylcholanthrene.
[b]EOC = efficiency of colony formation.
[c]NT = not tested; D = dominant expression of tranformed phenotype.
[d]DNA-mediated gene transfer using 20 µg DNA into NIH/3T3 (− = no colonies in agarose; + = colonies in agarose; NT = not tested).
[e]Results observed by Shih et al. (22) using 75 µg DNA (− = no foci, + = foci, NT = not tested).
[f]Variable with many small colonies observed in some experiments.
[g]Designated DMBA-Balb 3T3 in Shih et al. (22); foci observed with chromosome-transfer" but not with DNA transfection.
[h]Incidence of large, macroscopic colonies; additional tiny colonies also noted.

TABLE 4. Sensitivity of DNA to restriction enzymes[a]

| Restriction enzyme | Source of DNA (colonies per dish) | | | |
| | Clone H[b] | | | |
	Expt. 1	Expt. 2	Expt. 3	A31.DMBA
none	30.5	0.6	0.6	1.4
XhoI	21.8	2.6	2.4	NT[c]
SalI	11.1	1.6	1.4	NT
BamHI	1.1	0.8	0.5	2.8
EcoRI	0.2	0.1	<0.2	0.1
HindIII	0.4	<0.1	<0.2	NT
PvuII	NT	NT	NT	0.1

[a]Five to ten 60-mm dishes were transfected with 20 µg DNA/plate of treated or untreated DNA as in Table 3. SEts of 5 dishes were pooled separately for assay for Aga[+]. No colonies were observed on control plates (untransfected, transfected with salmon sperm, or normal mouse DNA).
[b]Three independent experiments were performed with a single DNA preparation over a 2-week period.
[c]NT = not tested.

BamHI had some effect on DNA from clone H but not on DNA from A31.DMBA. Whereas Shilo and Weinberg (23) classified BamHI as a "non-cutter', they noted that such enzymes occasionally reduced transfer by a factor of two to three.

As a prelude to attempted isolation of the cellular sequence responsible, we sought to verify that these carcinogen-transformed cells were free of transforming retroviruses. A31.DMBA cells were negative for production of focus-forming virus upon direct test and after infection with Moloney murine leukemia virus (MuLV). However, whereas clone H and its primary tranfectants produced no transforming virus, they produced readily detectible levels of virus upon infection with Moloney MuLV. Because such rescuability defined the virus as a putative MSV, we sought its identification by nucleic acid hybridization with known viruses. MSV (with MuLV helper) was prepared by sucrose gradient centrifugation. The RNA was extracted and analyzed by Northern blots with cloned onc sequences for rodent MSV (v-mos, v-ras-Ki, v-ras-Ha, and v-abl). A positive reaction was observed with the v-ras-Ki probe (HiHi-3). Furthermore, cDNA prepared with RNA from this virus preparation reacted with v-ras-Ki at high stringency and v-ras-Ha at low, but not high, stringency. Figure 1 shows a Northern blot containing rescued viral RNA and polyA containing RNA from clone H, clone H infected with MuLV, and a primary transfectant that had been reacted with HiHi-3 (7). Positive reaction is seen in all lanes, demonstrating the expression of a v-ras-Ki-related sequence in clone H. To distinguish between expression of endogenous onc sequences and exogenous KiSV, we took advantage of the presence of 30S rat sequences in KiSV. High-molecular-weight cellular DNA was prepared from clone H and a primary transfectant, digested individually with several different restriction enzymes, and analyzed by the Southern blot procedure. As probes, we used HiHi-3 for the ras sequence (and closely linked non-ras sequences) and I-1 for 30S rat sequences (6). For comparison, parallel Southern analyses were performed with normal mouse DNA (A31) and a known KiSV-transformed A31 (2). Figure 2 shows the results with EcoRI- and KpnI-digested DNAs. It is clear that clone H and its primary transfectants contain both 30S and ras, based on similar molecular weights and sequential hybridization of individual blots with both probes. These results are expected for the presence of exogenously introduced KiSV. We are in the process of definitively confirming this by direct analysis of cloned sequences from the rescued virus or clone H DNA. Although we anticipate that our conclusion is already quite unambiguous, some complexities remain in the data; most notably, that for the restriction enzyme sensitivities. A genomic map of KiSV has been published (24) and indicates sites for BamHI, EcoRI, and HindIII. BamHI cuts between the 5' long terminal repeat and ras; hence it would be expected to markedly reduce the transforming function. Indeed, some reduction was noted, although more might have been expected. The other two enzymes cut toward the 3' end of KiSV and would not be expected to reduce the transforming function to a considerable extent. [It has been reported that some reduction in transforming activity does occur when the 3' end is deleted in a cloned Moloney MSV genome (4)]. Analysis of the KiSV from

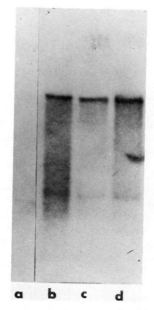

a   b   c   d

FIGURE 1. Northern blot analysis of "rescued" virion RNA from MuLV-infected clone H and cytoplasmic RNA from various cell lines. Virus from MuLV-infected clone H was purified on neutral sucrose gradients; virion RNA was isolated by phenol extraction and ethanol precipitation. Total cytoplasmic RNA was prepared from cells and polyA+-containing RNA was isolated by chromatography on oligo dT-cellulose. RNAs were electrophoresed through a 1.5% methyl mercury-agarose gel and transferred to nitrocellulose paper. The filters were incubated with 6 x 10^6 cpm of ^{32}P-labeled v-Kirsten-ras probe and exposed for autoradiography for 48 hr. (a) polyA+-RNA from WCT-L (MLV-infectaed rat cells); (b) virion RNA from MuLV-infected clone H; (c) polyA+-RNA from clone H, (d) polyA+-RNA from MuLV-infected clone H.

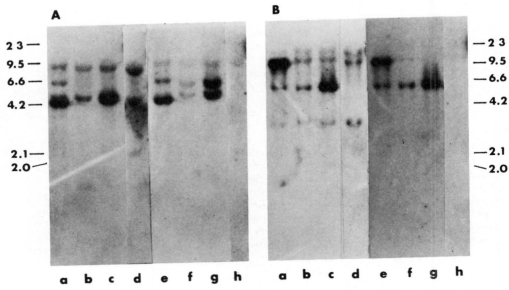

FIGURE 2. Southern blot analysis of cellular DNAs from (a) Kirsten MSV-3T3, (b) clone H, (c) primary transformant of NIH 3T3 generated by transfection with high-molecular-weight clone H DNA, (d) A31-DMBA 4-35. A and B are EcoRI and KpnI digests, respectively, of these DNAs fractionated by electrophoresis through a 0.7% agarose gel and transferred to nitrocellullose paper. The filters were incubated with 5 x 10^6 cpm of nick-translated ^{32}P-labeled v-Kirsten-ras probe (pHiHi-3) and exposed for auto-radiography for 48 hr (lanes a-d). The filters were dehybridized by washing at 65°C in 50% formamide and 5X SSPE, incubated with 5 x 10^6 cpm of nick-translated ^{32}P-labeled rat 30S DNA probe (pI-1), and exposed to autoradiography for 48 hr (lanes e-h).

clone H would, of course, verify whether rearrangements or other alterations in restriction enzyme sites had not occurred, explaining the presumed discrepancy. Indeed, the KiSV transformant used for comparison shows considerable alteration from the expected pattern. In any case, these results serve as a caveat in analyses that depend on restriction enzyme sensitivities for gene transfer of intergrated or cellular transforming sequences.

In conclusion, we have found that 3T3 cells transfomed either by virus or chemical agents consistently express the transformed phenotype in cell hybrids and by DNA-mediated gene transfer. This behavior is consistent with the genetic composition of these and other aneuploid rodent cell lines commonly used for transformation studies in vitro and may be dissimilar for multistep processes such as carcinogenesis in vivo. One would predict that such genetic alterations are particularly amenable to gene isolation methodologies. We are, therefore, currently attempting to isolate the responsible sequence(s) from A31.DMBA and other chemical transformants that are negative upon rescue.

ACKNOWLEDGEMENTS

This work was supported by NIH grants from the National Cancer Institute CA 23003 (H.L.O.), CA 30643 (H.L.O.), CA 24223 (D.D.) and RR 08176 funded by the Division of Research Resources and the National Institute of Arthritis, Metabolism, and Digestive Diseases. D.D. is the recipient of a Junior Faculty Research Award from the American Cancer Society. We thank Drs Ronald W. Ellis and Edward M. Scolnick of the laboratory of Tumor Virus Genetics, National Cancer Institute, for providing the molecular probes used in this study.

REFERENCES

1. Aaronson SA, Todaro GJ (1968): J Cell Physiol 72:141
2. Aaronson SA, Weaver CA (1971): J Gen Virol 13:245
3. Baker RM, Brunette DM, Mankovitz R, Thompson LH, Whitmore GF, Siminovitch L, Till JE (1974): Cell 1:9.
4. Blair DG, McClements WL, Oskarsson M, Fischinger PJ, Vande Woude GF (1980): Proc Natl Acad Sci USA 77:3504
5. Botchan M, Topp WC, Sambrook J (1976): Cell 9:269
6. Ellis RW, DeFeo D, Maryak JM, Young HA, Shih TY, Chang EH, Lowy DR, Scolnick EM (1980): J Virol 36:408
7. Ellis RW, DeFeo D, Shih TY, Gonda MA, Young HA, Tsuchida N, Lowy DR, Scolnick EM (1981): Nature 292:506
8. Graham FL, van der EB AJ (1973): Virology 52:456
9. Gurney EG, Gurney T (1979): J Virol 32:661
10. Jainchill JS, Aaronson SA, Todaro GJ (1969): J Virol 4:549
11. Jha, KK, Ozer HL (1976): Somatic Cell Genet 2:215
12. Jha KK, Cacciapuoti J, Ozer HL (1978): J Cell Physiol 97:147
13. Jha KK, Gurney EG, Feldman LA, Ozer HL (1979): Cold Spring Harbor Symp Quant Biol 44:689
14. Jha KK, Siniscalco M, Ozer HL (1980): Somatic Cell Genet 6:603
15. Krontiris TG, Cooper GM (1981): Proc Natl Acad Sci USA 78:1181
16. Lane M, Sainten A, Cooper GM 1981): Proc Natl Acad Sci USA 78:5185
17. Ozer HL, Jha KK (1977): Adv Cancer Res 25:53
18. Perucho M, Goldfarb M, Shimizu K, Lama C, Fogh J, Wigler M (1981): Cell 27:467
19. Quarles JM, Tennant RW (1975): Cancer Res 35:2637
20. Renger HC, Basilico C (1972): Proc Natl Acad Sci USA 69:109
21. Sen A, Todar GJ (1978): Proc Natl Acad Sci USA 75:1647
22. Shih C, Shilo BZ, Goldfarb MP, Dannenberg A, Weinberg RA (1979): Proc Natl Acad Sci USA 76:5714
23. Shilo BZ, Weinberg RA (1981): Nature 289:706
24. Tsuchida N, Kominami R, Hatanaka M, Uesugi S (1981): J Virol 38:797
25. Varmus HE, Bishop JM, Vogt PK (1973): J Mol Biol 74:613
26. Vogel A, Pollack R (1974): J Virol 14:1404
27. Wigler M, Pellicer A, Silverstein S, Axel R (1978): Cell 14:725
28. Yoshida MC, Sasaki M, Takeichi N, Boone CW (1976): Cancer Res 36:2235

Gene Transfer and Cancer, edited by M. L. Pearson
and N. L. Sternberg. Raven Press, New York © 1984.

DNA Methylation and Gene Activity

Walter Doerfler, [1]Lily Vardimon, [2]Inge Kruczek, Dirk Eick,
Birgitt Kron, and [3]Ingrid Kuhlmann

*Institute of Genetics, University of Cologne, 5000 Cologne 41,
Federal Republic of Germany*

ABSTRACT. We have investigated how DNA methylation affects gene expression in eucaryotic cells and have established an inverse correlation
between the extent of DNA methylation in specific segments of integrated
adenovirus type 12 (Ad12) and type 2 (Ad2) DNAs and the level of gene expression. In vitro methylation of the cloned E2a region of Ad2 DNA by
the HpaII DNA methyltransferase (5'-CCGG) leads to transcriptional inactivation on microinjection into nuclei of Xenopus laevis oocytes. Unmethylated DNA or DNA methylated at 5'-GGCC sites is readily expressed.
Thus methylation of certain genes at specific sequences has a regulatory
effect on gene expression. We have analyzed the state of methylation of
all 5'-CCGG sites in the early regions of integrated Ad12 DNA in three
lines of Ad12-transformed hamster cells. Methylation of the promoter
regions of integrated viral genes correlates with transcriptional inactivation, whereas active genes have unmethylated promoter regions. Ad12
DNA in Ad12-induced tumors is undermethylated at 5'-CCGG and 5'-GCGC
sites, although viral genes are minimally expressed. When Ad12-trans-
formed cells, in which late viral genes are completely methylated and
not expressed, are treated with azacytidine, some of the methylated 5'-
CCGG sites become unmethylated, but late genes are not activated.
Hence, the unmethylated state of a gene is a necessary but not a sufficient precondition for expression. Upon transfer of tumor cells into
culture the extent of methylation of integrated Ad12 DNA increases.

INTRODUCTION

A deeper understanding of many basic biological phenomena such as
differentiation or cancer is likely to be based on the elucidation of
the mechanisms involved in the regulation of gene expression in eucaryotes. It is likely, though unproven as yet, that the interaction of
specific proteins with certain regions of the genome plays an important
role in eucaryotic gene regulation. There are numerous examples in
which DNA-protein interactions are guided directly by specific DNA
sequences or indirectly by specific structures which are sequence
dependent. Recently, it has been recognized that DNA methylation,

-----

Present addresses: [1]Massachusetts Institute of Technology, Boston, Massachusetts; [2]Institute of Biochemistry, University of Munich, Munich, Germany; [3]Institute of Virology, University of Cologne, Cologne, Germany.

probably at specific sites, can serve as an important signal on the DNA molecule that somehow affects gene expression (for reviews, see references 7,9,10,18,26,27,43). It is unknown whether DNA methylation directly constitutes a signal modulating specific DNA-protein interactions or whether it does so by eliciting or stabilizing structural changes in DNA. In this context it is interesting to mention that an alternating poly(d^{m}CdG)poly(d^{m}CdG) polymer containing 5-methylcytosine (5-mC) has a high propensity for the transition from the B form of DNA to the Z form (1,2,24,42). The unmethylated polymer undergoes this transition only at unphysiologically high ionic strength. The ability to convert to the Z configuration of DNA (42) is presumably dependent on the strict alternation of purine and pyrimidine bases in such polymers. It has been shown recently that the sequence CCGG can convert to the A configuration of DNA (5). Consideration of methylated bases as regulatory signals raises the question as to whether modified bases exert their function in short-term or in long-term regulation.

We have used the adenovirus system, in particular adenovirus-transformed cells or adenovirus-induced tumor cells of rodent origin (for review, see reference 8), to study the regulation of gene expression. Many Ad12-transformed cells, although containing essentially the entire viral genome in multiple copies (8,21,22,29), express the early viral functions while late viral genes are permanently turned off (12,13,25, 28). An inverse correlation between the levels of methylation at 5'CCGG-3' sites in integrated Ad12 and Ad2 genes in transformed cells and the extent to which these genes are expressed has been established (32-34). Similar correlations have been documented in many other viral and nonviral eucaryotic systems (for review, see references 7,9). Ad2 or Ad12 DNA extracted from purified virions is not methylated (16, see also below and Figure 3). The inverse relationship between DNA methylation at 5'-CCGG-3' sites and gene activity has been studied in detail for the E2a region, which is the gene encoding the Ad2-specific DNA-binding protein (DBP), in the Ad2-transformed hamster cell lines HE1, HE2 and HE3 (4,34,37). Cell line HE1 expresses the DBP; cell lines HE2 and HE3 fail to do so (11,19,34). Interestingly, all 5'-CCGG-3' sites in the E2a region of cell line HE1 are unmethylated, while in cell lines HE2 and HE3 the same sites are completely methylated (34). Cell lines HE1, HE2, and HE3 all contain a late promoter/leader of the E2a region, and cell line HE1 utilizes this promoter (37,38). Thus, the absence of expression of the E2a region in cell lines HE2 and HE3 cannot be due to the lack of a functional promoter. DNA methylation, perhaps at specific sites, could be considered the cause for, or the consequence of, the absence of gene expression.

RESULTS AND DISCUSSION

DNA Methylation at Specific Sites is Causally Related
to Gene Inactivation

We have designed an experiment to distinguish between these alternatives (35,36). The possibility existed that DNA methylation had to occur at highly specific sites in a gene in order to be functionally significant. Different genes might still require methylation at different sites. The results of the analyses on the state of methylation of the E2a region of Ad2 DNA in transformed cell lines cited above suggested that the 5'-CCGG-3' sequences might constitute such specific sites at least for this particular gene. Thus, the 5'-CCGG-3' sites in the

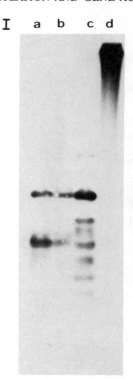

FIGURE 1. (I) Stability of the methylation pattern of the cloned
HindIII A fragment of Ad2 DNA on microinjection into nuclei of Xenopus
oocytes. The cloned DNA fragment was methylated in vitro (lanes c and
d) by using HpaII DNA methyltransferase or was left unmethylated (lanes
a and b). The DNA preparations were then microinjected into nuclei of
Xenopus oocytes and, 24 hr later, the total intracellular DNA was extracted. Subsequently, the DNA preparations were cleaved with MspI
(lanes a and c) or HpaII (lanes b and d). The fragments were separated
by electrophoresis on a 1.5% agarose slab gel, transferred to nitrocellulose filters, and visualized by hybridization to ^{32}P-labeled Ad2 DNA
followed by autoradiography. Failure of cleavage by HpaII indicated
methylation at the internal cytosine of 5'-CCGG-3' sequences. Reprinted
from (36). (Figure 1 continues on following pages.)

cloned E2a region of Ad2 DNA were methylated in vitro using the DNA-
methyltransferase from Haemophilus parainfluenzae (HpaII; 23). The HpaII
DNA methyltransferase methylates to completion the 5'-C*CGG-3' site at
the internal C-residue. Methylated or unmethylated, cloned E2a DNA was
microinjected into the nuclei of X. laevis oocytes, and the synthesis of
Ad2-specific RNA in these oocytes was monitored. Experimental details
have been published elsewhere (36). The data presented in Figure 1,
part I, demonstrate that the methylated or the unmethylated DNA maintains its state of methylation at least 24 hr after microinjection, in
that it is still refractory or suspectible, respectively, to cleavage by
the HpaII restriction endonuclease. Methylated Ad2 DNA (gene E2a) is
not transcribed in X. laevis oocytes; unmethylated DNA can be readily
expressed as mRNA (Figure 1, part II A, B). It has also been shown that
one of the late promoters of the E2a region of Ad2 DNA is used in
X. laevis oocytes (37; data not shown). Moreover, when unmethylated,

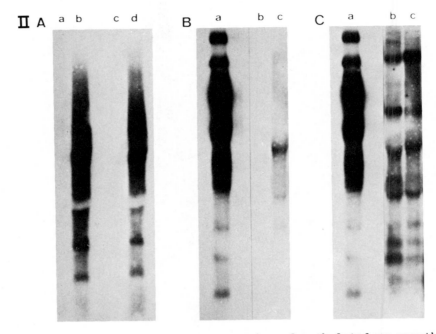

FIGURE 1, cont'd. (II). Test for expression of methylated or unmethylated cloned HindIII A fragment of Ad2 DNA or of unmethylated h22 DNA (histone gene from sea urchin) after microinjection into oocytes from Xenopus. Twenty-four hours after microinjection, the total intracellular RNA was extracted and fractionated by electrophoresis on 0.8% agarose slab gels containing 2.2 M formaldehyde. The RNA was then transferred to nitrocellulose filters. (A) The cloned HindIII A fragment of Ad2 DNA was methylated in vitro (lanes a and c) by using HpaII DNA methyltransferase or was left unmethylated (lanes b and d). The RNA blot was probed with ^{32}P-labeled Ad2 DNA. The RNA preparations analyzed in lanes c and d were treated with DNase. (B) Methylated cloned HindIII A fragment (lane b) or unmethylated DNA (lane c) was mixed with unmethylated recircularized h22 DNA before microinjection. RNA was analyzed as in A. HindIII-cleaved Ad2 DNA (lane a) was used as a size marker. (C) The blots obtained in B were rehybridized after autoradiography with ^{32}P-labeled h22 DNA from sea urchin. Reprinted from reference 36.

cloned histone genes from sea urchin and methylated, cloned E2a DNA from Ad2 were simultaneously injected into the same oocytes, histone mRNA was readily detectable and Ad2 DNA remained silent (Figure 1, part II C). These results demonstrate that DNA methylation is causally related to gene inactivation.

In a similar set of experiments, we have methylated the same cloned E2a region of Ad2 DNA with the DNA methyltransferase BsuRI from Bacillus subtilis (17). This DNA-methyltransferase specifically methylates the internal C-residue in the 5'-GGC*C-3' sequence. On microinjection of E2a DNA thus methylated or of unmethylated E2a DNA into nuclei of X. laevis oocytes, the DNA again maintains its methylated or unmethylated state for at least 24 hr after microinjection (data not shown). However, in this experiment, both the methylated and the unmethylated

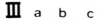

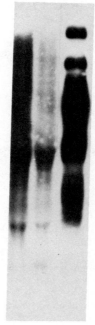

FIGURE 1 cont'd. (III). Methylation of the cloned HindIII-A fragment of Ad2 DNA by the BsuRI DNA-methyltransferase at 5'-GGCC-3' sites does not inhibit transcription after microinjection into X. laevis oocytes. (lane a) RNA from oocytes injected with methylated DNA (5'-GG^{m}CC-3'). (lane b) RNA from oocytes injected with unmethylated DNA (5'-GGCC-3'). (lane c) Ad2 marker DNA cleaved with HindIII. Reprinted from (38).

E2a DNA is equally expressed into mRNA (Figure 1, part III).

We conclude that in the E2a region of Ad2 DNA, methylation of the internal C-residues of the 5'-CCGG-3' sites leads to transcriptional inactivation of this gene. Methylation at the 5'-GGCC-3' sites, however, does not affect expression. Hence, DNA methylation at highly specific sites in specific genes can serve as a (long-term) signal for gene inactivation. Similar conclusions have been drawn for simiam virus 40 (SV40) DNA (14,41) and the thymidine kinase gene of herpes virus (41). The methylated sequence 5'-C*CGG-3' can probably serve as a signal in its own right and not via a local B form-Z form transition of DNA. Transition of the 5'-CCGG-3' sequence to the A form of DNA has been demonstrated (5).

Is Methylation at the Promoter/Leader and 5'- Regions of a Gene Decisive in Gene Regulation?

For DNA methylation at a specific sequence to signal gene inactivation, it may not be necessary to methylate all available sites in a particular gene; rather, it may be sufficient to limit methylation to the promoter/leader and/or 5'-regions of the gene. Methylation at the 5'-end of a gene may have a distinct regulatory meaning, and subsequent methylation events involving extended regions of the body of the gene may signal other specific modulating functions. We know next to nothing about these possibly very detailed signal values that depend on the precise locations of DNA methylation. It will be necessary to investigate whether there are significant differences in DNA methylation at intron or exon regions of a particular gene.

As a first attempt to decipher these possibly very complex signals, we have precisely mapped the methylated and the unmethylated 5'-CCGG-3' sites in integrated Ad12-DNA sequences in the three Ad12-transformed hamster cell lines T637, HA12/7, and A2497-3 (29) and correlated the state of methylation of these sites to viral gene expression in these cell lines. The experimental details have been published (20,32,33) and are not repeated here. By using a large number of cloned restriction endonuclease fragments of Ad12 DNA (39) as hybridization probes and blotted DNA from the three Ad12-transformed cell lines that had been cleaved with the isoschizomeric restriction endonucleases HpaII or MspI (40), we were able to derive the maps presented in Figure 2. We had previously shown which parts of the integrated viral genomes were expressed and which parts were permanently shut off (12,25,28). The horizontal arrows designate regions that are actually expressed in each of the three cell lines (Figure 2a,b). Interestingly, the 5'-CCGG-3' sites at the 5'-ends of the genes are unmethylated in all viral genes that are expressed. Methylated 5'-CCGG-3' sites are found at the 3' ends of the E1b, E2a, and E3 regions, although these regions are expressed. In cell line HA12/7, the E3 region is not expressed (12, 20,28), and accordingly the 5'-CCGG-3' sites at its 5' end are methylated, whereas some of the same sites toward its 3' end are unmethylated (20). From the same series of investigations there is evidence that the levels of methylation at the 5'-CGCG-3' (HhaI) sites in Ad12 DNA integrated in the three cell lines are similar to those at the 5'-GCGC-3' sites (20).

The following conclusions can be drawn from these results:

a) The use of highly specific hybridization probes has permitted the construction of detailed maps of the methylated and unmethylated 5'-CCGG-3' sites in integrated Ad12 DNA in cell lines T637, HA12/7, and A2497-3. Previous conclusions about an inverse correlation between the extent of DNA methylation of specific genes in integrated viral genomes and the levels of expression of these genes have been confirmed and refined.

b) The mapping data now suggest that the levels of methylation in the promoter/leader and/or 5'-regions of specific viral genes determine gene expression.

c) The data are consistent with the notion that most of the multiple copies of integrated Ad12 DNA persisting in cell lines T637 and A2497-3 conform to the same methylation pattern. This finding may suggest that any one of these multiple viral DNA copies is available for expression in the early regions. Which copies are eventually expressed may be determined by factors not exclusively related to DNA methylation.

d) The levels of methylation at 5'CCGG-3' and at 5'-GCGC-3' sites seem to be the same or very similar.

The Unmethylated State of a Gene Appears to be a Necessary but not Sufficient Precondition for Gene Activity

We have investigated the patterns of integration and of methylation of viral DNA in 39 different Ad12-induced hamster tumors and tumor cell lines established from some of these tumors (21,22). The striking observation has been made that the integrated Ad12 genomes in the tumors

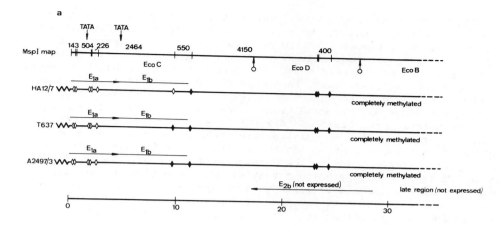

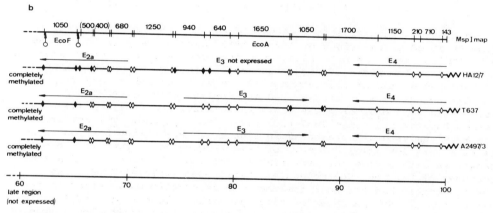

FIGURE 2. Functional maps of the left (a) and the right (b) parts of the Ad12 DNA molecules integrated in cell lines HA12/7, T637, and A2497-3. The horizontal lines represented the Ad12 genomes (———) integrated into the genomes of cell lines (∿) as indicated. The MspI maps of the left (a) and right (b) ends of Ad12 DNA are presented in the top lines. Vertical bars on and figures above the horizontal lines indicate the locations of the MspI sites and the sizes of some of the MspI fragments, respectively. The arrows (○) designate EcoRI sites. TATA marks the locations of presumptive Goldberg-Hogness signals in the E1a region (3,30).

The unmethylated (◊) and methylated (◆) 5'-CCGG-3' sites in the integrated Ad12 genomes in the lines HA12/7, T637 and A2397-3 are designated by open or closed symbols as indicated. The horizontal arrows indicate map positions and direction of transcription of the individual early regions in each of the cell lines. Presence of an arrow indicates expression of corresponding regions of the Ad12 genome.

MspI sites to the right of the EcoRI-D/B and to the left of the EcoRI-A/F junctions have not been mapped. These sites are all methylated. The early regions of Ad12 DNA (12,13,25) and a fractional length scale have also been indicated. The map of the E1 region of Ad12 DNA is as described (3). Reprinted from ref 20.

are undermethylated or not methylated at all at the 5'-CCGG-3' or the
5'-GCGC-3' sites, although there is very little Ad12-specific RNA detectable in these tumors (21). When tumor cells are explanted into
culture and passaged consecutively, an increase in the levels of DNA
methylation can be observed (21). We do not know the mechanisms responsible for this apparent shift in the levels of viral DNA methylation.
It could be caused by selection of cells with a higher level of DNA
methylation under culture conditions. Nevertheless, the data indicate
that the unmethylated state of Ad12 DNA integrated in Ad12-induced tumor
cells is not correlated to massive viral gene expression; additional,
unidentified factors must be lacking in the tumors for viral gene expression to proceed. Hence, the unmethylated state of integrated adenovirus DNA is a necessary but not a sufficient precondition for viral
gene expression. In cloned lines of tumor cells the patterns of methylation have been found to be remarkably stable. The tumor cell system
may provide an interesting tool to study in more detail parameters determining the levels of DNA methylation.

Levels of 5-Methylcytosine in Viral and Cellular DNAs

In previous investigations we have demonstrated that DNA extracted
from purified preparations of Ad2 or Ad12 contains very little if any
5-mC (16). There was no evidence for the occurrence of 6-methyladenine.
By using the technique of high pressure liquid chromatography (HPLC) and
an improved system of resolution (15), we have reexamined Ad2 virion DNA
for its actual content of 5-mC. DNAs from the plasmid pBR322, from
Drosophila melanogaster cells grown in culture, and from the Ad12-trans-
formed hamster cell line T637 (29) were also analyzed. The results of
the HPLC-analyses are presented in Figure 3. Ad2 virion DNA indeed contains a very low level, if any, of 5-mC (Figure 3a). Even this highly
sensitive method does not permit us to rule out the presence of a few
residues of 5-mC per DNA molecule. Virion DNA isolated from virus
particles that had not been treated with pancreatic DNase prior to the
extraction of Ad2 DNA revealed slightly higher amounts of 5-mC (Figure
3b). Thus, it is possible that at least a fraction of the low levels of
5-mC possibly detectable in Ad2 DNA could be due to trace contaminations
of purified virions with human cellular DNA. The DNA of plasmid pBR322
contains 12 residues of 5-mC per molecule (31), and this amount can
serve as an internal standard for quantitations of 5-mC when compared to
the surface area corresponding to 5-mC (Figure 3c). The DNA from
D. melanogaster cells grown in culture contains even less 5-mC than Ad2
DNA (Figure 3d). The best estimate for the limit of detectability using
this method of resolution is about one 5-mC residue per about 2000 C
residues. The presence of 5-mC in the DNA from T637 cells can be clearly
demonstrated (Figure 3e); the 5-mC/C content amounts to about 3.3%, a
value very close to that published earlier (16). It is concluded that
Ad2 virion DNA and DNA from _D. melanogaster_ cells contain very low amounts
of 5-mC, if any.

DNA Methyltransferase Activities in Uninfected
and in Ad2-infected KB Cells

The question arises how adenovirion DNA can avoid methylation in the
nucleus of human cells in which it replicates. It has been shown previously that human cellular DNA contains 3.6 to 4.4% 5-mC (16). Furthermore, adenovirion DNA can be readily methylated to completion in vitro

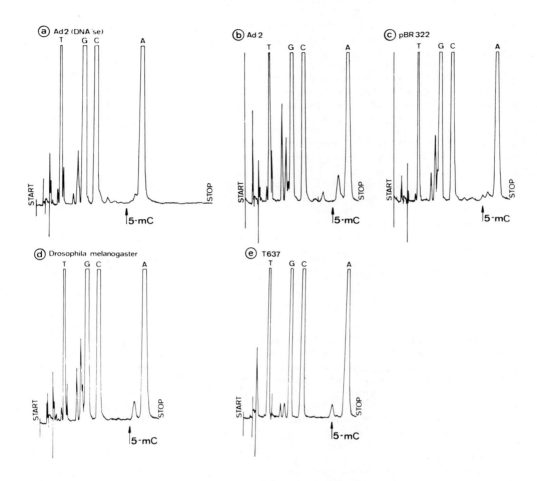

FIGURE 3. Determination of the 5-mC content of Ad2, pBR322, D. melanogaster, and hamster cell DNAs as determined by HPLC. Ad2 DNA was extracted from CsCl-purified Ad2 that had been treated with pancreatic
DNase (28) and had been repurified by equilibrium sedimentation prior to
DNA extraction (a). Ad2 DNA extracted from CsCl-purified virions untreated with DNase (b). pBR322 plasmid DNA (c). DNA extracted (29),33)
from D. melanogaster cells grown in culture (d). DNA extracted from
cells of the Ad12-transformed hamster line T637 (e). DNA preparations
were treated with 1N NaOH for 1 hr at 50°C, neutralized, and precipitated with two volumes of ethanol to remove traces of RNA. All DNA preparations were hydrolyzed in 90% formic acid for 0.5 hr at 170°C. Hydroly-
sis products were fractionated on a 3.9 mm x 30 cm µBondapak C_{18} column.
Mobile phase: 40% picB7 (Waters), 1.25% acetonitrile, 1 mN NaOH. A
Waters HPLC instrument was used.

Each graph was scanned and peaks were integrated by a Shimadzu
Integrator. Relative surface areas were calculated but not reproduced
here. The arrows designate the 5-mC peaks in each graph. A,C,G, and T
refer to the four bases.

using HpaII or BsuRI DNA methyltransferase (35,36,38). We have therefore started to investigate DNA methyltransferase activities that can be extracted from the nuclei of uninfected KB cells and of KB cells harvested at various times after infection with 30 plaque-forming units of Ad2. The preliminary data demonstrate that DNA-methyltransferase activity can be extracted from nuclei of KB cells. Thus far, no differences in DNA methyltransferase activities can be detected in extracts from nuclei of uninfected KB cells and extracts from nuclei of KB cells harvested at various times after infection with Ad2. The lack of methylation of adenovirion DNA cannot simply be accounted for by the absence or shut-off of DNA-methyltransferase activity after viral infection. More complicated mechanisms would have to be involved. It can be shown that the DNA methyltransferase activity extracted from uninfected or from infected cells is capable of methylating adenovirus DNA de novo. Conceivably, the DNA methyltransferase in KB cells does not have access to adenovirus DNA, which may be compartmentalized to some degree in the nucleus and which replicates at a very high rate. Perhaps most of the DNA-methyltransferase activity in the cell is bound to cellular DNA and thus not able to reach the newly synthesized viral DNA in the nucleus. Obviously, this tentative explanation is only one of several possible ones.

CONCLUSIONS

The data presented here and in previous publications (7,20,33,34-38) demonstrate that DNA methylation at highly specific sites, notably at 5'-CCGG-3' sequences, plays an important role in the long term inactivation of specific genes. Methylation of the sequence 5'-CCGG-3' leads to transcriptional inactivation of many viral genes. There is evidence that methylation of these sites at or close to the promoter/leader and/or 5'-regions of a gene is functionally most important (20).

It is not yet known how the methylated sequence 5'-C*CGG-3' can be recognized by specific proteins that could turn off certain genes by binding to specific sequences. Because the sequence 5'-CCGG-3' lacks strict alternation between pyrimidine and purine residues, methylation at these sites is not likely to lead to a local transition of the DNA from the B to the Z form (42). Perhaps, the A form of DNA could play a role (5). The results gleaned from Ad12-induced tumors suggest that DNA methylation may serve as a long-term signal for gene inactivation and that the absence of methylation of integrated viral DNA alone does not necessarily lead to gene expression.

Adenovirion DNA and intracellular viral DNA (16,34) are not methylated or are methylated to a very limited extent, although Ad2 DNA can be readily methylated in vitro by procaryotic DNA methyltransferases and by DNA methyltranserase activities extracted from human KB cells. The results of HPLC analyses also suggest that the DNA of D. melanogaster cells contains very little, if any 5-mC. The way in which adenovirus DNA escapes being methylated in human cells cannot be completely explained at this time. DNA methyltransferase activities extractable from uninfected and Ad2-infected KB cells appear to be very similar. In any event, it would be inopportune for an obligatorily parasitic genome to succumb to a long-term shut-off mechanism of the host cell.

ACKNOWLEDGEMENTS

We thank Linda Bautz, Heidelberg, for a gift of D. melanogaster

cells and Hans-Jochen Fritz for help and advice with the HPLC analyses.
I.K. was supported by a fellowship of the Friedrich-Ebert Foundation.
This research was made possible by the Deutsche Forschungsgemeinschaft
through SFB 74-C1 and by a grant of the State Ministry for Science and
Research, Northrhine-Westfalia (IIB5-FA8381).

REFERENCES

1. Behe M, Felsenfeld G (1981): Proc Natl Acad Sci USA 78:1619
2. Behe M, Zimmermann S, Felsenfeld G (1981): Nature 293:233
3. Bos JL, Polder LJ, Bernards R, Schrier PI, van den Elsen PJ, van der Eb AJ, van Ormondt H (1981): Cell 27:121
4. Cook JL, Lewis AM Jr. (1979): Cancer Res 39:1455
5. Conner BN, Takano T, Tanaka S, Itakur K, Dickerson RE (1982): Nature 295:294
6. Creusot F, Acs G, Christman JK (1982): J Biol Chem 257:2041
7. Doerfler W (1981): J Gen Virol 57:1
8. Doerfler W (1982): Curr Top Microbiol Immunol 100:127
9. Doerfler W (1983): Annu Rev Biochem 52:93
10. Ehrlich M, Wang RYH (1981): Science 212:1350
11. Esche H (1982): J Virol 41:1076
12. Esche H, Siegmann B (1982): J Gen Virol 60:99
13. Esche H, Schilling R, Doerfler W (1979): J Virol 30:21
14. Fradin A, Manley JL, Prives CL (1982): Proc Natl Acad Sci USA 72:5142
15. Fritz H-J, Eick D, Werr W (1982): In: Chemical and Enzymatic Gene Synthesis of Gene Fragments - A Laboratory Manual (Gassen HG, Lang A, eds), Weinheim: Verlag Chemie, p 199
16. Gunthert U, Schweiger M, Stupp M, Doerfler W (1976): Proc Natl Acad Sci USA 73:3923
17. Gunthert U, Jentsch S, Freund M (1981): J Biol Chem 256:9346
18. Hattman S (1981): In: The Enzymes (Boyer PD, ed), Vol 14, New York: Academic Press, p 517
19. Johansson K, Persson H, Lewis AM, Pettersson U, Tibbetts C, Philipson, L (1978): J Viol 27:628
20. Kruczek I, Doerfler W (1982): EMBO J 1:409
21. Kuhlmann I, Doerfler W (1982): Virol 118:169
22. Kuhlmann I, Achten S, Rudolf R, Doerfler W (1982): EMBO J 1:79
23. Mann MB, Smith HO (1977): Nucleic Acids Res 4:4211
24. Nickol J, Behe M, Felsenfeld G (1982): Proc Natl Acad Sci USA 79:1771
25. Ortin J, Scheidtmann KH, Greenberg R, Westphal M, Doerfler W (1976): J Virol 20:355
26. Razin A, Riggs AD (1980): Science 210:604
27. Razin A, Friedman J (1981): Prog Nucleic Acids Res Mol Biol 25:33
28. Schirm S, Doerfler W (1981): J Virol 39:694
29. Stabel S, Doerfler W, Friis RR (1980): J Virol 36:22
30. Sujisaki H, Sugimoto K, Takanami M, Shiroki K, Saito I, Shimojo H, Sawada Y, Uemizu Y, Uesugi S, Fuginaga K (1980): Cell 20:777
31. Sutcliffe JG (1978): Cold Spring Harbor Symp Quant Biol 43:77
32. Sutter D, Doerfler W (1979): Cold Spring Harbor Symp Quant Biol 44:565
33. Sutter D, Doerfler W (1980): Proc Natl Acad Sci USA 77:253
34. Vardimon L, Neumann R, Kuhlmann I, Sutter D, Doerfler W (1980): Nucleic Acids Res 8:2461
35. Vardimon L, Kuhlmann I, Cedar H, Doerfler W (1981): Eur J Cell Biol 25:13

36. Vardimon L, Kressmann A, Cedar H, Maechler M, Doerfler W (1982):
     Proc Natl Acad Sci USA 79:1073
37. Vardimon L, Renz D, Doerfler W (1982): Recent Results in Cancer
     Res 84:90
38. Vardimon L, Gunthert U, Doerfler W (1982): Mol Cell Biol 2:1574
39. Vogel S, Brotz M, Kruczek I, Neumann R, Eick D, Winterhoff U,
     Doerfler W (1981): Gene 15:273
40. Waalwijk C, Flavell RA (1978): Nucleic Acids Res 5:4631
41. Waechter DE, Baserga R (1982): Proc Natl Acad Sci USA 79:1106
42. Wang AH-J, Quigley GJ, Kolpak FJ, Crawford JL, van Boom JH, van
     der Marel G, Rich A (1979): Nature 282:680
43. Wigler MH (1981): Cell 24:285

Gene Transfer and Cancer, edited by M. L. Pearson
and N. L. Sternberg. Raven Press, New York © 1984.

Concerted Hypermethylation and Stable Shutdown of a Cluster of Thymidine Kinase Genes

*Stephen C. Hardies, **David E. Axelrod, *Marshall H. Edgell, and *Clyde A. Hutchison III

*Department of Microbiology and Immunology, University of North Carolina, Chapel Hill, North Carolina 27514; and **Waksman Institute of Microbiology, Rutgers University, Piscataway, New Jersey 08854*

ABSTRACT. A mouse L cell line with a cluster of 200 tandem herpes simplex virus thymidine kinase (tk) genes was established using DNA-mediated gene transfer. By alternatively selecting against and for TK expression in this cell line, we have observed genetic events that alter the expression of the entire tk cluster. This cell line was named HM for "hypermethylater" because it is unusually prone to produce TK⁻ variants that are methylated in all of their tk genes. Methylation was monitored either as alteration of HpaII/MspI cleavage patterns or as blockage of a single EcoRI site per gene. The EcoRI assay, which proved to be particularly sensitive, also detected a gradual increase in methylation of the tk cluster, even in cells under selection for TK expression. Experiments with other cell lines showed that hypermethylation to produce HM TK⁻ variants is genetically distinct from this gradual increase in methylation. Hypermethylation was a reproducible result in HM TK⁻ variants after selection with either bromo-deoxyuridine or acycloguanosine [Acyclovir or 9-(2-hydroxyethoxymethyl) guanine]. Rare revertants to TK⁺ did not demethylate their tk genes, but instead amplified them an additional 10-fold. So we have distinguished three genomic changes affecting cellular phenotype: a) a gradual increase in methylation, b) hypermethylation, and c) amplification.

INTRODUCTION

Genes introduced into cells in culture by gene transfer can be used to probe cellular gene regulation. This paper describes the control exerted over a newly introduced tk gene cluster by an L cell. One clone is described that produces TK⁻ variants in which the tk cluster has had a significant number of its CpG sequences converted to 5Omethyl CpG. The behavior of this cell line is contrasted to that of several others with independently derived tk clusters. Variability in the expression of genes introduced into cells in culture is usually considered a nuisance. We will put forward a perspective in which this variability can be a valuable probe into mechanisms of eucaryotic gene regulation.

249

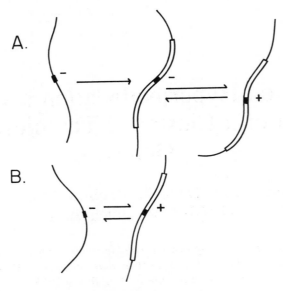

FIGURE 1. Regional activation during gene regulation. A) A model in which the region surrounding a gene must first be activated before subsequent steps can cause expression. B) A constitutive gene that is expressed as soon as the surrounding region becomes activated. The gene in panel B acts as a probe into the state of the surrounding chromatin.

Models for Regional Control Mechanisms

The rationale for these experiments is based on the idea that regional changes in chromatin structure are involved in gene regulation. Models for the behavior of an inducible gene and a noninducible gene are illustrated in Figure 1. The model for activation of the inducible gene is taken from studies of chicken α and βglobin (25,30), and ovalbumin (15). Before these genes are expressed, a change in the state of the surrounding chromatin is observed. In the cases cited, the change is detected by an increase in DNase I sensitivity. As a result, genes in the affected region, called a domain (25), acquire the potential to be expressed. Subsequent events induce the expression of specific genes within the domain. A cell culture system featuring strong positive and negative selection on such an inducible gene could be used to study the changes occurring during these latter steps.

An alternate model allows the study of the regional activation or inactivation events (Figure 1B). Here a gene is pictured whose expression is more directly tied to the state of the surrounding chromatin. This gene is constitutive in the sense that if it resides in a region that has acquired the potential for gene activity, then it will be expressed. A cell culture system with strong positive and negative selection on such a constitutive gene would allow analysis of regional control mechanisms.

We propose that the tk gene from herpes simplex virus can act as such a constitutive gene. To establish a model system, we transferred purified tk genes into mouse L cells by the calcium phosphate precipitation method (31). TK+ clones were isolated that were shown to have acquired a cluster of tk genes. Southern blot analyses were then used to examine the state of the tk gene cluster in survivors of selection against TK expression. The presence of multiple tk genes in the same region enhanced the probability of selecting for regional changes. To the extent that tk genes are treated like cellular genes, this allowed us to observe the reverse of regional activation.

The tk Gene Cluster in HM

The arrangement of the tk gene cluster in one of the L cell TK transformants named HM was deduced from Southern blot analyses (Figure 2). There are over 200 copies of the tk gene in HM, mostly arranged in perfect head-to-tail tandem repeats. The repeat unit consists of 7 kb containing the tk gene and its Escherichia coli plasmid vector. The 200 copies are distributed in some unknown way over approximately six subclusters which are presumed to be interspersed with carrier DNA. TK⁻ derivatives can be obtained from HM that lose all 200 copies, indicating that the subclusters are not dispersed through the genome. In cell lines examined by in situ hybridization (22), stable transformants are generally found to have integrated the new genes into the chromosomal complement. Although HM has not yet been examined by in situ hybridization, its stability suggests that its tk cluster is integrated into the genome.

The tk cluster in HM is an unusual arrangement for the L cell. It contains a total of about 1.4×10^6 bp of DNA that is not of mouse origin. Although the carrier, which is mouse DNA, is probably interspersed at a few positions, the tandemly repeated subclusters consist of hundreds of contiguous kilobases of purely viral and E. coli sequences. The tk genes inside these subclusters will have to be silent in TK⁻ variants. So to survive the selection, the cell must control multiple genes in long stretches of sequence with which it has had no previous experience.

RESULTS

The changes that we do, in fact, see occurring in HM are collected in the Southern blot in Figure 3. These altered fragment patterns are interpreted in the following paragraphs to represent changes in the modification and copy number of genes in the tk cluster.

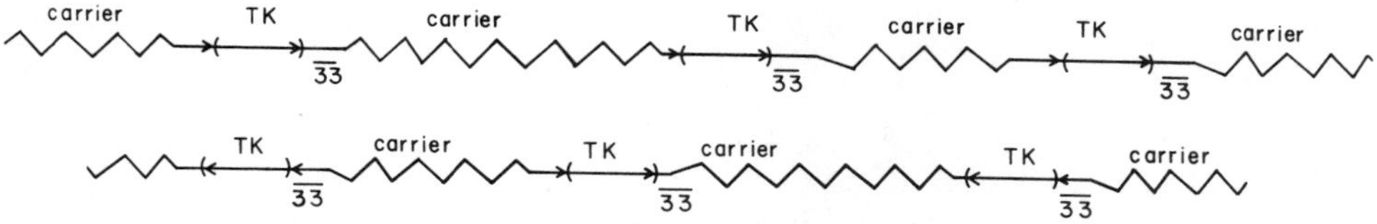

FIGURE 2. A possible arrangement of the tk genes in L cell line HM. The second line is a continuation of the first. HM was constructed by DNA-mediated gene transfer according to the procedure of Wigler (31) of circular pX1 (6: a clone of HSV tk in pBR322) plus carrier into tk⁻ L cells (31). The gene arrangement was deduced from Southern blots like that shown in Figure 3. The same fragmentation pattern as for circular pX$_1$ occurs in EcoRI-cut HM DNA at an intensity of 200 copies per cell. Since circular pX1 is not detected in uncleaved HM DNA, the 200 copies exist in head-to-tail tandem 7 kb repeats. Long exposures of Southern blots with EcoRI reveal 11 single-copy bands with pX1 homology. So the perfect tandem repeats must be interrupted five to nine times. A possible arrangement incorporating these features is shown.

Because of the tandem gene arrangement, the restriction pattern of the
tk genes in HM illustrated in this Southern blot is simple (Figure 3, lane
marked HM). EcoRI produced mainly the same tk fragments from HM DNA as
from the circular tk plasmid pX1 (5 kb, 2.4 kb, and 0.8 kb). Since only
fragments occurring in multiple copies are visible in Figure 3, changes
in the band pattern must reflect events that affected multiple sites.

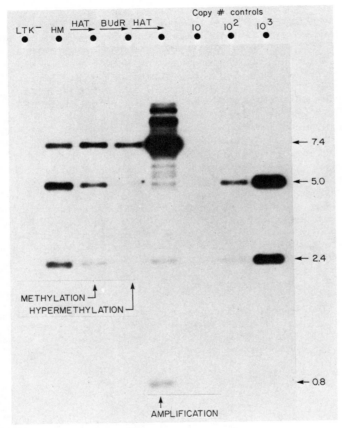

FIGURE 3. Southern blot analysis of HM and derivatives with restriction
endonuclease EcoRI. All of pX1 was used as probe. The right 3 lanes
contain pX1 mixed with tk⁻ DNA from L cells to simulate the numbers of
copies per cell indicated. Fragment sizes are expressed in kilobases.
The other lanes from left to right contain 5 µg apiece of DNA from:
a) tk⁻ L cells before transfer, b) the tk⁺ clone named HM after the
original HAT selection (the selective agent for TK expression), c) HM
after additional time in HAT, d) population of survivors after HM was
plated in bromodeoxyuridine (BUdR, a selective agent against TK), and
e) TK⁺ clone recovered after that TK⁻ population was plated in HAT.
Prior to digestion, the DNA in each lane was mixed with bacteriophage
lambda DNA. The filter shown in this figure subsequently was washed
and reprobed with lambda to verify complete digestion.

Methylation in HM

An extra multicopy band appears in HM, even while it is still growing in hypoxanthine/aminopterin/thymidine (HAT, the selective agent for TK$^+$). The appearance of this new band at 7.4 kb is accompanied by an equal decrease in intensity of the bands at 5.0 and 2.4 kb. We interpret this shift to represent blockage of the EcoRI site between the 5-kb and 2.4-kb fragments. The blockage is seen to increase with time in culture until just over half of the sites are not cut (Figure 3, lane marked methylation). When HM is plated in bromodeoxyuridine (a selective agent against TK expression) about 1 in 10^3 cells survives. The survivors are found to have lost all or nearly all of these EcoRI sites. This is true whether one looks at the total surviving population (Figure 3, lane marked hypermethylation) or at clones, although, clones with no remaining tk genes are also found. Therefore, the EcoRI site blockage reflects a change occurring throughout the cluster and is correlated with a transition to the TK$^-$ phenotype.

There are several circumstantial reasons to associate blockage of the EcoRI site with methylation. The sequence of this site is known to be CGAATTCG (29). Therefore, the recognition sequence (GAATTC) for the enzyme is flanked by the dinucleotide CG which is known to be frequently converted to 5-methyl CpG in eucaryotes (4,7). HpaII sites are also blocked in the tk cluster of TK$^-$ variants, whereas MspI sites are not (Figure 4). Both of these enzymes recognize CCGG. HpaII is known to be blocked by a methyl group on the second C residue, whereas MspI is known not to be blocked by methylation at this position (27). We found similar results with other enzymes that are affected by 5-methyl CpG. Since we also found enzymes that show no difference in their cleavage patterns, the cluster has not been rearranged. These results definitely establish an increase in modification of the tk gene cluster in the TK$^-$ variants of HM.

The mechanism for association of EcoRI blockage with 5-methyl CpG is less clear because no direct evidence is available that GAATTm^{5}C is not a substrate for EcoRI. EcoRI is able to cleave bacteriophage T4 DNA when all of its cytosines are 5-hydroxy methylated (13). However, two DNAs which are laden with 5-methyl C are not cleaved by EcoRI: bacteriophage XP12 DNA (11) and Chlamydomonas chloroplast DNA (21). (In the former case, the presence of EcoRI sites is only inferred from the size of the phage genome.) These results taken together leave it unclear whether the EcoRI site is blocked directly by steric hindrance from the methyl group or whether some less direct mechanism is involved. Also, it is not impossible that some other modification is correlated with methylation at C residues and blocks the EcoRI site. So, we could phrase our observations in terms of "modification" and "hypermodification". Instead, we prefer to conclude that the EcoRI site is blocked by 5-methyl CpG because the only EcoRI site that we see blocked is surrounded by CG sequences.

Methylation Versus Hypermethylation

By contrasting the behavior of HM to other transformants, we have concluded that the hypermethylation of TK$^-$ variants of HM is not a simple continuation of the methylation observed during growth in HAT. Two other clones and two populations with similar tk gene clusters were carried through the same series of treatments. While growing in HAT, all of these showed a gradual increase in methylation leveling off at an extent similar to that of HM. None of these others, however, produced any hypermethylated

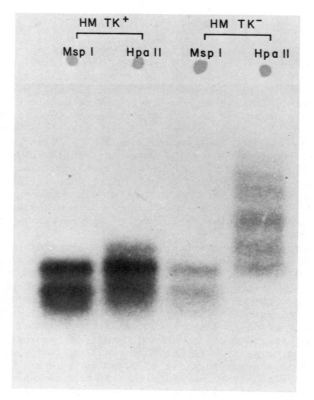

FIGURE 4. Southern analysis of HM and a TK⁻ variant with restriction
endonuclease HpaII or MspI. The 2 lanes at left contain the same DNA
as in Figure 3, lane HM. The 2 lanes at right contain DNA from a TK⁻
variant isolated with acycloguanosine. The lanes are not equally loaded.
Lambda DNA was mixed with each DNA prior to digestion to act as a control
for complete digestion. Whole pX1 was used as probe. Most of the fragments from pX1 are too small to transfer under the conditions used.

variants when challenged with bromodeoxyuridine. HM, on the other hand,
reproducibly produced hypermethylated TK⁻ variants at about 10^{-3} with
either bromodeoxyuridine or acycloguanosine [Acyclovir or 9-(2-hydroxy-
ethoxymethyl) guanine, (5)] as the selective agent.
    The hypermethylated HM variants were stably TK⁻ with only one cell in
10^6 surviving when the variants were plated back into HAT medium. In contrast, the other cell lines did not produce stable TK⁻ variants except
for those that had lost all of their tk genes. The HAT sensitivity of
the HM TK⁻ variants shows that they could not have arisen prior to the
lifting of the original HAT selection. Consequently, the shutdown of the
tk cluster and presumably the completion of the methylation occurred in
the short time between lifting of the HAT selection and application of
the negative selection. For this reason we propose that hypermethylation
in HM is a concerted event over the tk cluster in contrast to the gradual
methylation exhibited by all of these cells. That is, during hypermethylation in HM multiple sites are methylated and multiple genes are shut down.

Amplification

The rare TK$^+$ back revertants of HM tk$^-$ variants do not simply reverse the hypermethylation. These clones show an amplification of the tk cluster of about 10-fold (Figure 3, lane marked amplification). Much rearrangement is evident in association with the amplification. Since one fully active tk gene can produce the positive phenotype, we cannot rule out the possibility that it is the rearrangement or demethylation of one gene that causes the reversion. However, based on the fact that 4 of 4 revertants are amplified and none are rearranged without amplification, we favor the interpretation that amplification of the basal expression of the genes is rendering the cells TK$^+$. In either case, the lack of restoration of the 5-kb and 2.4-kb bands shows that there is not demethylation on a regional scale.

DISCUSSION

Our experiments demonstrate that L cells, and by implication other cells, have the molecular machinery to shut down at one time very large clusters of genes. This mechanism functions even when the sequences in the cluster are novel to the cell and might not themselves have any special sites for this purpose. Methylation is associated with this process.

Methylation at CpG has been proposed as a general mechanism to generate a heritable indicator of expression state (10,20). The key element of the proposed system is that a maintenance methylase exists with a specificity for hemimethylated CpG created by replication of fully methylated CG sites. Once put in place, the 5-methyl CpG would be propagated through replication, continuing to mark the DNA inactive. Conversely, if the CpG is demethylated, then that state will also be passed on through replication. So the decision to activate or inactivate would be propagated even though the original mechanism for placing or removing the methyl group may have been dismantled.

The regional inactivation that we have observed can be added to the domain activation model in several ways. One way is to consider the regional shutdown as the reverse of domain activation. Then there are some contrasts that need to be exlained between our region of tk genes and the domains described for chicken ovalbumin (15) and globin (25,30). Those domains are only 50 to 100 kb, smaller than the region observed during the shutdown of the tk cluster in HM. The size of the inactivated region in HM could be unnaturally large because of the number of tk genes the cell was forced to shut down, or the size difference between our observed region and domains could reflect an intrinsic difference in the scope of activation versus inactivation processes.

Active domains are usually observed as contiguous regions of DNase I-sensitive chromatin. Although DNase I-sensitive chromatin is, on average, less methylated (18), all sites in active domains are not uniformly hypomethylated. Loss of methylation at specific sites has been associated with gene expression for globin (9,16,17,24,28,30; see, however, ref. 23), ovalbumin (14,16), conalbumin (14,16), ovomucoid (16), metallothionein I (3), δcrystallin (12), ribosomal RNA genes (1), latent herpes simplex virus (33), and endogenous retroviruses (8). In many of these cases, only some of the assayable sites become hypomethylated during gene activation. The hypomethylation appears not to be spread throughout the domain and may be confined to smaller subdomains around the genes (24, 25,30).

This model, then, must consider regional shutdown and domain activation as two opposing processes rather than a single reversible one. Shutdown would proceed over many contiguous domains, with methyl groups appearing at many sites whether or not they are relevant to regulation. Domain activation would consist of reactivation of smaller units coupled with a selective removal of methyl groups from sites relevant to regulation. By opposing the two processes in this way, there is no need to propose that they both have the same specificity for sites in the DNA. This would be parallel with the observation that HM has the capability to shut down the tk region but lacks the capability to reverse the shutdown.

A second way to add the process we observed to the domain activation model is to propose a separate, irreversible inactivation process. In this model, genes are shut down, not by reversing the activation process, but by switching them to a new state that is permanently inactive. Also, genes that had not yet gone through domain activation could be committed to permanent silence by the same process. This model also fits the observation that HM apparently does not reactivate its tk cluster once it is shut down.

It is clear in only a few cases that a heritable inactivation of previously active genes occurs in normal cells. An alternative model, applicable in most cases, proposes that domains inherit their inactive state from the germ line and can undergo only activation, not inactivation. This is not true for the X chromosome, in which inactivation does occur at a set developmental stage. Methylation has been implicated in that process (see other papers in this volume; see ref. 32 for a contrasting opinion). Endogenous retroviruses are an example of nonsexlinked genes that were subjected to a shutdown involving methylation (8). The shutdown and methylation of these genes occurred in the germ line of animals rather than in cell culture. This inactivation happened on an evolutionary rather than a developmental time scale and may have been a natural analogy to what happened to the tk genes in HM.

The reason that HM can hypermethylate in contrast to the other cells studied is not known. However, we will comment on one plausible model. If the difference among these cell lines depends on site of integration in the genome, then cis-acting effects from the adjacent chromatin are responsible. Since the cluster is at least 1.4×10^6 bases long, this would imply the existence of a long range cis-acting influence to shut down the genes in the middle of the cluster.

Now consider the variability in behavior among different transformants with respect to the hypothesis that it reflects the site of integration. Not only do the four other lines studied here differ from HM, they also differ one from another in ways we have not discussed here. Other examples of differences in behavior among TK transformants can be found in the literature (2,19, Christy and Scangos, this volume, Davies et al., this volume). At this point, it seems entirely possible that every transformant is going to have at least some subtle individualistic streak. This variability can be a source of good fortune if, rather than trying to use the L cell to study the tk gene, we think of tk as a probe of the L cell. If a tk gene will co-regulate with whatever region it falls into, then this kind of experiment will shed light on a range of different control mechanisms working in the cell.

Clearly the application of other methods of analysis of TK variants may provide useful information. Methods involving DNase I sensitivity have been exploited (Davies et al., this volume). The amplified genes in the TK[+] back-revertants of HM present an unusual opportunity. The bulk of these genes are hypermethylated and in an inactive or basal expression state. These cells may produce enough of this DNA without cloning in bacteria to allow a direct purification of the tk DNA and a biochemical analysis of the modification pattern on it.

Finally, if a tk gene behaves differently depending on its environment, then cellular genes probably also do. This leads to important considerations in terms of a) the arrangement of genes within their clusters, b) the understanding of mutations involving rearrangements, and c) the role of such mutations in the evolution of gene clusters.

ACKNOWLEDGEMENTS

This work was supported by grants (A108998 and GM21313) from NIH. D.E.A. was supported by NSF-PCM78-05462. S.C.H. was supported by an NIH fellowship.

REFERENCES

1. Bird AP, Taggart MH, Gehring CA (1981): J Mol Biol 152:1
2. Clough DW, Kunkel LM, Davidson RL (1982): Science 216:70
3. Compere SJ, Palmiter RD (1981): Cell 25:233
4. Doskocil J, Sorm F (1962): Biochim Biophys Acta 55:953
5. Elion GB, Furman PA, Fyfe JA, DeMiranda P, Beauchamp L, Schaeffer JH (1977): Proc Natl Acad Sci USA 74:5716
6. Enquist L, Vande Woulde GF, Wagner M, Smiley JR, Summers WC (1979): Gene 7:335
7. Grippo P, Iaccarino M, Parisi E, Scarano E (1968): J Mol Biol 36:195
8. Groudine M, Eisenman R, Weintraub H (1981): Nature 292:311
9. Groudine M, Weintraub H (1981): Cell 24:393
10. Holliday R, Pugh JE (1975): Science 187:226
11. Huang LH, Farnet CM, Ehrlich KC, Ehrlich M (1982): Nucleic Acids Res 10:1579
12. Jones RE, DeFeo D, Piatigorsky J (1981): J Biol Chem 256:8172
13. Kaplan DA, Nierlich DP (1975): J Biol Chem 250:2395
14. Kuo MT, Mandel JL, Chambon P (1979): Nucleic Acids Res 7:2105
15. Lawson GM, Knoll BJ, March CJ, Woo SLC, Tsai MJ, O'Malley BW (1982): J Biol Chem 257:1501
16. Mandel JL, Chambon P (1979): Nucleic Acids Res 7:2081
17. McChee JD, Ginder GD (1980): Nature 280:419
18. Naveh-Many T, Cedar H (1981): Proc Natl Acad Sci USA 78:4246
19. Ostrander M, Vogel S, Silverstein S (1982): Mol Cell Biol 2:708
20. Razin A, Riggs AD (1980): Science 210:604
21. Royer HD, Sager R (1979): Proc Natl Acad Sci USA 76:5794
22. Scangos G, Ruddle FH (1981): Gene 14:1
23. Sheffery M, Rifkind RA, Marks PA (1982): Proc Natl Acad Sci USA 79:1180
24. Shen CJ, Maniatis T (1980): Proc Natl Acad Sci USA 77:6634
25. Stalder J, Larsen A, Engel JD, Dolan M, Groudine M, Weintraub H (1980): Cell 20:451
26. Van der Plaeg LHT, Flavell RA (1980): Cell 19:947
27. Waalwijk C, Flavell RA (1978): Nucleic Acids Res 5:3231
28. Waalwijk C, Flavel RA (1978): Nucleic Acids Res 5:4631
29. Wagner MJ, Sharp JA, Summers WC (1981): Proc Natl Acad Sci USA 78:1441
30. Weintraub H, Larsen A, Groudine M (1981): Cell 24:333
31. Wigler M, Pellicer A, Silverstein S, Axel R (1978): Cell 14:725
32. Wolf SF, Migeon BR (1982): Nature 295:667
33. Youssoufian H, Hammer SM, Hirsch MS, Mulder C (1982): Proc Natl Acad Sci USA 79:2207

Gene Transfer and Cancer, edited by M. L. Pearson
and N. L. Sternberg. Raven Press, New York © 1984.

DNA Methylation Controls Expression of Transferred Genes in a Mouse L Cell Derivative

Barbara Christy and George Scangos

Department of Biology, The Johns Hopkins University, Baltimore, Maryland 21218

ABSTRACT. The role of methylation in the control of gene expression in mouse L cells was examined. The herpes simplex virus (HSV) gene for thymidine kinase (tk) was introduced into Ltk⁻ cells by calcium phosphate precipitation in the absence of carrier DNA. Line 101 is a TK⁺ derivative of Ltk⁻ that contains multiple copies of the tk gene at a unique chromosomal site. A derivative of 101 which retained but which no longer expressed the HSV tk genes (termed 101BU1), and derivatives of 101BU1 which reexpressed the genes were selected. The tk genes in 101BU1 were hypermethylated relative to those in line 101 and those in the reexpressors, as determined by digestion of cell DNA with the methylation-sensitive enzymes HpaII, SmaI and AvaI. Two lines of evidence support a causal role for methylation in the elimination of tk gene expression. First, growth of 101BU1 in the presence of the methylation inhibitor 5-azacytidine resulted in a 6- to 23-fold increase in the number of TK⁺ reexpressors, suggesting that a decrease in the extent of DNA methylation results in increased gene expression. Second, although DNA isolated from line 101 and from TK⁺ reexpressors was active in secondary gene transfer experiments, 101BU1 DNA was inactive. The only detectable difference between the tk genes in 101 and in 101BU1 is the extent of methylation, indicating that methylation of the gene sequences is sufficient to abolish gene expression. Finally, all TK⁺ reexpressors examined exhibited DNA rearrangements involving tk DNA, suggesting that DNA rearrangement might be involved in the demethylation process.

INTRODUCTION

Although active and inactive genes have been shown to differ in chromatin structure (15), in the extent of DNA methylation (1,6,10,13), and in association with nonhistone chromosomal proteins (16), it has been difficult to translate these correlations into causal relationships and to understand the sequence of events necessary for gene activation/inactivation. Recently, Groudine et al. (5) demonstrated that inhibition of DNA methylation by growth of cells in the presence of 5-azacytidine resulted in the hypomethylation and transcriptional activation of endogenous viral genomes, and Compere and Palmiter (2) demonstrated that growth of cultured cells in the presence of 5-azacytidine resulted in hypomethylation and activation of the metallothionein-I gene. These studies suggested a causal role for DNA methylation in the reduction of gene expression, but they could not conclusively demonstrate that reexpression of the genes resulted directly from demethylation of gene sequences induced by 5-azacytidine and not from undefined secondary effects.

To elucidate some of the mechanisms involved in the control of gene expression, we have transferred the HSV gene for TK into tk-deficient mouse Ltk⁻ cells. The powerful selections for and against expression of tk allowed the isolation first of TK⁺ derivatives of Ltk⁻, second of derivatives of those in which the tk genes were turned off, and finally, of derivatives of those in which the genes were reexpressed. The use of the cloned tk gene as a nucleic acid probe and the use of cellular DNA in secondary gene transfer experiments demonstrated precise correlations between the state of the tk DNA and the expression of the tk gene.

The experiments described here characterize one TK⁺ cell line, termed 101, and its derivatives and demonstrate that the extent of methylation of the tk DNA is correlated inversely with gene expression. Furthermore, growth of a TK⁻ derivative of 101 in the presence of 5-azacytidine resulted in an increase in the number of TK⁺ reexpressing derivatives, and DNA isolated from 101 and from all TK⁺ reexpressors was active in secondary gene transfer, whereas DNA isolated from a TK⁻ derivative of 101, in which the tk genes were heavily methylated, was inactive. These data suggest that methylation/demethylation of tk gene sequences directly affects gene expression.

Finally, each of three independently isolated TK⁺ derivatives of a cell line with methylated, inactive tk genes had alterations in the structure of the tk and flanking DNA, raising the possibility that DNA rearrangement might be a mechanism of demethylation.

RESULTS AND DISCUSSION

An outline of the experiments described here is shown in Figure 1. Plasmid pTKx-1 consists of a 3.5-kb BamHI fragment of HSV DNA containing the tk gene inserted into the unique BamHI site of pBR322 (3). The plasmid has 2 BamHI sites, a unique HindIII site, and no sites for XbaI. Plasmid pTKx-1 was introduced into Ltk⁻ by calcium phosphate coprecipitation in the absence of carrier DNA, and positive colonies were isolated using HAT selection (8,12). Several TK⁺ cell lines were isolated and characterized (7), and one such cell line, termed 101, is described here. TK⁻ derivatives of 101 in which the tk genes no longer were expressed were selected in medium containing the toxic thymidine analog bromo-deoxyuridine (BrdU), and derivatives of those in which the tk genes were reexpressed again were selected in HAT medium. DNA was isolated from 101, from a TK-deficient derivative of 101 termed 101BU1, and from three TK⁺ reexpressing derivatives of 101BU1, termed 101H1, 101Hc, and 101HG. The DNA of these cell lines was analyzed by restriction enzyme digestion and Southern-blotting-filter hybridization experiments to identify changes in the state of the DNA that correlated with changes in the pattern of gene expression.

DNA from 101 and from 101BU1 was digested with XbaI, HindIII, BamHI, and PvuII, which recognize 0, 1, 2, and 3 sites in pTKx-1, respectively. DNA samples were electrophoresed through 0.8 to 1.2% agarose gels, blotted onto nitrocellulose, and hybridized with ³²P-labeled pTKx-1 as a probe. One band was visualized after digestion with XbaI, suggesting that pTKx-1 was present at a unique site in the genome. Multiple bands were seen after HindIII, BamHI, and PvuII digestion, and in each case

EXPERIMENTAL DESIGN

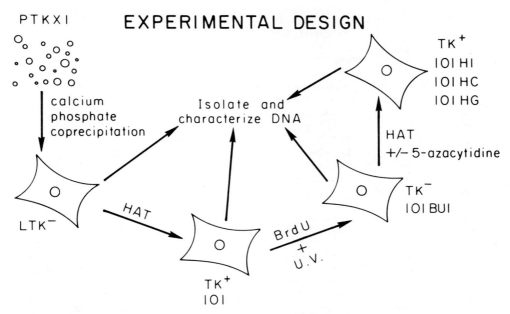

FIGURE 1. Experimental design. Plasmid pTKx-1, containing a 3.5-kb fragment of HSV DNA including the gene for TK inserted into the unique BamHI of pBR322 (3), was precipitated onto TK-deficient mouse fibroblast Ltk⁻ cells. A TK⁺ derivative of Ltk⁻, termed 101, was selected in HAT medium (8,12), and a TK⁻ derivative of 101, termed 101BU1, was selected by growth in the presence of the toxic thymidine analog BrdU and exposure to ultraviolet light. TK⁺ reexpressing derivatives of 101BU1 again were selected in HAT medium with or without prior treatment with the methylation inhibitor 5-azacytidine. DNA was isolated from all cell lines and analyzed by Southern blotting and filter hybridization with either pTKx-1 or the purified 3.5-kb fragment of viral DNA as a probe.

the predominant bands were the same size as those obtained from pTKx-1 alone. These data indicate that line 101 contained multiple copies of pTKx-1 in a tandem structure at a unique site in the genome. No differences in the intensity or pattern of tk-specific bands in lines 101 and 101BU1 were detected after digestion with any of the enzymes. Enzymatic assays demonstrated that 101BU1 had no detectable TK activity, demonstrating that while the tk genes were present in the DNA of 101BU1, they were not expressed.

HpaII and MspI are isoschizomers that recognize and cleave the same nucleotide sequence, CCGG, but although HpaII fails to cut restriction sites in which the internal C is methylated, MspI is insensitive to methylation at that site (11). Since 5-methylcytosine is the only detectable methylated base in mammalian DNA, and more than 90% of methylcytosine occurs as part of the dinucleotide CpG (4,17), a comparison of the band patterns obtained with these two enzymes provides an indication of the extent of DNA methylation. In totally unmethylated DNA, the pattern of bands generated by the two enzymes is identical. In methylated DNA, the failure of HpaII to cleave sites at which MspI does cleave results in higher-molecular-weight fragments after HpaII digestion than after MspI digestion.

DNA from 101, 101BU1, 101HI, 101HC, and 101HG was digested with HpaII and MspI and analyzed by electrophoresis through 1.2% agarose gels and filter hybridizaiton with the 3.5-kb tk fragment as a probe. MspI and HpaII recognize more than 40 sites in pTKx-1 to generate fragments of 9 to 600 bp (9,14). MspI digestion of 101 DNA generated a number of low-molecular-weight bands which were not resolved well on the agarose gels. HpaII digestion generated the same low-molecular-weight bands and a number of high-molecular-weight bands, indicating that the tk genes in 101 were partially methylated, but that at least one copy contained unmethylated HpaI sites. Digestion of 101BU1 DNA with MspI yielded the same pattern of low-molecular-weight bands, while HpaII digestion generated only the high-molecular-weight bands; the low-molecular-weight region indicative of unmethlated HpaII sites within the tk gene was absent. HpaII digestions of DNA of each of the reexpressing cell lines generated the low-molecular-weight bands, indicating that at least 1 copy of the TK gene in these lines contained unmethylated HpaII sites.

The above data indicated that one or more of the tk genes were hyper-methylated in 101BU1. To ascertain the region of the gene in which the methylation pattern was altered, the DNA of 101, 101BU1, and each of the reexpressors was digested with the methylation-sensitive enzymes SmaI and AvaI. SmaI digestion of pTKx-1 generates bands of 1.6 and 0.8 kb, which represent the 5' and 3' ends of the tk gene, respectively. AvaI digestion generates 2 bands of 0.78 kb, one each from the 5' and 3' ends of the gene, and a 0.64-kb band composed entirely of coding sequences (Figure 2). Digestion of 101 DNA with SmaI generated bands of 1.6 and 0.8 kb that hybridized to the tk probe. These bands were not detected in 101BU1 DNA and reappeared in the DNA of all of the reexpressors. Similarly, the 0.64- and 0.78-kb bands were seen after AvaI digestion of DNA from 101 and the reexpressors but were not detected in 101BU1 DNA. These data demonstrate that the methylation/demethylation involved sites on the 5' and 3' ends of the gene as well as within the structural gene sequences. They do not, however, indicate which of the sites are important for the control of gene expression. Further experiments to determine which of the sites of methylation are important for gene expression are in progress.

To determine whether DNA methylation was causally related to gene expression, 101BU1 cells were grown in the presence of 2, 5, and 10 µM concentrations of the methylation-inhibitor 5-azacytidine. These concentrations decreased the extent of total DNA methylation as judged by the extent of HpaII digestion of treated and untreated whole cell DNAs. The number of Tk$^+$ reexpressing derivatives was increased 6-, 11-, and 7-fold over untreated controls after treatment with 2, 5, and 10 µM 5-azacyti-dine, respectively. We believe that the smaller increase induced by 10 µM 5-azacytidine was a result of toxicity and increased cell death. These data indicated that decreasing the extent of DNA methylation led to an increase in the frequency of TK reexpression and therefore, suggested a causal relationship between DNA methylation and the reduction of gene expression.

Further support for a causal relationship between DNA methylation and gene expression was derived from secondary gene transfer experiments in which DNA isolated from 101, 101BU1, and each of the reexpressors was used to transfer TK activity to Ltk$^-$ cells. DNA from 101 and from each of the reexpressors was active in these experiments; these DNAs were able to transfer TK activity to Ltk$^-$ cells. DNA from 101BU1 was inactive; no TK$^+$ colonies were obtained after treatment of Ltk$^-$ cells under conditions where 101DNA generated 355 colonies. Since DNA-mediated gene transfer

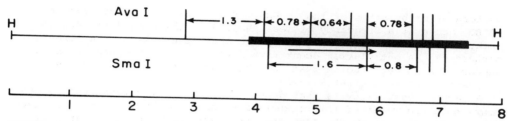

FIGURE 2. Partial restriction map of pTKx-1. The 3.5-kb HSV DNA fragment is depicted as a heavy line and the region and direction of transcription of the tk gene are depicted by the arrow (9). The sites of AvaI and SmaI cleavage are from M. Wagner and W. C. Summers (personal communication). SmaI cleaves the tk insert 5 times and pBR322 not at all and generates a 1.6-kb fragment representing the 5' portion of the insert and a 0.8-kb fragment representing the 3' end of the insert. AvaI yields a 1.3-kb fragment derived from cleavage within pBR322 and at a site within the 5' end of the insert, two 0.78-kb fragments, one each from the 5' and 3' ends of the structural gene, and a 0.64-kb fragment, composed entirely of coding sequences. All of the SmaI- and AvaI-derived bands were present in the DNA of 101 and of all TK⁺ reexpressors, but were absent from the DNA of 101BU1, indicating that the sites which generated these bands were unmethylated in TK⁺ lines and methylated in the TK⁻ derivative.

separates the active gene from other cell constituents and from most of the rest of the genome, these results indicate that it is methylation of tk gene sequences themselves or of closely linked sequences that affects their expression.

Each of the reexpressors had alterations in the pattern of tk-specific bands compared to 101 and 101BU1 DNA after digestion with HindIII, BamHI, and PvuII. HindIII digestion generated six bands (17.5, 15.25, 13, 7.9, 6.5, and 3.5 kb) in the DNAs of 101 and 101BU1. In 101H1, the 17- and 3.5-kb bands were missing, but two new bands of 4.8 and 3.0 kb appeared. In 101HG, all of the bands except for the 7.9- and 3.5-kb bands were missing. In 101HC DNA, all of the bands were visible, but as judged from the intensity of the bands, there was a 5-fold amplification of the tk sequences. Thus, two of the reexpressing cell lines had deletions and/or rearrangements and one had an amplification of the tk sequences.

Since each of the reexpressors was a subclone of 101BU1, we wanted to determine whether the rearrangements were correlated with the change in TK gene expression or were merely random changes existing in subpopulations of 101BU1. To differentiate between these two possibilities, 12 subclones of 101BU1 were isolated randomly and without selection, and the pattern of tk-specific bands found in their DNA was compared to the pattern in 101BU1. DNA from 7 of the 12 was indistinguishable from 101BU1 DNA, and DNA from 5 subclones possessed rearrangements of tk DNA. These data indicate that rearrangement within the region of the transferred tk genes was a common event but do not determine whether the rearrangements are correlated with changes in expression.

One plausible hypothesis is that the pattern of methylation of the tk DNA in the initial TK⁺ line is influenced by the pattern of the DNA into which it has integrated. Thus in 101, the DNA which flanks the tk genes may be partially methylated. The most common mechanism of demethylation might be rearrangements that bring a structurally intact but methylated tk gene adjacent to hypomethylated flanking DNA and thus disrupt the pattern of methylation of the tk DNA. Since the TK$^+$ derivatives of 101BU1 arose at a frequency of less than 10^{-6}, this would imply that methylation is a very tight control and that reversals of the normal pattern of DNA methylation occur very rarely. This interpretation is supported by other studies that indicate that demethylation and gene activation are rare events. (2,5).

A second possibility is that demethylation and structural rearrangements both are required for reexpression and occur independently of each other. Finally, it may be that the DNA rearrangements occur randomly and without regard to gene expression or that demethylation sometimes involves a large region and is lethal. Experiments to determine the nature of the rearrangements in the TK$^+$ reexpressors are in progress.

In summary, in 101, expression of the transferred tk genes is inversely correlated with methylation. The tk DNA of the initial cell line was hypomethylated while the DNA of a TK$^-$ derivative was hypermethylated. Reexpressing derivatives again had low levels of methylation of the tk genes. 5-Azacytidine reactivation and gene transfer experiments support a causal role for methylation in the elimination of gene expression, and it may be that DNA demethylation is effected through rearrangements which bring the hypermethylated tk genes adjacent to unmethylated or hypomethylated DNA.

REFERENCES

1. Bird A, Tagart M, Macleod D (1981): Cell 26:381
2. Comperi SS, Palmiter RD (1981): Cell 25:233
3. Enquist LW, VandeWoude GF, Wagner M, Smiley JR, Summers WC (1979): Gene 1:335
4. Grippo P, Iacarino M, Parisi E, Scarano E (1970): J Mol Biol 35:195
5. Groudine M, Eisenman R, Weintraub H (1981): Nature 292:311
6. Groudine M, Weintraub H (1981): Cell 24:393
7. Huttner KM, Barbosa JA, Scangos, GA, Pratcheva DD, Ruddle FH (1981): J Cell Biol 91:153
8. Littlefield JN (1964): Science 145:709
9. McKnight SL, Gavis ER, Kingsbury R, Axel R (1981): Cell 25:385
10. Naveh-Many T, Cedar H (1981): Proc Natl Acad Sci USA 78:4246
11. Roberts R (1980): Gene 8:329
12. Szybolski Y, Szybalska EM, Ragni G (1962): Natl Cancer Inst Monogr 1:75
13. VanderPloeg LHT, Flavell RA (1980): Cell 19:947
14. Wagner MJ, Sharp JA, Summers WE (1981): Proc Natl Acad Sci USA 78: 1441
15. Weintraub H, Groudine M (1976): Science 193:848
16. Weisbrod S, Weintraub H (1979): Proc Natl Acad Sci USA 76:630
17. Wyatt GR (1951): Biochem J 48:584

Gene Transfer and Cancer, edited by M. L. Pearson
and N. L. Sternberg. Raven Press, New York © 1984.

Gene Inactivation and Reactivation at the *emt* Locus in Chinese Hamster Cells

Ronald G. Worton, Stephen G. Grant, and Catherine Duff

*Genetics Department and Research Institute, Hospital for Sick Children;
and Department of Medical Genetics, University of Toronto,
Toronto, Ontario M5G 1X8 Canada*

ABSTRACT. The ability to detect gene inactivation and reactivation in animal cells is severely hampered by the presence of two copies of auto-somal genes in diploid cells. In heterozygotes (m/+) carrying a recessive mutant allele (m) and a wild-type allele (+) it is possible to specifically monitor the activity of the single wild-type allele; however, studies of gene expression require that cells with an inactive + gene remain viable. Heterozygous cells meeting this condition are difficult to obtain. We have created a series of somatic cell hybrids of Chinese hamster ovary (CHO) cells that fulfill these conditions. The hybrids are heterozygous at the emt locus and were created by fusing emetine-resistant cells carrying a single recessive emt^r allele with wild-type CHO carrying a single dominant emt^+ allele. The emt^r/emt^+ hybrids have a wild-type phenotype (sensitive to emetine), but "segregants" that reexpress the Emt^r phenotype occur at high frequency. Some of these are due to loss of the chromosome carrying the emt^+ gene but a few appear to be due to loss of expression of the emt^+ gene. Two criteria suggest that these are the result of gene inactivation. First, transfer of the chromosome carrying the putative null emt (emt^ϕ) allele into a cell where it should be expressed fails to reveal any gene expression. Second, treatment of the putative inactivants with 5-azacytidine results in reexpression of the emt^+ gene in 15 to 20% of cells. This suggests the possibility that the original gene inactivation event involves DNA methylation or perhaps some other mechanism sensitive to reversal by this cytidine analog.

INTRODUCTION

Over the past few years our laboratory has studied the genetic events responsible for segregation of recessive phenotypes in intraspecies somatic cell hybrids. Our basic approach has been to construct CHO hybrids that are heterozygous for one or more recessive drug-resistance markers, and then to examine segregants that have reexpressed the recessive (drug-resistance) phenotype.

The recessive marker utilized in many of these studies was emetine resistance (emt^r) (11,13,15). Emetine inhibits protein synthesis (11), and emetine resistance has been associated with an alteration in a ribosomal protein (2,14). The emt gene maps to the long arm of Chinese hamster chromosome 2 (27) and in the CHO line it is opposite a major deletion such that in CHO there is only a single copy of this gene (27,28,29). Hybrids formed by fusing an emetine-resistant line with a wild-type line are therefore heterozygous ($\underline{emt^r}/\underline{emt^+}$), and segregants that are resistant to emetine must have lost or inactivated the $\underline{emt^+}$ allele.

In an attempt to determine the nature of the genetic events responsible for segregaton, we have utilized CHO cell lines and hybrids with multiple genetic and cytogenetic markers on chromosome 2 so that we could follow the fate of the chromosomal arms through the segregation process. Our results have indicated that the most common segregation event is loss of the chromosome carrying the $\underline{emt^+}$ allele and that in most cases this is accompanied by duplication of the homolog carrying the $\underline{emt^r}$ allele (5). In a few segregants, chromosome loss was not involved and, in at least some of these segregants, a mechanism involving gene inactivation has been postulated (4,5). Mitotic recombination (somatic crossing-over), which might have accounted for some segregants was not observed (5).

One of our concerns was that the use of cytogenetically abnormal chromosomes in these experiments might inhibit some of the events (mitotic recombination, gene inactivation) that we were trying to detect. In this paper, therefore we describe segregation studies in hybrids containing a pair of chromosomes 2 with cytogenetically normal long arms. We report that in such hybrids there is an increased proportion of segregation not involving chromosome loss and, in at least some segregants, the mechanism appears to be inactivation of the $\underline{emt^+}$ gene. Furthermore, the inactive gene coding for wild-type sensitivity can be reactivated by treatment of the cells with 5-azacytidine (5-azaCR), suggesting that DNA methylation may have been responsible for the original inactivation event.

RESULTS AND DISCUSSION

Construction of $\underline{emt^r}/\underline{emt^+}$ Hybrids

The SLA hybrids utilized in this study are of genotype $\underline{mtx^{RIII}emt^r}/\underline{emt^+}$ $\underline{emt^{rI}}$ and were created by fusion of the methotrexate-resistant line $\underline{Mtx^{RIII}}$ (9) with the emetine-resistant line EOTC5 (4,28). The hybrids are resistant to methotrexate because $\underline{mtx^{RIII}}$ is a dominant marker (9) but are sensitive to emetine because $\underline{emt^{rI}}$ is recessive (15). Both markers are on Chinese hamster chromosome 2: $\underline{mtx}$ is on the short arm (28) and $\underline{emt}$ is on the long arm (27,28). Both parent lines are derived from CHO cells and therefore have the large interstitial deletion of 2q (q=long arm) opposite the $\underline{emt}$ locus (Figure 1). Hybrids are therefore heterozygotes with one copy of each of the $\underline{emt^{rI}}$ and $\underline{emt^+}$ alleles.

Also significant for this study is the fact that the Mtx^{RIII} line has no normal chromosome 2. In addition to the chromosome 2 with the deleted long arm, it has another abnormal chromosome 2 (called 2p$^-$) whose short arm (p) is reduced in length due to a translocation between 2p and 5q (Figure 1). Thus, the karyotype and genotype of the hybrids is 2p$^-$ ($\underline{mtx^{RIII}emt^+}$)/2($\underline{mtx^+emt^{rI}}$).

Mechanisms of Reexpression of the Recessive Emt^r Phenotype

Figure 2 is a schematic diagram illustrating four possible mechanisms by which the hybrid cells could reexpress the recessive Emt^r phenotype. As Figure 2 shows, segregants that become resistant to emetine by loss of the 2p$^-$ chromosome, whether or not they duplicate the remaining normal chromosome 2, can be easily distinguished by a karyotype analysis. Two

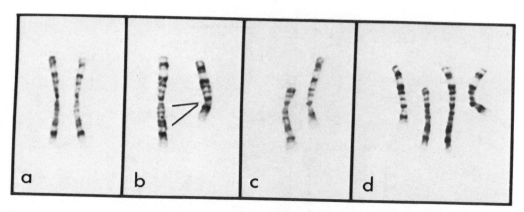

FIGURE 1. (a) Chinese hamster chromosome 2 pair as they appear in a diploid cell. (b) The chromosome 2 pair of the CHO cell line. The chromosome on the right is called Z2 and has an extensive deletion from the long arm as indicated. (c) The chromosome 2 pair of the MtxRIII mutant line. The 2p⁻ chromosome on the left has a normal long arm, but more than half of the short arm is missing because it had been translocated onto a chromosome 5 (not shown). The chromosome on the right is the Z2 characteristic of all CHO lines. (d) The four chromosomes 2 of the SLA hybrids used in this study. From left to right Z2, 2p⁻, 2, Z2. The 2p⁻ carries mtxRIII on the short arm and emt⁺ on the long arm. The 2 carries mtx⁺ on the short arm and emtrI on the long arm.

other mechanisms that might also give rise to the Emt^r phenotype include gene inactivation, which does not affect the karyotype, and mitotic recombination, which involves an exchange of chromosomal arms that is not detectable by karyotype analysis. Karyotype analysis of Emt^r segregants therefore does not distinguish these two mechanisms from one another but does distinguish them from chromosome loss or from chromosome loss and duplication.

Selection of Emt^r Segregants

In the first experiment, independent segregants were selected by plating hybrid cells in medium containing emetine. The independent origin of each was assured by selecting only one colony from each of several minicultures, each of these started from an inoculum of about 100 hybrid cells.

Thirteen Emt^r colonies were picked and karyotyped. Seven of these had the parental 2p⁻/2 karyotype suggesting a gene inactivation or mitotic recombination event. The remaining six had lost the 2p⁻ chromosome or had undergone deletion of the long arm carrying the emt gene; all six of these had duplicated the normal chromosome 2.

In a second experiment, hybrid minicultures were plated in medium containing both emetine and methotrexate. The purpose of the double selection was to eliminate chromosome loss or chromosome loss and duplication events from consideration since segregants arising by these mechanisms would have lost the mtxRIII gene (Figure 2) and would die in the double selection

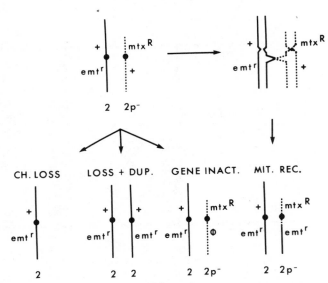

FIGURE 2. Diagram of four possible segregation mechanisms. In the upper
left corner are the 2 and 2p$^-$ chromosomes of the SLA hybrids used in this
study. Emetine-resistant segregants may arise by loss of the 2p$^-$ chromosomes, by loss of the 2p$^-$ coupled with duplication of the chromosome 2, by
inactivation of the emt$^+$ gene, or by a mitotic recombination event, with
the crossover occurring between the centromere and the emt loci (upper
right) followed by segregation of the first and third chromatids to the
same cell (lower right). A fifth mechanism that would produce emetine-
resistant cells is new mutation at the emt$^+$ locus, but segregants arising
by this mechanism are expected to be rare in comparison with the high frequencies at which our segregants arise.

medium. Eighteen independent segregants were picked. Eleven had a 2p$^-$/2
karyotype consistent with gene inactivation or mitotic recombination. The
remaining 7 had undergone deletion of the long arm of the 2p$^-$ chromosome
but retained the short arm portion carrying the mtx^{RIII} gene; all seven of
these had also duplicated the normal chromosome 2.

In the two experiments combined, 18 of the 31 segregants were considered
to have arisen by either mitotic recombination or gene inactivation. The
experiments described below were designed to determine which of these two
mechanisms might be responsible for the Emt^r phenotype.

Transfer of the 2p$^-$ Chromosome into an Emt^{rII} Host

Examination of Figure 2 reveals that segregants arising by gene inactivation would have an inactive or emtϕ allele at the emetine locus on the
2p$^-$ chromosome, whereas segregants arising by somatic crossing-over would
have an emt^{rI} allele at this position. To determine which is the case for
our segregants, we utilized the microcell-mediated chromosome transfer
technique (10,26) to transfer the 2p$^-$ chromosome from putative gene inactivation or mitotic recombination segregants into another cell type where
the emt^{rI} gene would be detectable if it were present on this chromosome.

The recipient cell chosen for the transfer was the multiply marked line
EOHM2C2. This line is also resistant to emetine but it is a second-step

mutant with a higher level of emetine resistance (rII level) (16). In somatic cell hybrids, this rII level resistance is recessive to both wild-type and to rI level resistance (16). Conversely, rI resistance is dominant to rII so that transfer of the 2p$^-$ chromosome from an emetine-resistant segregant into EOHM2C2 should, if it carries the emt^{rI} allele, convert this cell from an Emt^{rII} phenotype to the less resistant Emt^{rI} phenotype. However, if the segregant arose by gene inactivation, the 2p$^-$ chromosome would carry an emtϕ allele, producing one of two possible results upon transfer. Either the inactive allele will remain inactive in the new host and the phenotype of the transferant will remain Emt^{rII}, or the inactive allele will be reactivated to the emt$^+$ form in which case the transferant will acquire wild-type sensitivity. These two possibilities are distinguishable from each other and from the rI phenotype which results from transfer of a recombinant chromosome.

To transfer the 2p$^-$ chromosome, we utilized the mtx^{RIII} marker on the short arm, selecting for transfer of the dominant methotrexate-resistance phenotype. Such transfers have been done previously in this laboratory and have been shown to transfer the 2p$^-$ marker chromosome either alone or together with a few other chromosomes (28).

Therefore, microcells were prepared from each of several different segregants and were fused to intact EOHM2C2 cells with polyethylene glycol. Microcell hybrids (transferants) were selected in medium containing methotrexate. Colonies were picked, karyotyped, and tested for growth in methotrexate and in two different levels of emetine. Four transferants were examined in detail, 2 from each of 2 different segregants. The results, shown in Table 1, demonstrate that all four transferants carried the 2p$^-$ marker, all four were resistant to methotrexate as expected, and all four were fully resistant to the rII level of emetine. This suggests that the transferred 2p$^-$ chromosome carries a null allele and the segregants from which they were derived had therefore arisen by a process of gene inactivation.

Reactivation of the Inactive emt Gene by 5-azaCR

More definitive proof for inactivation of the emt locus in our segregants depended on the successful reactivation of the emt$^+$ state. As the above experiments were in progress, reports began to appear demonstrating the ability of the demethylating agent, 5-azaCR (7,18) to activate previously inactive genes coding for differentiated gene products (6,7,17,23,25), viral gene products (1,12,22), or products of the inactive X chromosome (19,21). We therefore tested 5-azaCR for its potential to reactivate the emt$^+$ state in our emetine-resistant segregants.

In the first type of experiment, putative inactivants (segregants with karyotype 2p$^-$/2) were exposed to medium containing 2 µM 5-azaCR for 24 hr, allowed a 3-day expression time in nonselective medium, and were then plated in nonselective medium and in medium containing emetine. If the 5-azaCR treatment had reactivated the emt$^+$ gene in a significant proportion of cells, these cells would have become sensitive to emetine and would exhibit a drop in the plating efficiency only in the emetine-containing plates. The results of many experiments of this type are summarized in Table 2, and clearly demonstrate a 15 to 22% reduction in the relative plating efficiency (in emetine) after treatment with 5-azaCR. Control experiments showed that without 5-azaCR treatment these same cells had an identical plating efficiency in medium with or without emetine, and that segregants whose karyotype was not consistent with gene inactivation failed to show any effect of 5-azaCR treatment. We conclude that the

TABLE 1. Phenotypic testing of transferants after transfer of the 2p$^-$ marker chromosome into an Emt^{rII} host cell

Name of segregant[a]	Transferant[b]	Transferant[b] karyotype	Relative plating efficiency in drug[c]		
			MTX(RIII)	EMT(rI)	(EMT(rII)
SLA2-E5	1	2/2p$^-$	0.88	1.19	0.31
	2	2/2p$^-$	0.82	0.96	0.51
SLA2-EM7	1	2/2p$^-$	1.00	1.02	0.88
	2	2/2p$^-$	0.17	–	0.27
CHO (wild-type)			0	0	0
EOTC5			0	0.83	0
EOHM2C2			0	0.99	1.04

a SLA2 is the name of the parental hybrid while SLA2-E5 and SLA2-EM7 are independent segregants of this hybrid. EOTC5 is the Emt^{rI} line used in the construction of the SLA2 hybrid and EOHM2C2 is the Emt^{rII} line used as recipient for transfer of the 2p$^-$ marker chromosome.
b Transferants are microcell hybrids formed by fusion of SLA2-E5 or SLA2-EM7 microcells with intact EOHM2C2 cells. Transferants were selected in medium containing methotrexate and methylglyoxal bis guanylhydrazone (MBG). Since the EOHM2C2 line is resistant to MGB, a recessive marker resulting in altered polyamine transport (20) this drug was used in the selective medium to select against intact donor cells or hybrids formed with intact donor cells. The only cells to survive are EOHM2C2 cells that have received the dominant mtx^{RIII} marker but not the wild-type mbg$^+$ marker.
c Plating efficiencies were measured by plating 200 cells in each of two dishes containing methotrexate (MTX) (10^{-6}M), rI levels (.15 µM) or rII levels (3.0 µM) of emetine (EMT). Relative plating efficiency was obtained by dividing each value by the plating efficiency in nonselective medium.

5-azaCR treatment of two putative inactivants resulted in the reactivation of the emt$^+$ state in 15 to 22% of cells.

With this high frequency of reactivation, it was clear that one should be able to isolate clones of reactivated cells, even though one could not select for them directly. To this end, putative inactivants were treated with 5-azaCR for 24 hr and after a 3-day expression period, cells were plated at low density (fewer than 1 viable cell/well) into multiwell Linbro trays. Wells were examined after 1 to 2 days, and wells with single tiny colonies were marked. Many days later these clones were picked and tested for their ability to grow in emetine. Of 79 clones picked and tested, 64 (81%) grew equally well in medium with or without emetine; 15 (19%) grew in nonselective medium but not in medium with emetine. These latter clones presumably are sensitive to emetine as a result of 5-azaCR-induced reactivation of the emt$^+$ gene.

The combined results of the chromosome transfer experiments and the 5-azaCR experiments provide strong evidence, we believe, that certain of our Emt^r segregants are the result of a process of gene inactivation and that this inactivation is reversible by 5-azaCR. If we consider the emt gene, coding for a ribosomal protein, to be a good example of a housekeeping gene, then we must conclude that in long-term cell cultures such genes are subject to apparently random events resulting in their loss of expression.

TABLE 2. Relative plating efficiency in medium containing emetine
after treatment with 5-azaCR

Segregant name	Segregant type	No. of experiments	Relative plating efficiency (+EMT/-EMT)	
			Untreated	5-azaCR-treated
SLA2-E5	GI or MR[a]	6	1.0	0.78[c]
SLA2-E3	GI or MR[a]	3	1.0	0.85[c]
SLA2-C1	Chr loss[b]	2	0.96	1.0
SLA2-C4	Loss & dup[b]	2	0.96	0.98
EOTC5	EMT[rI] Parent	2	0.99	0.95

[a] Segregants SLA2-E5 and SLA2-E3 had a 2 and 2p$^-$ chromosome and had therefore arisen by gene activation (GI) or mitotic recombination (MR).
[b] Two segregants used as controls included SLA2-C1 which had a single
chromosome 2 (derived by chromosome loss (Chr loss)) and SLA2-C4 with a
pair of normal 2's (derived by chromosome loss and duplication (Loss &
dup)).
[c] Reduction significant ($P < 0.05$) in each of the 9 individual experiments.

Only in a heterozygote, such as the emt$^+$/emt^{rI} cells described here, would
such a loss in gene expression be detectable. Furthermore, considering
that 5-azaCR might be acting to disrupt an inherited DNA methylation pattern (7,18), it appears that methylation of cytosine may be one type of
event responsible for this loss of gene expression.

The existence of gene inactivation in cultured cells may have considerable significance in somatic cell genetics. For example, in trying to
explain the ease with which recessive mutants are isolated in CHO cells,
Siminovitch (24) has suggested that the genes involved may have only a
single functional copy. Extensive methylation might account for such
functional hemizygosity at some loci. For other genes, such as the adenosine phosphoribosyl transferase (aprt) gene in CHO, there appears to be
two functional copies. Bradley and Letovanec (3) have recently presented
evidence that mutation to the aprt$^-$/aprt$^-$ homozygous state involves two
events, one of which occurs at low frequency and is stable, the other of
which occurs at higher frequency and is unstable. The latter event, they
suggest, is a gene inactivation. Here again, DNA methylation may be a
good candidate for this high frequency event. Whether these events are
peculiar to long-term cultures or whether they are events that occur in
diploid cells in vivo remains to be determined. Certainly, if they do
occur in vivo it would be of utmost importance to determine their effect
on cell phenotype, especially with regard to the irreversible alterations
leading to malignancy or cell aging.

ACKNOWLEDGEMENTS

This work was supported by a grant from the Medical Research Council
of Canada. The authors are grateful to Dr. Christine Campbell for initiating the segregation studies and the chromosome transfer approach to
test for inactivation, to Sandra Toth for excellent technical assistance,
and to Dr. L. Siminovitch for critical reading of the manuscript.

REFERENCES

1. Ben-Sasson SA, Klein G (1978): Int J Cancer 28:131
2. Boersma D, McGill SM, Mollenkamp JW, Roufa DJ (1979): Proc Natl Acad Sci USA 76:415
3. Bradley WEC, Letovanec D (1982): Somatic Cell Genet 8:51
4. Campbell CE, Worton RG (1980): Somatic Cell Genet 6:215
5. Campbell CE, Worton RG (1981): Mol Cell Biol 1:336
6. Compere SJ, Palmiter RD (1981): Cell 25:233
7. Creusot F, Acs G, Christman JK (1982): J Biol Chem 257:2041
8. Farrell SA, Worton RG (1977): Somatic Cell Genet 3:539
9. Flintoff NF, Spindler SM, Siminovitch L (1976): In Vitro 12:749
10. Fournier REK (1981): Proc Natl Acad Sci USA 78:6349
11. Grollman AP (1966) Proc Natl Acad Sci USA 56:1867
12. Groudine M, Eisenman R, Weintraub H (1981): Nature 292:311
13. Gupta RS, Siminovitch L (1976): Cell 9:213
14. Gupta RS, Siminovitch L (1977): Cell 10:61
15. Gupta RS, Siminovitch L (1978): J Biol Chem 253:3978
16. Gupta RS, Siminovitch L (1978): Somatic Cell Genet 4:77
17. Ivarie RD, Morris JA (1982): Proc Natl Acad Sci USA 79:2967
18. Jones PA, Taylor SM (1980): Cell 20:85
19. Lester SC, Korn NJ, DeMars R (1982): Somatic Cell Genet 8:265
20. Mandel J-L, Flintoff WF (1978): J Cell Physiol 97:335
21. Mohandas T, Sparkes RS, Shapiro LJ (1981): Science 211:393
22. Niwa O, Sugahara T (1981): Proc Natl Acad Sci USA 78:6290
23. Sager R, Kovac P (1982): Proc Natl Acad Sci USA 79:480
24. Siminovitch L (1976): Cell 7:1
25. Taylor SM, Jones PA (1979): Cell 17:771
26. Worton RG, Duff, C (1981): Cytogenet Cell Genet 29:184
27. Worton RG, Duff C, Campbell CE (1980): Somatic Cell Genet 6:199
28. Worton R, Duff C, Flintoff W (19891): Mol Cell Biol 1:330
29. Worton RG, Ho CC, Duff C (1977): Somatic Cell Genet 3:27

Gene Transfer and Cancer, edited by M. L. Pearson
and N. L. Sternberg. Raven Press, New York © 1984.

Inhibition of DNA Methylation by 5-Azacytidine and Chemical Carcinogens

Peter A. Jones, Shirley M. Taylor, and Vincent L. Wilson

*Division of Hematology-Oncology, Childrens Hospital of Los Angeles,
Los Angeles, California 90027*

ABSTRACT. The nucleoside analog 5-azacytidine (5-aza-CR) has marked effects on the differentiated state of cells and induces the formation of myocytes, chondrocytes and adipocytes in treated 10T1/2 or 3T3 cells. These effects are probably due to the ability of 5-aza-CR to inhibit the methylation of newly replicated DNA.

Cellular DNA synthesized in the presence of the analog was hemimethylated and served as an efficient substrate for a crude extract of mouse spleen methyltransferase in a cell-free assay. Methyl groups were transferred specifically to cytosine residues located in the undermethylated strand of the duplex hemimethylated DNA, suggesting that the activity measured represented the spleen "maintenance" methylase. The methylase exhibited several of the properties of a processive enzyme, and its ability to methylate the hemimethylated substrate was impaired by increasing levels of 5-azacytosine residues in DNA. The presence of apurinic sites or single-strand breaks, but not double-strand breaks or thymine dimers, impeded the progress of the enzyme. A wide variety of ultimate chemical carcinogens inhibited the action of the methylase after incubation with DNA. Although these carcinogens also induced alkali-labile sites, the degree of enzyme inhibition was greater than that which could be ascribed to this damage alone. The presence of carcinogen adducts may therefore be inhibitory to the scanning of the DNA template by the maintenance methylase. Thus agents which damage DNA in vivo may change methylation patterns in DNA and ultimately alter gene expression in treated cells.

INTRODUCTION

One of the mechanisms by which cells control the expression of their genetic information is by the methylation of cytosine residues within DNA. The expression of globin (15,25), metallothionein (6) and J chain (29) genes among others has been shown to be inversely correlated with the state of methylation of specific cytosine residues within or around the gene sequences. Correlations between the expression of viral information and hypomethylation have also been found in many cases, including adenovirus (23), endogenous chicken viruses (9) and mouse mammary tumor virus (5). The expression of adenovirus information can be inhibited by the enzymatic application of methyl groups to the DNA (26) and

evidence for a cause and effect relationship has also come from the use
of the methylation inhibitor, 5-aza-CR (12).

The original hypotheses of Holliday and Pugh (11) and Riggs (19)
suggested that the methylation patterns in parent cells might be copied
due to the substrate specificity of a DNA maintenance methylase enzyme.
The function of such an enzyme would be to apply methyl groups to cytosine residues located opposite methylated CG doublets. Hemimethylated
CG sites would therefore be converted to symmetrically methylated sites
ensuring the heritability of the original methylation pattern.

Recent experiments involving transfected DNA molecules with known
modification patterns have shown that the pattern can be inherited after
several rounds of replication (10,22,27), implying the existence of maintenance methylase enzymes. Tissue-specific methylation patterns are
probably also perpetuated by such an enzyme(s). However, the arrangement
of methyl groups is not necessarily invariable and changes in the methylation state at specific sites have been observed (27). The heritability
of the methylation pattern after DNA synthesis is one of the attractive
features of models, suggesting that DNA modification may be involved in
controlling gene expression, since it would immediately explain how
differentiated cells breed true.

There have been suggestions that certain types of cancer should be
regarded as diseases of differentiation (14,17). Transformed cells may
not express unique products, but may rather be characterized by the
inappropriate expression of normal cellular genes. Included in these
would be the oncogenes, whose derepression may be associated with transformation in certain instances. If DNA methylation patterns control
gene expression in normal cells, it follows that changes in these modification patterns might be associated with the aberrant gene expression
or activation of oncogenes seen during neoplastic transformation.

We have investigated the possibility that various chemical carcinogens
that react with DNA inhibit DNA maintenance methylation. Many carcinogens, after activation to their ultimate electrophilic forms, react with
guanine residues in DNA, to form adducts, and to induce other DNA damage
such as single-strand breaks. Alteration of the DNA substrate may interfere with the action of the methylase, leading to heritable hypomethylation in subsequent cell generations.

We have therefore developed an assay for the action of maintenance
methyltransferases using hemimethylated DNA substrates extracted from
mouse cells exposed to 5-aza-CR. The abilities of ultimate chemical
carcinogens to interact with these substrates and inhibit maintenance
methylase activity were then measured to determine whether a range of
carcinogens could influence methylation in vitro.

RESULTS

Preparation and Characterization of DNA Substrates

Progress in understanding the action of maintenance methylases has
been hampered by the lack of adequately defined hemimethylated DNAs that
represent the natural substrates of the enzymes. DNA extracted from
eucaryotic cells would be expected to contain symmetrically modified
sites, whereas that obtained from procaryotic cells would contain either
no 5-methylcytosine (5mC), and therefore no hemimethylated sites, or
symmetrically modified sequences. Other investigators have prepared
hemimethylated substrates by nick translation in the absence of

methylase (1), or have used 5-methyl-2'-deoxycytidine triphosphate as a substrate for DNA polymerase in vitro (2). Alternatively, DNA has been extracted from ethionine-treated cultures (4) or from cells dividing in the absence of methionine (24). In this study, we utilized the ability of 5-aza-CR to induce a hypomethylation of newly synthesized DNA to prepare hemimethylated DNA substrates (13).

Transformed mouse embryo cells (MCA CL-15-C), which are a derivative of the C3H/10T1/2 CL8 line (18), were grown in roller bottles and treated with 5-aza-CR at various concentrations in the presence of medium containing 5 µg/ml of 5-bromodeoxyuridine (BUdR) in a darkened room. The cells were harvested by trypsinization after a 20-hr exposure time exposure time, and the DNA was extracted and banded on cesium chloride density gradients. The fractions containing heavy-light (HL) DNA were pooled and used for further analysis. This DNA contained bromouracil (BU) in the newly synthesized strand and represented the duplex molecule that had been synthesized in the presence of 5-aza-CR.

The DNAs were lyophilized and hydrolysed in 88% formic acid for 25 min at 180°C (21). The hydrolysates were then analyzed for 5mC and cytosine contents by high pressure liquid chromatography and the bases were detected and quantitated by their absorbances at 280 nm. The ratio of 5mC to total cytosine in the HL DNA extracted from untreated control samples was 3.36% (Table 1). The HL DNAs synthesized in the presence of 5-aza-CR showed dose-dependent decreases in the levels of 5mC. Since the parental light strands in these HL DNAs would be expected to contain the normal levels of 5mC, we also calculated the percentage decrease in 5mC contents of the H-strands (i.e., the strands synthesized in the presence of the drug). These values, shown in Table 1, were in close agreement with our earlier determinations for the percentage inhibition of DNA methylation using radioactive precursors (12).

The HL DNAs were therefore hemimethylated and were characterized further for their abilities to accept methyl groups from S-adenosyl-methionine in the presence of a crude extract of methylase enzyme from mouse spleen. Nuclei were prepared from the spleens of female BDF_1 mice essentially as described by Simon et al. (20), except that 1 mM DTT and 10 mM Tris HCL, pH 7.8, were included in all buffers, and nuclei were

TABLE 1. 5-mC content of DNA substrates[a]

Treatment	$\dfrac{5mC}{5mC + C}$ x 100 in HL DNA	5mC in H strand % Control
None	3.36	100
2-µM 5-aza-CR	2.36	38
3-µM 5-aza-CR	2.08	21
10-µM 5-aza-CR	1.70	0

[a] DNAs prepared from cultures treated as indicated in the presence of BUdR were banded on CsCl density gradients. The ratio of 5mC/5mC + C in these DNAs was determined by high pressure liquid chromatography, and the percentage decrease in the 5mC content of the H strand was calculated.

centrifuged through a 2.4 M sucrose cushion. The DNA methyltransferase
was extracted from these nuclei as described previously (13) and a 35 to
60% ammonium sulfate fraction used for further characterization. The
enzyme was assayed by its ability to transfer ^{3}H-methyl groups into
alkali and protease-insensitive, acid-precipitable material (13).

Our initial studies showed that the HL DNAs synthesized in the
presence of 2 or 3 μM 5-aza-CR were 6- to 7-fold more efficient in
accepting methyl groups in vitro than equivalent DNAs extracted from
untreated control cultures (13). These methyl groups were transferred
specifically to the hypomethylated (i.e., the BU-containing) strand so
that the activity measured represented that expected for a maintenance
methylase enzyme. Although increasing concentrations of 5-aza-CR led
to the formation of increasing numbers of hemimethylated sites (Table 1),
the percentage of these sites which were modified subsequently by the
maintenance methylase decreased with increasing 5-aza-CR levels (Table 2).
Thus, whereas 7.3% of the available sites were methylated per hr in the
DNA extracted from cells treated with 2 μM 5-aza-CR, only 3.5% of the
potential sites were methylated in DNAs extracted from cells treated
with 10 μM 5-aza-CR. The presence of increased levels of 5-azacytosine
in the DNA therefore appeared to be inhibitory to the action of the
enzyme. More recent experiments have suggested that this might be due
to a strong binding reaction between the methyltransferase and a potential modification site containing the fraudulent base.

Further experiments were therefore conducted using DNAs synthesized
in the presence of 2 μM 5-aza-CR which contained hemimethylated sites
but low levels of incorporated azacytosine.

Inhibition of Methyltransferase Activity by DNA Damage

The pioneering studies of Drahovsky and Morris (8) suggested that the
DNA methyltransferase might bind strongly to duplex DNA and might subsequently scan the molecule for potential modification sites. The methylase
should therefore be considered a processive enzyme, and it is conceivable
that aberrations, such as single-strand breaks, might impede its progress

TABLE 2. Methyl accepting capabilities of HL DNAs[a]

Treatment	pMol of hemimethylated sites available/μg DNA	% available sites methylated in vitro/hr
2 μM 5-aza-CR	7.3	7.3
3 μM 5-aza-CR	9.5	6.9
10 μM 5-aza-CR	12.4	3.5

[a] Duplex HL DNAs were extracted from cells treated with the indicated
concentrations of 5-aza-CR in the presence of BUdR. The number of
potential methylation sites was calculated from the data in Table 1
and the abilities of these DNAs to accept methyl groups from sites
available for methylation in the presence of DNA methyltransferase
determined.

and inhibit the methylation reaction. Since BU-containing DNA is known to be very sensitive to ultraviolet radiation damage, we took advantage of the fact that the HL substrate contained BU to introduce single-strand breaks into the substrate molecule.

The number of single-strand breaks was determined by alkaline sucrose gradient centrifugation (28) and the effect of these breaks on the substrate efficiency of the DNA determined. Single-strand breaks inhibited the action of the enzyme and the degree of inhibition was proportional to the number of breaks induced by ultraviolet light. The substrate DNA had an average length of 11.5 kb pairs and approximately one break per strand resulted in a 3% decrease in methyl acceptor ability. Methylation was inhibited by 26% in DNA containing 20 single-strand breaks per 11.5 kb, and control experiments using substrate DNA which contained no BU showed that the ultraviolet radiation by itself had no effect on the ability of the DNA to serve as a substrate. Thus, the inhibition observed was not due to the formation of other DNA aberrations such as thymine dimers.

Alkylation of Hemimethylated DNAs by Chemical Carcinogens Inhibits Maintenance Methylation

Many chemical carcinogens are converted intracellularly to active electrophiles which interact with DNA to form adducts, whose size varies with the nature of the carcinogen, and DNA damage, which can be detected as alkali-labile sites. The substrate HL DNA was therefore reacted with a series of alkylating agents and the abilities of these modified DNAs to accept methyl groups from the mouse spleen enzyme determined in vitro (Table 3).

All of the agents tested caused substantial inhibitions in the abilities of the treated DNAs to accept methyl groups from S-adenosyl-methionine. The number of alkali labile breaks induced by these same concentrations of ultimate carcinogens was also determined by alkaline sucrose gradient centrifugation (results not shown). Although all of the

TABLE 3. Inhibition of DNA methyltransferase activity by chemical carcinogens[a]

Carcinogen	Concentration (r_B)[b]	% Inhibition of DNA methylation[c]
ENNG	16.1	72.0
ENU	92.6	44.4
BCNU	18.2	70.7
Melphalan	0.43	87.6
NAAAF	2.0	71.1

[a] Duplex HL DNAs were treated with the indicated concentrations of ultimate carcinogens.
[b] r_B is the molar ratio of agent to DNA base pairs.
[c] Abilities of these DNAs to accept methyl groups in vitro compared to control untreated DNA.

active agents induced some formation of alkali-labile sites, the degree
of inhibition observed in Table 3 was greater than that which could be
ascribed only to the presence of these lesions. Thus, the formation of
adducts with the bases or sugar phosphate backbone of the hemimethylated
substrate may also impede the activity of the methyltransferase.

Chemical carcinogens therefore can inhibit enzyme-mediated DNA
methylation by a variety of mechanisms linked to their abilities to alter
the suitability of duplex DNA for methyltransferase activity. Other
experiments have shown that certain carcinogens, such as N-methyl-N-
nitro-nitrosoguanidine, may be able to alter the enzyme directly, thus
inhibiting the reaction by alternative additional mechanisms (28).

DISCUSSION

The results of the present experiments, using defined hemimethylated
DNA substrates to measure maintenance methylation, demonstrate that a
wide range of chemical carcinogens can inhibit enzymatic DNA modification
by several mechanisms. They extend the earlier studies of others using
less-well-defined substrates (7,16) and show the importance of adduct
formation, DNA damage and direct enzyme modification in the inhibition
of maintenance methylation. It remains to be seen whether the carcinogens inhibit cytosine modification in living cells, but Boehm and
Drahovsky (3) have found that MNU can inhibit methylation in Raji cells
and preliminary experiments in our laboratory have shown that benzo[a]-
pyrene can inhibit DNA methylation in 3T3 cells.

The inhibition of DNA maintenance methylation, which we have observed
in vitro, may lead to heritable changes in methylcytosine distribution
in living cells. Thus, the abilities of chemical carcinogens to interfere with the arrangement of methyl groups on the genome by various
mechanisms, including adduct formation, single-strand breaks and enzyme
inactivation, may result in heritable changes in gene expression. It
is tempting to speculate that this may, in some cases, result in the
expression of suppressed oncogenic information.

ACKNOWLEDGEMENTS

Supported by Grants GM25739 and 1-T32-CA90320 from the National Institutes
of Health.

REFERENCES

1.   Adams RLP, McKay EL, Craig LM, Burdon RH (1979): Biochim Biophys
     Acta 561:345
2.   Behe M, Felsenfeld G (1981): Proc Natl Acad Sci USA 78:1619
3.   Boehm TLJ, Drahovsky D (1981): Carcinogenesis 2:39
4.   Christman JK, Weich N, Schoenbrun B, Schneiderman N, Acs, G (1980):
     J Cell Biol 86:366
5.   Cohen JC (1980): Cell 19:653
6.   Compere SJ, Palmiter RD (1981): Cell 25:233
7.   Cox R (1980): Cancer Res 40:60
8.   Drahovsky D, Morris NR (1971): J Mol Biol 57:475
9.   Groudine M, Eisenman R, Weintraub H (1981): Nature 292:311
10. Harland RM (1982): Proc Natl Acad Sci USA 79:2323
11. Holliday R, Pugh JE (1975): Science 187:226
12. Jones PA, Taylor SM (1980): Cell 20:85
13. Jones PA, Taylor SM (1981): Nucleic Acids Res 9:2933

14. Markert CL (1968):   Cancer Res 28:1908
15. McGhee JD, Ginder ED (1979):   Nature 280:419
16. Pfohl-Leszkowicz A, Salas C, Fuchs RPP, Dirheimer A (1981):
    Biochemistry 20:3020
17. Pierce GB (1974):   In: Developmental Aspects of Carcinogenesis and
    Immunity (King TJ), New York: Academic Press
18. Reznikoff CA, Brankow D, Heidelberger C (1973):   Cancer Res 33:3231
19. Riggs AD (1975):   Cytogenet Cell Genet 14:9
20. Simon D, Grunert F, Acken U, Doring HP, Kroger H (1978):   Nucleic
    Acids Res 5:2153
21. Singer J. Stellwagen RM, Roberts-Ems J, Riggs AD (1977):   J Biol
    Chem 252:5509
22. Stein R, Gruenbaum Y, Pollak Y, Razin A, Cedar H (1982):   Proc
    Natl Acad Sci USA 79:61
23. Sutter D, Doerfler W (1980):   Proc Natl Acad Sci USA 77:253
24. Turnbull JF, Adams RLP (1976):   Nucleic Acids Res 3:677
25. Van der Ploeg LHT, Flavell RA (1980):   Cell 19:947
26. Vardimon L, Kressmann A, Cedar H, Maechler M, Doerfler W (1982):
    Proc Natl Acad Sci USA 79:1073
27. Wigler M, Levy D, Perucho M (1981):   Cell 24:33
28. Wilson VL, Jones PA (1983):   Cell 32:239
29. Yagi M, Koshland ME (1981):   Proc Natl Acad Sci USA 78:4907

Gene Transfer and Cancer, edited by M. L. Pearson
and N. L. Sternberg. Raven Press, New York © 1984.

DNA Methylase-Dependent Transcription of the Phage Mu *mom* Gene

Stanley Hattman

Department of Biology, University of Rochester, Rochester, New York 14627

ABSTRACT. The phage Mu mom gene controls an unusual DNA modification. Expression of the mom function requires an active host (dam⁺) DNA adenine methylase; in dam⁻ hosts, Mu development is normal except that the viral DNA does not undergo the mom modification. The present communication compares transcription of the mom gene in dam⁺ versus dam⁻ cells.
^{32}P-labeled probes were prepared by nick-translation of a purified mom gene-containing restriction fragment and of virion DNA, respectively. These probes were hybridized with various RNAs blotted onto nitrocellulose filters (after fractionation by agarose gel electrophoresis). The salient findings are summarized as follows: a) mom specific RNA was readily detected in dam⁺ lysogenic cells, but only after induction of the Mu prophage; b) the level of mom RNA was at least 20-fold lower in induced dam⁻Mu lysogens; c) little difference, if any, was observed between dam⁺ versus dam⁻ cells with respect to total Mu transcripts produced following prophage induction. These results are in accord with the known pattern of mom gene expression and Mu development. They show that the host dam⁺ methylase activity is required for transcription of the mom gene. This represents a unique example where a DNA methylase exerts a positive regulatory role in mRNA transcription; alternative mechanisms for this process will be discussed.

INTRODUCTION

Escherichia coli bacteriophage Mu specifices a protein that modifies DNA to resistance against various restriction nucleases (1,17). The modification is under control of the mom gene (17), which is located at the right-most end of the Mu genome (17,19) flanked on the left by the Mu gin gene (5,12) and on the right by a variable length of bacterial DNA (2,3,6,7). Another phage gene(s) appears to be involved in the modification (4). It is most interesting that the host E. coli dam⁺ DNA-adenine methylase activity (16) is also required for mom modification (13,18). For example, Mu mom⁺ phages induced in dam⁻ strains are unmodified. In this regard, the efficiency of modification is highly dependent on the manner in which the phage has been propagated (1,17); e.g., phages produced after thermal or spontaneous induction of lysogenic strains are effectively modified, in contrast to lytic infection which produces poorly modified phages.

The chemical nature of the modification has been under intensive study in my laboratory and in collaboration with J. McCloskey's group at the

University of Utah. In my original reports (8,9), I showed that modification occurs in specific sequences and that about 15% of the adenine
residues were modified to some new unusual form, designated A_x. Recently,
we have identified A_x to be N^6-carboxymethyladenine; however, A_x is derived from a more highly modified residue that is acid-labile. We have purified this form and characterized it by mass spectrometric analysis (16b).

The role of the host dam$^+$ methylase in the mom modification process
has remained an intriguing mystery. Several models have been tested and
ruled out. For example, the specificity and frequency of the mom modification is very different from that for dam$^+$ methylation (GATC → Gm^{6}ATC
[10,15]) sugesting that N^6-methyladenine (m^{6}A) residues are not modified
to a new form. Moreover, the specificty of the dam$^+$ methylase is not
altered by the mom protein (8). These and other results led me to test
the possibility that the dam$^+$ methylase is required for transcription
of the Mu mom gene. In the present report, I present evidence demonstrating this requirement to be the case. This finding represents the
only known instance in which a DNA methylase is involved in positive
regulation of transcription.

RESULTS

In order to test whether transcription of the Mu mom gene is DNA-
methylase dependent, I first isolated RNA from induced and uninduced Mu
lysogens of dam$^+$ and dam$^-$ bacteria. The strategy was then to determine
whether mom specific mRNA was detectable in dam$^+$, but not dam$^-$, cells.
Furthermore, since modification occurs only after induction, one would
expect that no mom mRNA would be detected in RNA preparations from uninduced cells. To screen for mom specific transcripts it was essential to
have a labeled probe derived from the mom gene. This was made possible
by taking advantage of the fact that various recombinant plasmids have
been produced containing a cloned Mu mom gene. Figure 1 is a diagram of
the physical map of one such plasmid, pDK XXV-3 (14), from which the mom
gene can be excised on a 1.4-kb PvuI fragment (along with some bacterial
DNA). After digestion with PvuI and agarose gel electrophoresis, this
fragment was purified and nick translated to make ^{32}P-labeled probe.
As a control, total Mu genomic probe was separately prepared by nick
translation of virion DNA.

The RNA isolated from uninduced and prophage-induced dam$^+$ and dam$^-$
E. coli lysogens was electrophoresed through agarose gels, blot transferred to nitrocellulose filters and then hybridized with the ^{32}P-labeled
probes. As shown in Figure 2, the ^{32}P-labeled mom probe hybridized only
with RNA from the induced dam$^+$ Mu lysogen. The low level of mom mRNA
in uninduced dam$^+$ lysogens is consistent with poor mom expression in
the absence of prophage induction (1,17).

Although phage Mu production is normal in dam$^-$ hosts, it was necessary
to verify the presence of other Mu specific mRNAs in these gels. In a
parallel analysis, it was shown that ^{32}P-labeled total Mu probe hybridized equally with RNA from induced dam$^+$ and dam$^-$ lysogens (Figure 3).
Under the hybridization conditions, little or no Mu mRNA was detected
in the uninduced cells. These results are consistent with the fact that
Mu development is normal in a dam$^-$ host, and they preclude the possibility of extensive degradation of Mu mRNAs.

In order to rule out the trivial possibility of differential mRNA
transfer in the two blots, the same filter was taken for sequential
hybridization with ^{32}P-labeled mom and ^{32}P-labeled total Mu probes.
In Figure 4 (left panel) it is again evident that mom mRNA is present

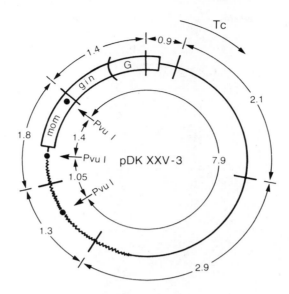

FIGURE 1. Schematic diagram of the physical map of plasmid pDK XXV-3. The outer arrows represent distances between restriction sites for HindII (D. Kwoh, personal communication); the arrows pointing to filled circles indicate PvuI sites (S. Hattman, unpublished data). The wavy line represents bacterial DNA, the box represents Mu genes and the remainder is plasmid DNA. The relative amounts of Mu mom and bacterial DNAs in the 1.4-kb PvuI fragment are not accurately known. That one PvuI site is in bacterial DNA was deduced in a separate experiment; another plasmid containing an independently cloned Mu mom-gin-G segment was cut only once by PvuI presumably in the mom gene (S. Hattman, unpublished data).

at a much lower concentration in the induced dam⁻ lysogen; I estimate that the dam⁺ host contained at least 20-fold more mom RNA than the dam⁻ strain. In the secondary hybridization with ^{32}P-labeled total Mu probe, both dam⁺ and dam⁻ cells exhibited similar patterns of hybridization (Fig. 4, right panel). In this experiment, a reduced amount of total Mu probe was used and, consequently, one can discern distinct mRNA bands.

In conclusion, the results show that an active E. coli dam⁺ methylase is essential for transcription of the phage Mu mom gene after prophage induction. The implications of this finding are discussed below.

DISCUSSION

It has been known for some time that expression of the Mu mom modification is blocked following prophage induction in dam⁻, but not dam⁺, hosts (13,18). The present report provides evidence that this block is due to a marked reduction in the level of mom gene transcription in the dam⁻ host, while synthesis of other Mu transcripts appears normal. Although formally possible, mom mRNA is probably not subject to selective degradation in dam⁻ cells. The presence of an active dam⁺ methylase is

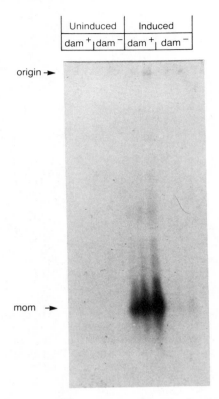

FIGURE 2. Hybridization of ^{32}P-labeled mom probe to RNA from uninduced
and induced Mu lysogens. RNA was isolated by hot phenol-sodium dodecyl
sulfate extraction and samples of 4, 8, and 16 µg were subjected to
agarose gel electrophoresis. Following transfer to nitrocellulose
filters, Northern hybridization with the mom probe was carried out.

a necessary, but not sufficient, condition for mom gene expression.
This conclusion is based upon the fact that mom modification is not
constitutively expressed by plasmids containing a cloned mom gene (4);
however, infection by a Mu mom phage results in 'transactivation' of mom
modification expression. Thus, there are additional elements of mom
regulation that are yet to be elucidated (4,19).

   How does the E. coli dam$^+$ methylase exert a positive regulatory function in transcription of the Mu mom gene? I should like to discuss two
related but alternative mechanisms: a) the enzyme acts only by methylating
a specific site(s) on Mu DNA; or b) the enzyme acts by virtue of its
binding to a specific site(s) on the Mu DNA. Thus, both models require
a specific target site(s) which serves either as a methylation or a
binding substrate for the E. coli dam$^+$ methylase. There is, in fact,
evidence supporting the existence of such a site(s); viz. certain Mu
deletions allow mom expression independent of dam$^+$ activity (10a, 11a).
Since site-specific methylation presumably also involves site-specific
binding, the distinction between the two models should be made clear.
In the first model, once DNA methylation has occurred, the methylase

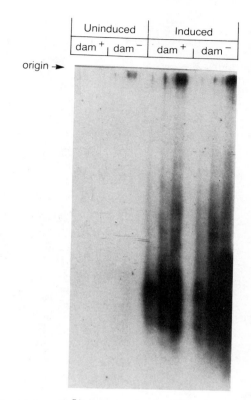

Uninduced		Induced	
dam$^+$	dam$^-$	dam$^+$	dam$^-$

origin →

FIGURE 3. Hybridization of ^{32}P-labeled total Mu probe to RNA from uninduced and induced Mu lysogens. See legend to Figure 2.

is no longer required; in the second model, the bound methylase serves as a regulatory element. According to the first model, the presence of m^{6}A residues in a GATC sequence(s) upstream, downstream or within a mom promoter is the recognition signal; in this model, the positive regulatory role could be to promote initiation or to prevent termination of mRNA transcription. In contrast, the second model requires presence of a bound E. coli dam$^+$ methylase at the target site, most likely to promote mRNA initiation in a manner analogous to the CAP protein involvement in transcription of the lac operon.

At the present time there are no unequivocal data ruling out either alternative. However, the following result leads me to favor the first model. We have molecularly cloned a functional phage T4 DNA-adenine methylase gene (16a). The T4 methylase is capable of replacing the E. coli dam$^+$ methylase in promoting Mu mom$^+$ modification (S. Hattman, unpublished result). Based on what we know about the E. coli and phage T2 dam$^+$ proteins, we expect that the phage T4 enzyme will also be very different from E. coli dam$^+$ methylase (although the phage enzymes are also capable of methylating GATC). The E. coli dam$^+$ gene codes for a polypeptide of MW 31,000 (11) compared to only about 15,000 for the T2 dam$^+$ polypeptide (M. Masurekar and S. Hattman, unpublished data). Thus, for the present, it seems more likely that the T4 and E. coli enzymes

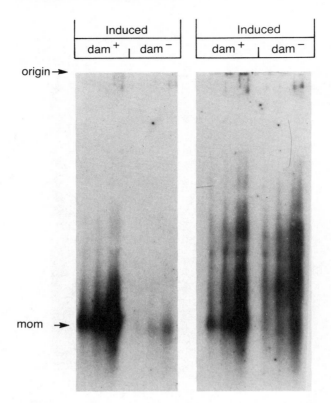

FIGURE 4. Sequential hybridization of ^{32}P-labeled probes to RNA from induced Mu lysogens. See legend to Figure 2. The primary hybridization was with ^{32}P-labeled <u>mom</u> probe (left panel). After autoradiography, the filter was taken for secondary hybridization with ^{32}P-labeled total Mu probe (right panel).

act by virtue of their ability to methylate a common tetranucleotide sequence, rather than by sharing a common binding sequence. Nevertheless, experiments are in progress attempting to reach a definitive distinction between the two models. If my current view is correct, it will be very interesting to see whether <u>E. coli</u> RNA polymerase alone is capable of distinguishing between the unmethylated and the methylated target site(s). Whatever the outcome, phage Mu has provided us with an exciting regulatory system.

Finally, it is also interesting to speculate as to whether other pro-caryote genes are positively (or negatively) regulated by <u>dam</u>[+] or <u>dcm</u>[+] methylation (or methylases). The fact that DNA methylation-defective mutants are viable and propagate phages suggests that no essential host or viral gene is positively regulated. Nevertheless, it would be worthwhile to screen nonessential genes for such a regulatory control.

ACKNOWLEDGEMENTS

This work was supported by a Public Health Service grant No. GM-29227.

The author is most grateful to D. Pederson and F. Calzone for their many helpful discussions, suggestions and advice on methods. The author gratefully acknowledges the suggestion of R. Plasterk to use PvuI to cut the pDK XXV-3 plasmid. I thank D. Kwoh for generously providing strains and detailed information on various Mu clones, and H. Smith for his critical comments.

REFERENCES

1. Allet B, Bukhari AI (1975): J Mol Biol 92:529
2. Bukhari AI, Froshauer S, Botchan M (1976): Nature 264:580
3. Bukhari AI, Taylor AL (1975): Proc Natl Acad Sci USA 72:4399
4. Chaconas G, de Bruijn FJ, Casadaban M, Lupski JR, Kwoh TJ, Harshey RM, DuBow MS, Bukhari AI (1981): Gene 13:37
5. Chow LT, Kahmann R, Kamp D (1978): J Mol Biol 113:591
6. Daniell E, Abelson J, Kim JS, Davidson N (1973): Virology 51:237
7. Daniell E, Kohne DE, Abelson J (1975): J. Virol 15:739
8. Hattman S (1979): J Virol 32:468
9. Hattman S (1980): J Virol 34:277
10. Hattman S, Brooks JE, Masurekar M (1978): J Mol Biol 126:367
10a. Hattman S, Goradia M, Monaghan C, Bukhari AI (1982): Cold Spring Harbor Symp Quant Biol 47:647
11. Herman GE, Modrich P (1982): J Biol Chem 257:2605
11a. Kahmann R (1982): Cold Spring Harbor Symp Quant Biol 47:639
12. Kamp D, Kahmann R, Zipser D, Broker T, Chow LT (1978): Nature 271:577
13. Khatoon H, Bukhari AI (1978): J Bacteriol 136:423
14. Kwoh DY, Zipser D, Erdmann DS (1980): Virology 101:419
15. Lacks S, Greenberg B (1977): J Mol Biol 114:153
16. Marinus MG, Morris NR (1973): J Bacteriol 114:1143
16a. Schlagman S, Hattman S (1983): Gene 22:139
16b. Swinton D, Hattman S, Crain PF, Cheng C-S, Smith DL, McCloskey JA (in press): Proc Natl Acad Sci USA
17. Toussaint A (1976): Virology 70:17
18. Toussaint A (1977): J Virol 23:825
19. Toussaint A, Desmet L, Faelen M (1980): Mol Gen Genet 177:351

Gene Transfer and Cancer, edited by M. L. Pearson and N. L. Sternberg. Raven Press, New York © 1984.

High Frequency Alterations of Transfected Thymidine Kinase Gene Expression Are Mediated by Changes in Chromatin Structure

Robin L. Davies, Stelia Fuhrer-Krusi, and [1]Raju Kucherlapati

Department of Biochemical Sciences, Princeton University, Princeton, New Jersey 08544

ABSTRACT. A bacterial plasmid containing the herpes simplex virus (HSV) thymidine kinase (tk) gene was introduced into mouse fibroblasts by DNA-mediated transfer. When stable cell lines containing integrated plasmid sequences were exposed to medium containing 5-bromodeoxyuridine (BrdU), cells which lost the tk expression were obtained at a high frequency. These cells did not lose their tk gene sequences and were capable of rereversion to a TK+ phenotype at high frequency. This modulation of gene expression appears to be mediated by changes at the transcriptional level. We failed to detect any DNA rearrangements which would explain the modulation in gene activity. Experiments designed to examine changes in the methylation patterns of DNA also did not reveal any differences. However, examination of the chromatin structure of the TK- and TK+ cells showed that the chromatin containing the HSV tk sequences in the TK+ cells was considerably more sensitive to digestion with DNase I than chromatin in the TK- cells. These results show that exogenously introduced sequences are subject to modulation mediated by changes in chromatin structure.

INTRODUCTION

Several methods are now available to introduce purified DNA into mammalian cells. These can be classified into direct and indirect methods. The most prominent among the direct methods of gene transfer is microinjection. Anderson et al. (2) and Capecchi (5) have shown that a relatively large proportion of somatic cells, into which DNA of a selectable gene such as the HSV tk gene is injected, become stably transformed by it. Gordon and Colleagues (8,9) and Wagner et al. (26) have shown that similar injections into fertilized mouse embryos result in incorporation of the foreign DNA sequences into all tissues of the organism that develops from it. The most widely used indirect method of gene transfer is that mediated by calcium-phosphate coprecipitation. After the initial observation by Bacchetti and Graham (3) that a calcium phosphate precipitate enhances the transfection of adenoviral DNA, Maitland and McDougall (16) and Wigler et al. (28) showed that restriction-enzyme-digested DNA or a fragment

---

[1] Present address: Center for Genetics, University of Illinois at Chicago, 808 S. Wood St., Chicago, IL 60612.

purified from such a digest of HSV DNA can effectively transfer the TK$^+$
phenotype to TK$^-$ mouse fibroblasts. Since these observations were made,
numerous other genes have been successfully introduced into mammalian
cells (for a review see 13). For these gene transfer systems to be of
general utility in correlating DNA structure to function, the mechanisms
of DNA uptake, the fate of the DNA in the cell, and the cellular features
or properties that affect the foreign gene expression must be understood.
    Loyter et al. (15) have studied the mechanism of DNA uptake and pro-
vided evidence that DNA is not taken up by any active transport mechanism
and that calcium phosphate may provide protection against degradation of
DNA. A number of investigators (e.g., 19,20) have shown that a relatively
large proportion of cells may express the foreign genes transiently. Only
a fraction of the cells that transiently express the genes become stably
transformed by the foreign DNA. Examination of the foreign DNA in recipient cells revealed its integration into high-molecular-weight DNA.
Scangos et al. (23) and Perucho et al. (21) have shown that when carrier
DNA is used in the transfer, the selectable DNA becomes complexed with
the carrier DNA, and Robins et al. (22) have shown that such complexes
integrate into chromosomal sites in a random fashion. Since only a subset of genes in any given cell are expressed, it is reasonable to propose
that the expression or regulation of the foreign DNA may, at least to
some extent, be dictated by its site of integration. We have obtained
evidence to support this view which will be presented here.

RESULTS

DNA Transfection

    We have introduced a circular plasmid pHSV106, containing pBR322 and
a 3.4-kb HSV1 DNA carrying the tk gene (17,18) into mouse LMtk$^-$ cells
by the calcium phosphate coprecipitation method described by Wigler et
al. (28). TK$^+$ colonies that are capable of growing in medium containing
hypoxanthine, aminopterin, and thymidine (HAT) were isolated (11). Several such cell lines were examined for pHSV106 sequences by the blot-
hybridization method developed by Southern (24). All of the cell lines
tested contained pHSV106 sequences in multiple copies and integrated
into high-molecular-weight DNA. We have chosen one of these cell lines,
LGC22c, for further study. This cell line contained two copies of the
plasmid, at least one of which contains an intact HSV tk gene sequence.
We have derived a stable derivative of this cell line. When this cell
line was plated into medium containing 30 µg/ml of BrdU, 3 to 10% of
the cells were able to form revertant colonies. When examined for pHSV106
sequences, these revertant colonies fell into two categories: those that
lost the pHSV106 sequences and those that retained these sequences. When
a population of the BrdU^R cells were passaged in nonselective medium and
plated into HAT medium, a high proportion (1 to 10%) were found to be
capable of rereversion to a TK$^+$ HAT^R phenotype. We have observed that
these cells retain this capacity to modulate their TK phenotype through
additional rounds of selection and counterselection. Cells that behave
in a similar fashion were observed by other investigators (e.g., 7,20).
We have examined the molecular basis for this modulation of HSV tk gene
expression.

Basis of Gene Modulation

We have tested the possibility that the tk gene is active in BrdU^R

cell lines, although at a reduced level. Cell extracts from BrdU[R] and HAT[R] cells were examined for TK-specific enzyme activity by the method of Adelstein et al. (1). While the HAT[R] cells contained high levels of TK activity, the BrdU[R] cells contained no detectable levels of TK. We then examined whether TK mRNA is produced in the two cell types. Total cellular RNA from the cells was fractionated on denaturing formaldehyde agarose gels (14), transferred to nitrocellulose, and hybridized with a labeled TK-specific DNA fragment. The HAT[R] cells showed a 14S species of RNA that hybridized to the probe and that corresponded to the authentic TK mRNA. No such hybridization was detected in RNA from the BrdU[R] cells. The method we have employed is sensitive enough to detect two to five copies of TK-specific RNA/cell and as such we have concluded that the level of accumulated TK mRNA in the BrdU[R] cells is less than 2 copies per cell. We concluded that the tk gene expression in these cells is modulated at the transcriptional level.

Examination of DNA

The modulation of gene expression we observed in LGC22c subclones is possibly mediated by DNA rearrangement. To test this possibility, DNA from the revertants and rerevertants was cleaved with each of five different restriction endonucleases (EcoRI, BamHI, HindIII, KpnI and BglII) and blot-hybridized using pHSV106 as the probe. If DNA rearrangements play a role in the alterations of gene expression observed in these cell lines we should have noted differences in the patterns of bands revealed by one or more of these enzymes. We were unable to detect any such differences between the two classes of cells. We estimate that we examined 20- to 25-kb span of DNA using these enzymes. That DNA rearrangement does not play any major role in the observed modulation is substantiated by the fact that purified DNA from each of the cell lines is capable of acting as donor in secondary transfer of the TK phenotype to TK⁻ cells.

Examination of DNA Modification

The major modification of DNA in mammalian cells is the methylation of cytosine residues and a majority of this modification is restricted to the palindromic dinucleotide sequence CpG. A number of investigators (e.g., 4,25) have shown that gene activity can be correlated with hypomethylation of DNA. Accordingly, we have tested whether the TK DNA sequences are hypermethylated in the BrdU[R] cells. We have initially used the isoschizomers MspI and HpaII to examine this question. Both of these enzymes recognize the tetranucleotide sequence CCGG, but HpaII fails to cleave at this sequence if the internal C is methylated. Since there are numerous recognition sites for these enzymes in pHSV106, DNA from the two classes of cells was digested with MspI or HpaII, fractionated on polyacrylamide gels and blot-hybridized as described before. Although there was some methylation of the sequences, we failed to detect any differences in the methylation patterns between the revertant and rerevertant cell DNA.

The role of methylation was also tested by treating the revertants with 2 to 10 μM 5-azacytidine (a nucleotide analog whose incorporation into DNA results in reduction in CpG methylation levels) and testing their plating efficiency in medium with or without HAT. Treatment with azacytidine did not result in any measurable increase in rereversion. Thus, both a biological and molecular biological test showed that DNA methylation does not play any appreciable role in the gene modulation we observed.

Chromatin Structure

Weintraub and Groudine (27) have shown that chromatin containing active genes or genes with a history of activity exhibits a greater sensitivity to digestion by the enzyme DNase I. We have conducted experiments to test whether the two classes of cell lines exhibit such differences. To prepare for such a test, we needed to determine whether the exogenously introduced HSV tk genes acquire a nucleosome-like structure. Isolated nuclei from HAT[R] cells were subjected to limited digestion with micrococcal nuclease. DNA was isolated, fractionated on agarose gels, and stained with ethidium bromide. A ladder of bands representing the nucleosome monomer and oligomers was observed. This DNA was denatured, transferred to nitrocellulose, and hybridized with labeled pHSV106. The pattern of hybridization correlated precisely with the ethidium bromide staining. This observation permitted us to conclude that the pHSV106 sequences are organized into nucleosome-like structures. We then examined the DNase I sensitivity of these sequences. Nuclei from the revertants and rerevertents were subjected to increasing levels of mild digestion with DNaseI.

In these experiments, isolated nuclei were treated with pancreatic DNase (2U/1O.D. unit) for periods ranging from 0 to 60 minutes at 26°C. Following digestion, DNA was isolated, digested with each of several restriction endonucleases, and blot-hybridized. Labeled pHSV106 was used as a probe. We obtained the following results. EcoRI digestion of revertant and rerevertant cell DNA revaled, among others, a 4.6-kb and a 2.2-kb band that hybridize with pHSV106. The 4.6-kb band contains almost exclusively pBR322 DNA, whereas the 2.2-kb band contains exclusively HSV DNA and encompasses all of the coding sequences for the tk gene. We noted that in the HAT[R] cells, the 2.2-kb band was digested by DNase I at 15 minutes of digestion, whereas the 4.6-kb band remained intact even after 45 minutes of digestion. In the BrdU[R] cells, neither of these bands were sensitive to DNase I digestion at any time point up to 45 minutes. In addition, we noted a gradual loss of high-molecular-weight bands with increasing levels of DNase I digestions. We concluded that a sequence containing the tk structural gene was more sensitive to DNase I digestion in the HAT[R] cells than in the corresponding BrdU[R] cells. Apparently the modulation of gene expression we have observed is mediated by changes in chromatin structure. The results we have described are summarized in Table I.

TABLE 1. Comparison of Revertant and Rerevertant Cell Lines

	HAT[R]	BUdR[R]
TK activity	+	−
TK mRNA	+	−
TK DNA	+	+
Transfectability	+	+
Rearrangements	−	−
Methylation	+	+
TK activity after azacytidine	+	−
Nucleosome structure	+	+
DNase I sensitivity	+	−

DISCUSSION

We have observed that the expression of an exogenously introduced tk gene is modulated in mouse fibroblasts. Davidson and colleagues (7) have noted a similar modulation in cells transfected with HSV that had been inactivated by ultraviolet radiation. Pellicer et al. (20) have reported similar observations with purified HSV tk, and Hanahan et al. (10) noted that SV40 T-antigen expression is also subject to fluctuation in cells transfected with SV40 DNA. It is, however, necessary to note that TK⁻ revertants obtained in these various experiments fall into two categories. The first class is characterized by a very low rate (10^{-6}) of rereversion, and the second class (described in this report) exhibits a very high rate of change (1 to 10%). Furthermore, the first class of alteration seems to be mediated by hypermethylation of tk DNA (6; Christy and Scangos and Hardies et al., this volume), whereas the modulation we observed is mediated by changes at a different level. Since the donor DNA, the recipient cells, and the methods of transfer resulting in these two classes of gene modulation are the same, it must be concluded that the sites of integration may determine the fate of the gene expression. Genes may become integrated into inactive regions (these will not be detected in our system because we select for gene expression) or into active regions, and they may be subject to hypermethylation or may exhibit alterations in chromatin structure at high frequency. Indeed, Jaenisch and colleagues (12) have found evidence that the sites of integration of foreign DNA does influence its expression.

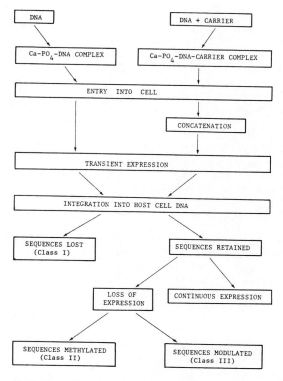

FIGURE 1. A view of the fate of the DNA and its expression in transfected cells.

The observations reported here as well as several other reports provide a picture of the events in DNA-mediated gene transfer (Fig. 1). When DNA is presented to cells, only some cells will be able to acquire it. The DNA that enters the cytoplasm may or may not enter the nucleus, where it exists as an autonomous expressing entity in a transient fashion. If carrier DNA is present, the DNA may become associated into high-molecular-weight structures, the mechanism of which is ill understood. These "pekelasomes" or transgenomes" are integrated into cell DNA at random locations. The sites of integration may permit continuous expression or may result in modulation of gene expression mediated by several alternate mechanisms. If this picture is fairly accurate, the exogenously introduced sequences may act as windows that permit examination of cellular features or phenomena which have been hitherto inaccessible. Examination of other cell lines in which gene expression is modulated may thus prove fruitful.

ACKNOWLEDGEMENTS

This work was supported by a grant from the NIH. R.L.D. was supported by a predoctoral training grant from NIH. S.F.K. was supported by the Swiss National Science Foundation. We thank Mr. Ray Roginsky and Dr. A. Skoultchi for many discussions and sharing their knowledge of RNA blotting procedures. We appreciate the help of Ms. Noel Mann in preparing this manuscript.

REFERENCES

1. Adelstein SJ, Baldwin C, Kohn HI (1971): Dev Biol 26:537
2. Anderson WF, Killos L, Sanders-Haigh L, Kretschmer PJ, Diacumakos EG (1980): Proc Natl Acad Sci USA 77:5399
3. Bacchetti S, Graham FL (1977): Proc Natl Acad Sci USA 74:1590
4. Bird AP, Southern EM (1978): J Mol Biol 118:27
5. Capecchi MR (1980): Cell 22:479
6. Clough DW, Kunkel LM, Davidson RL (1982): Science 216:70
7. Davidson RL, Adelstein SJ, Oxman MN (1973): Proc Natl Acad Sci USA 70:1912
8. Gordon JW, Ruddle FH (1981): Science 214:1244
9. Gordon JW, Scangos GA, Plotkin DJ, Barbosa JA, Ruddle FJ (1980): Proc Natl Acad Sci USA 77:7380
10. Hanahan D, Lane D, Lipsich L, Wigler M, Botchan M (1980): Cell 21:127
11. Hsiung N, Warrick H, DeRiel JK, Tuan D, Forget BG, Skoultchi A, Kucherlapati R (1980): Proc Natl Acad Sci USA 77:4852
12. Jaenisch R, Jahner D, Nobis P, Simon I, Lohler J, Harbers K, Grotkopp D (1981): Cell 21:529
13. Kucherlapati R (1982): In Advances in Cell Culture (Maromorosch, ed) Vol 2, New York: Academic Press, p 69
14. Lehrach M, Diamond D, Wozney JW, Boedtker H (1977): Biochem 16:4743
15. Loyter A, Scangos GA, Ruddle FH (1982): Proc Natl Acad Sci USA 79:422
16. Maitland NJ, McDougall JK (1977): Cell 11:233
17. McKnight SL (1980): Nucleic Acids Res 8:5949
18. McKnight SL, Croce C, Kingsbury R (1979): Carnegie Inst Wash Yearbook 78:56
19. Milman G, Herzberg M (1981): Somatic Cell Genet 7:161
20. Pellicer A, Robins D, Wold B, Sweet R, Jackson J, Lowy I, Roberts JM, Sim GK, Silverstein S, Axel R (1980): Science 209:1414
21. Perucho M, Hanahan D, Wigler M (1980): Cell 22:309
22. Robins DM, Ripley S, Henderson AS, Axel R (1981): Cell 23:29

23. Scangos GA, Huttner KM, Juricek DK, Ruddle FH (1981): Mol Cell Biol 1:111
24. Southern EM (1975): J Mol Biol 98:503
25. Sutter D, Doerfler W (1980): Proc Natl Acad Sci USA 77:253
26. Wagner EF, Stewart TA, Mintz B (1981): Proc Natl Acad Sci USA 78:5016
27. Weintraub H, Groudine M (1976): Science 193:848
28. Wigler M, Silverstein S, Lee L-S, Pellicer A, Cheng Y, Axel R (1977): Cell 11:223

Gene Transfer and Cancer, edited y M. L. Pearson
and N. L. Sternberg. Raven Press, New York © 1984.

Structural and Functional Analysis of the Glucocorticoid-Regulated MMTV Transcriptional Promoter

Michael C. Ostrowski and Gordon L. Hager

*Laboratory of Tumor Virus Genetics, National Cancer Institute,
Bethesda, Maryland 20205*

ABSTRACT. We have demonstrated previously (4) that transfection of
NIH/3T3 cells with chimeric plasmids containing the mouse mammary tumor
virus long terminal repeat (MMTV LTR) fused to v-ras, the transforming
gene of Harvey murine sarcoma virus (HaMuSV), results in transformed
foci. The synthesis of p21 (the v-ras gene product) and of MMTV LTR-
initiated p21 mRNA in these cells is regulated by the synthetic glucocorticoid, dexamethasone. More recently, we have found that the frequency with which these chimeric plasmids induce the transformation of
cells in culture can be increased 1000-fold by insertion of a fragment
containing the 72-bp direct repeats of the HaMuSV LTR 5' proximal to the
MMTV LTR in the hybrid plasmid. This enhancement of transfection efficiency suggests a) that the MMTV LTR requires the presence of such an
"enhancer" sequence for efficient expression, or b) that a host-range
phenomenon exists for transcriptional expression.

To analyze the regulation of MMTV-promoted transcription in the absence of unforeseen interactions between the LTR and cellular DNA sequences, we hae used bovine pappilloma virus (BPV) as a vector to introduce the MMTV LTR-v-ras fusions in mouse cells as extrachromosomal
elements. We have now developed cell lines transformed with BPV-LTR-
v-ras chimeras that stably contain as many as 200 copies per cell of
episomal molecules. These episomes retain the same physical organization
as the input DNA, indicating that the BPV-mobilized fusions have not
undergone rearrangement. Furthermore, the level of p21 MMTV LTR-initi-
ated mRNA is regulated by dexamethasone. Preliminary experiments indicate
that substantial enrichment of these BPV minichromosomes may be obtained
from nuclear preparations. These partially purified minichromsomes will
be useful in exploring the interaction of hormone receptor complex with
the MMTV LTR, especially with regard to in vitro reconstitution of transcriptional regulation.

INTRODUCTION

The expression of MMTV RNA and proteins is induced by glucocorticoid
hormones (14,17). Investigations concerning the mechanism of hormone
action in the MMTV system have demonstrated that the rate of transcription of MMTV RNA in chronically infected cell lines is increased 10 to
15 minutes after addition of hormone to the culture medium (11,17).

These results strongly suggest that glucocorticoid hormones directly
stimulate transcription of MMTV. Our goal is to utilize the MMTV system
as a general model for studying the molecular mechanisms by which glucocorticoid hormones regulate gene expression. With this goal in mind, we
first wished to define the portion of the MMTV genome that confers
hormone-regulated transcription. To accomplish this, we constructed
chimeras consisting of the 1300-bp LTR of MMTV fused to v-ra, the transforming region of Harvey sarcoma virus (HaSV), and introduced them into
NIH/3T3 cells via calcium-phosphate precipitation (4). Transformed foci
were generated from these experiments with efficiencies 1000-fold lower
than those obtained from transfection of authentic HaSV. However, synthesis of p21, p21 mRNA that is initiated within the MMTV LTR, and the
transformed phenotype of these NIH/3T3 cells are regulated by the presence of the synthetic glucocorticoid dexamethasone in the culture medium.
Lee et al. have obtained similar results by fusing MMTV LTR to mouse dihydrofolate reductase (6).

RESULTS

Addition of an "Enhancer" to MMTV-v-<u>ras</u> Chimeras

The next set of experiments we wished to perform using the MMTV-v-ras
chimeras involved deletion analysis of the LTR. However, given the low
efficiencies of transformation we obtain with these recombinants (4),
meaningful deletion analysis is impossible. Therefore, experiments were
designed to correct this deficiency in the system. These experiments
involved adding part of HaSV LTR to the MMTV LTR-v-ras chimeras (Figure 1).
The section of the HaSV LTR added contains 74-bp direct repeats, the
so-called transcription enhancer sequences (2,7,13), but not the more
conventional promoter elements such as the TATAA or CAT (1) sequences.
The recombinant plasmid was engineered in such a fashion that two orientations of the HaSV repeats relative to initiation of transcription within
the MMTV LTR (designated pA9⁻R⁺ or pA9R⁻) were obtained. Transfection of
recombinant plasmid pA9⁻R⁺ results in foci formation with the same efficiency as HaSV, around 1000 foci per μg of DNA, when the transfection
assay is performed in the presence of hormone; when hormone is absent,
or when pA9⁻R⁻ is transfected, focus formation is no more efficient
than for the original chimera discussed above. Both p21 and MMTV LTR-
initiated p21 mRNA levels are regulated by dexamethasone in the pA9⁻R⁺-
transformed cells; no 5' RNA ends are mapped to the HaSV sequences. From
these experiments we conclude that either: a) the MMTV LTR requires a
cis-acting regulatory element for efficient initiation of transcription
in the presence of hormone or, b) a tissue specific host-range exists
for MMTV LTR-promoted transcription.

Deletion Analysis of the MMTV LTR

The addition of the enhancer sequences to the hybrid recombinants thus
allow an easy assay to screen deletion mutants of the MMTV LTR, namely
the ability to form high numbers of transformed foci in the presence, but
not absence of steroid hormone. Using this system, we have tested LTR
mutants made by cleavage with specific restriction endonucleases. Cleavage
of the LTR with <u>ClaI</u>, <u>RsaI</u> or <u>HaeIII</u> eliminates the 5' portions of the LTR
located beyond positions -855, -365 or -225, respectively, in relation to
the MMTV RNA cap site. These mutants produce foci as well as a complete
LTR only in the presence of hormone. <u>SstI</u>-deleted LTR, which is missing

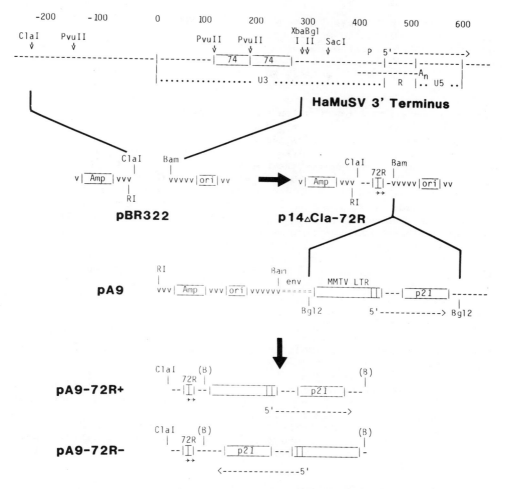

FIGURE 1. Addition of HaMuSV 74-bp direct repeat sequences to MMTV LTR-v-ras fusion.

all sequence information beyond position -105, generates foci whether hormone is present or absent. We can therefore assign a role in hormone-regulated transcription to the sequences located between -105 and -225 from the MMTV cap site. Additionally, the fact tht removing these sequences results in the conversion of the regulated MMTV promoter into a constitutive promoter may indicate that these sequences act as a re-pressor of MMTV transcription, and that this repression is relieved by the presence of steroid-receptor complex. This interpretation is clouded by the fact that the directly repeated 74-bp enhancer sequence is moved approximately 1 kb closer to the MMTV cap site in the SstI mutant than in pA9⁻R⁺. Thus, that the MMTV promoter becomes active in the absence of hormone in the SstI mutant may only reflect a positional effect of the enhancer element (10).

Mobilization of MMTV LTR on a Eucaryotic Plasmid Vector

Although the experiments discussed so far define the region of the

MMTV LTR that is important for hormone regulation of gene expression, they do not address the mechanisms by which hormone-receptor complex, MMTV LTR, RNA polymerase II and other nuclear components interact to produce the observed biological phenomenon, i.e., elevated rates of transcription. Ultimately, the only way to approach an understanding of this complex problem is to reconstitute accurate hormone regulated transcription in vitro. We believe epigenetic chromatin structure will be very important in such reconstitution attempts; however, assembly of such structures in vitro pose major technical problems. Therefore, we decided to use vectors that persist as plasmids to introduce MMTV LTR into eucaryotic cells so that we could attempt to isolate LTR as native nucleoprotein minichromosomes. The vector that we chose is BPV, a virus capable of nonproductive transformation of mouse cells in culture (8). BPV remains a plasmid while present at up to 200 copies per transformed cell (5).

We have made recombinant pBR322 derivatives that contain the 5.4-kb transforming region of BPV (8) and the MMTV LTR-v-ras fusion (4). Transfection of these plasmids onto mouse C127 cells yields approximately 8000 foci/pmol DNA. Tranformed cell lines that stably contain up to 200 copies of plasmid DNA have been identified. These plasmids retain the same physical arrangement as the input DNA. S1 mapping of RNA shows that MMTV-initiated p21 RNA levels are increased by dexamethasone. The amount of RNA present in these cells is consistent with the amount of plasmid template available, i.e., about 10-fold higher than in the NIH/3T3 transformed cells described above. However, by this analysis we can not rule out the possibility that a few integrated copies of MMTV LTR-v-ras are responsible for transcription of this RNA, or that only a subpopulation of the minichromosomes are transcriptionally active.

Initial attempts at making minichromosomes from nuclear preparations using published techniques (12,16) have been successful. 25 to 50% of the minichromosomes present have been enriched at least 100-fold using these procedures. We are currently studying these enriched BPV-MMTV LTR nucleoprotein preparations by transcription run-off analysis and nuclease digestion experiments to insure that the MMTV LTR remains transcriptionally active when mobilized on BPV plasmids.

DISCUSSION

We have previously shown that the MMTV LTR contains sequences required for glucocorticoid regulation of transcription (4). The low efficiencies with which the chimeras used to demonstrate this property transform cells in culture make it difficult to more precisely map by in vitro mutagenic techniques the control region(s) of the LTR responsible for this regulation. However, we have found that adding a transcriptional enhancer element derived from the LTR of HaSV to the MMTV LTR chimeras resolves this problem. This observation also yields a system for assaying mutant MMTV LTRs by taking advantage of the biological phenomenon of cellular transformation in the presence of glucocorticoid hormones. Utilizing this approach, we defined a 120-bp region, located between sequences -105 and -225 relative to the MMTV RNA cap site, that contains sufficient information to cause hormone regulation of transcription. Experiments are presently under way to further mutate this region in order to generate smaller, more discrete and/or insertions, and thereby more precisely define sequences important in hormone regulation.

Another side to the phenomonen of hormone-controlled gene expression is the interaction of hormone-receptor complex with its DNA target so that specific transcription is stimulated (or repressed). In vitro reconstitution of hormonally regulated transcription is one approach to understanding this interaction. To do this type of experiment, we have decided to introduce the MMTV LTR into eucaryotic cells as a plasmid by using BPV as a vector. In this way, we hope to be able to isolate the LTR as a nucleoprotein particle with its epigenetic structure intact. By taking this approach, we believe that we can overcome the major problem associated with current in vitro transcription systems i.e., that the in vitro situation does not accurately reflect the in vivo situation (2,3,9, 15). As shown above, this BPV vector system has been useful: we have been able to isolate enriched minichromosomes that contain MMTV LTR under conditions that should preserve native chromatin structure. The further usefulness of this system to obtain faithful, hormone-regulated transcription in vitro remains to be determined.

ACKNOWLEDGEMENTS

We acknowledge Dr. Alex Lichtler for his contributions to the MMTV LTR deletion studies and Ronald Wolford and Diana Berard for their excellent technical assistance.

REFERENCES

1. Benoist C, O'Hare R, Breathnach R, Chambon P (1980): Nucleic Acid Res 8:127
2. Benoist C, Chambon P (1981): Nature 290:304
3. Grosschedl R, Birnstiel ML (1980): Proc Natl Acad Sci USA 77:7102
4. Huant AL, Ostrowski MC, Berard D, Hager GL (1981): Cell 27:245
5. Law MF, Lowy DR, Dvoretzky I, Howley Pm (1981): Proc Natl Acad Sci USA 78:2727
6. Lee F, Mulligan R, Berg P, Ringold G (1981): Nature 294:228
7. Levinson B, Khoury G, Vande Woude G, Gruss P (1982): Nature 295:568
8. Lowy Dr, Dvoretzky I, Shober R, Law MF, Engel L, Howley PM (1980): Nature 287:70
9. McKnight SL, Gavis ER, Kingsbury R, Axel R (1981): Cell 25:385
10. Moreau P, Hen R, Wasylyk B, Everett R, Gaub MP, Chambon P (1981): Nucleic Acid Res 9:6047
11. Ringold GM, Yamamoto KR, Bishop JM, Varmus HE (1977): Proc Natl Acad Sci USA 74:2879
12. Su RT, DePamphilis ML (1978): J Virol 28:53
13. Tyndall C, LaMantra G, Thacker CM, Favaloro J, Kamen R (1981): Nucleic Acid Res 9:6231
14. Varmus HE, Ringold GM, Yamamoto KR (1979): Monogr Endocrinol 12:253
15. Wasylyk B, Derbyshire R, Guy A, Molko D, Roget A, Teoule R, Chambon P (1980): Proc Natl Acad Sci USA 77:7024
16. Wilhelm J, Brison O, Kedinger C, Chambon P (1976): J Virol 19:61
17. Young HA, Shih T, Scolnick E, Parks W (1977): J Virol 21:139

Gene Transfer and Cancer, edited by M. L. Pearson and N. L. Sternberg. Raven Press, New York © 1984.

Are Glucocorticoid Receptor Binding Domains Regulatable "Enhancer" Elements?

Vicki L. Chandler, Bonnie A. Maler, and Keith R. Yamamoto

Department of Biochemistry and Biophysics, University of California, San Francisco, San Francisco, California 94143

ABSTRACT. The rate of transcription of integrated mammary tumor virus (MTV) genes in cultured cells is selectively stimulated by glucocorticoid receptor protein complexed with an appropriate hormone ligand; consistent with this selectivity in vivo, purified hormone receptor complexes specifically recognize discrete regions within MTV proviral DNA in vitro. To determine whether a receptor binding fragment of MTV DNA can confer hormone responsiveness upon a promoter that is not normally regulated, we fused such fragments to the herpes simplex virus (HSV) thymidine kinase (tk) promoter and structural gene. In one construction, paPS1, a receptor binding fragment that maps 106 bp upstream from the MTV transcription initiation site was fused to the intact tk promoter 120 bp from the tk initiation site. It was found that dexamethasone, a synthetic glucocorticoid, increases the efficiency of recovering TK^+ transformants in rat $XCtk^-$ cells transfected with paPS1, whereas transformation with the tk plasmid alone was not stimulated by the hormone. Direct assays confirm that hormone treatment increases tk mRNA levels and enzymatic activity in cell populations and clones that have incorporated paPS1 DNA. The increased tk mRNA production appears to originate exclusively from the normal tk initiation sites. These results demonstrate that MTV receptor binding fragments have certain properties in common with recently described enhancer elements; by this view, the enhancement phenomenon in this case depends upon an identified diffusable regulator, the glucocorticoid receptor protein.

INTRODUCTION

In vitro mutation and recombination of defined DNA fragments, together with methods for introducing these molecules into intact cells, provide a powerful approach to the identification and functional analysis of genetic elements that specify and regulate transcription in eucaryotic cells. Such studies have revealed a novel class of DNA sequences, termed "enhancers", that reside upstream of the transcription start sites of some but not all genes. Enhancer elements are required for full activity of their corresponding promoters, and also act in cis to activate or enhance transcription from unrelated promoters when recombined in vitro and introduced into cells (1). The most striking characteristic of enhancers is their capacity to act in either orientation over large distances, even when placed distal to the affected gene (1,11,20).

The prevailing view is that enhancers increase transcriptional efficiency, but present experiments do not distinguish between the many molecular events, direct and indirect, that could potentially bring about
this effect. It should be emphasized that enhancer elements have been
recognized and defined solely on the basis of their ability to yield
increased expression of DNA that has been experimentally introduced into
cultured cells. That is, the activity of these elements in transfection
assays may relate indirectly or not at all to their normal function.
For example, it is conceivable that enhancers actually are involved in
mediating selectivity and regulation of transcription, rather than simply
elevating promoter activity in a nonspecific way. The isolation of polyoma virus host range mutants whose defects map within enhancer regions
(4,7) could be interpreted according to this view. Moreover, the nucleotide sequences of enhancers from different genes do not display obvious
homologies, consistent with the speculation that they may normally respond
to distinct signals.

Cloned MTV DNA apparently lacks a "simple" enhancer element of the type
described (8). However, transcription of the proviral sequences in mammary tumor cells and in heterologous infected cells in culture is under
strong regulation by glucocorticoid hormones, such as dexamethasone
(reviewed in ref. 14). Molecular analyses of the MTV transcripts suggest
that glucocorticoids stimulate the rate of viral RNA synthesis by increasing the efficiency of MTV promoter utilization (18).

Biochemical (15) and genetic (5) data have established that the intracellular glucocorticoid receptor protein mediates the transcriptional
stimulation. In vitro experiments with highly purified components reveal
that the receptor selectively recognizes several distinct regions on MTV
DNA (12,13); moreover, cultured cells stably transfected with cloned receptor binding fragments display hormone-responsive expression of the
associated plasmid vector sequences (12). One interpretation of these
results is that DNA fragments containing receptor binding sites identified
in vitro can act as complex, i.e., glucocorticoid-regulable enhancer elements upon introduction into intact cells. To examine this possibility,
and to investigate the mechanisms by which the hormone receptor:DNA complex might modulate promoter utilization, we fused fragments of MTV DNA
bearing receptor binding sites to a well-characterized promoter that is
not normally under hormonal control and assessed transcription from these
recombinants in stable transformants. Our initial results are briefly
summarized here.

RESULTS

Transfection of glucocorticoid receptor-containing cells with cloned
MTV DNA fragments that include both the MTV promoter region (18,19) and
a receptor binding domain (12) yields stable transformants in which
transcription from the introduced sequences is hormonally regulated (13,
22). When such fragments are fused to the coding sequence for dihydrofolate reductase (8) or to a retroviral oncogene (6), transformants are
recovered in which the selectable characteristic is conditionally expressed. Unexpectedly, certain transformants containing receptor binding
domains but lacking the MTV promoter also display dexamethasone-respon-
sive expression (12), suggesting either that these viral DNA fragments
contain hormone-responsive promoters that are cryptic in the intact
provirus, or that they enhance transcription from nearby cellular or
vector promoters. In the latter case, enhancement would occur only in

the presence of the hormone, presumably reflecting association of the receptor:hormone complex with the binding domain.

A prediction of the notion that receptor binding domains might be regulable enhancers is that they should act in cis to confer hormonal regulation on promoters other than the one specified by MTV. Accordingly, receptor binding fragments of MTV DNA were inserted into plasmids carrying either the intact HSV tk promoter and structural gene, or into derivatives with defined deletions that reduce or eliminate the promoter function while leaving the coding sequence intact (9).

McKnight and coworkers (10) have identified three distinct regions within the 105 bp upstream of the tk transcription initiation site that are required for full expression from that promoter. S. McKnight (9) generously provided a series of tk plasmids in which deletions 5' to the tk coding sequence had been generated in vitro, ligated to synthetic BamHI restriction site linkers and mapped by DNA sequencing. We constructed a corresponding series of BamHI-linked MTV DNA fragments, thereby facilitating construction of fusion plasmids.

Figure 1 diagrams the configuration of paPS1, an example of one such recombinant. In this case, the 1079-bp PstI-SacI fragment of MTV DNA, which maps within the MTV LTR upstream of the MTV transcription initiation site, was isolated and linked to BamHI, then inserted into a pBR322-tk plasmid (see Figure legend) that we have denoted patK. As shown in Figure 1, patK contains a BamHI linker attached 109 bp upstream of the tk trancription initiation site (9); the tk promoter is fully functional in this derivative (9). The open bars on the diagram (Figure 1) denote two contiguous restriction subfragments that contain specific binding sites for highly purified glucocorticoid receptor protein as asessed by nitrocellulose filter binding (12,23); electron microscopic measurements suggest that the receptor recognizes three discrete sites within the binding domain (23; see Figure 1). In the final construction, the MTV insert in paPS1 is situated 120 bp upstream of the tk transcription initiation site, whereas it normally resides 106 bp from the MTV transcription initiation site.

Fusion plasmids were introduced into tk⁻ cultured cell lines by standard calcium phosphate precipitation methods (21). In a few early experiments, mouse Ltk⁻ cells (21) were employed, but XCtk⁻, a rat line obtained from G. Hager, subsequently served as the recipient. The transfection efficiency of XCtk⁻ is low relative to Ltk⁻; however, the rat genome is free of endogenous MTV proviral sequences, thus facilitating detection of transformants and interpretation of the results. Furthermore, we found that dexamethasone severely inhibits growth of Ltk⁻ cells, and that the recovery of tk⁺ transformants in hormone-containing HAT medium is drastically reduced compared to selection in HAT medium alone. This unexplained phenomenon also occurs in XCtk⁻ (see below), but is much less prominent.

In principle, an effect of dexamethasone on tk promoter activity in paPS1 might result in more efficient transfection of XCtk⁻ to the TK⁺ phenotype. Whether this would be detected in practice likely depends upon factors such as the sensitivity of the selection to TK enzyme concentration, the threshold of "TK toxicity" that may occur at high levels of expression, and the magnitude of growth inhibition by the combined presence of HAT and dexamethasone (see above).

The results summarized in Table 1 suggest that dexamethasone increases the transfection efficiency of paPS1 DNA. In these experiments, XCtk⁻ cells were transfected with either paPS1 or patK plasmid DNA, and phenotypic TK⁺ transformants were selected in HAT medium in the presence or absence of dexamethasone. It can be seen that patk and paPS1 yield transformants with equal efficiency in the absence of dexamethasone, and that 1-μM

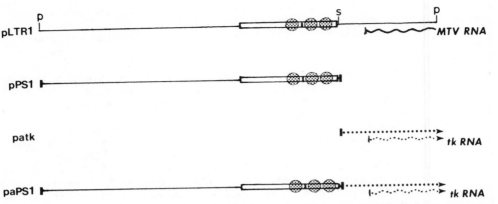

FIGURE 1. Fusion of a receptor binding fragment of MTV DNA to the promoter region and coding sequence of the HSV tk gene. The diagrams depict only the recombinant inserts, or relevant portions thereof, in the plasmids designated at left; all are cloned into pBR322 (pLTR1 at the PstI site and the others at the BamHI site). pLTR1 contains a 1453-bp PstI-PstI restriction fragment of MTV DNA that includes the lefthand MTV LTR; the transcription initiation site resides 1182 bp from the lefthand PstI (P) site (18). Three recognition sites for purified glucocorticoid-receptor complexes (⊙) have been detected within two contiguous restriction sub-fragments (open bars) proximal to a SacI (S) site 101 bp upstream of the initiation site (13,23). To construct the fusion, the 1079 bp Pst1-SacI fragment of pLTR11 was isolated, the tetranucleotide overhanging ends removed using the 3'-5' exonuclease activity of T4 DNA polymerase, and the flush termini ligated to 10 bp synthetic BamHI restriction site link-ers (▮) using T4 DNA ligase; insertion into the BamHI site of pBR322 yielded plasmid pPS1. This linked fragment was also inserted into the BamHI site of patK, a pBR322 derivative containing the intact HSV tk gene and 109 bp of HSV DNA upstream of the start site of transcription; a synthetic BamHI linker was ligated at this terminus by McKnight et al. (9). Plasmid paPS1 contains the pPS1 insert in the same orientation, but 14 bp further upstream of the tk initiation site than it normally resides from the MTV initiation site.

TABLE 1. Transfection of XCtk⁻ cells

Plasmid DNA	TK⁺ colonies per 10^6 cells cultured	
	without dexamethasone	with dexamethasone
None	0	0
0.5 μg patK	6	1
1.0 μg patK	19	5
0.5 μg paPS1	7	30
1.0 μg paPS1	21	34

Transfections were carried out according to the calcium phosphate precipi-tation protocol of Wigler et al. (21) using 20 μg of salmon sperm car-rier DNA per 10^6 cells. Two 100-mm dishes containing a total of 2 x 10^6 rat XCtk⁻ were employed for each condition; 24 hr after addition of DNA, transfected cultures were shifted to HAT selective medium either with or without 1 μM dexamethasone. Colonies were counted 9 days later.

dexamethasone appears to inhibit the appearance of patK transformants by about 4- to 6-fold. In contrast, transfection by paPS1 is 2- to 4-fold more efficient in the presence of dexamethasone, yielding 7- to 30-fold more TK$^+$ colonies than are detected after transfection with patK under the same conditions.

It seemed likely that the hormone effect on the transfection efficiency of paPS1 reflects a stimulation of tk mRNA and enzyme production and activity. These parameters were therefore monitored in transfected cell populations that had been selected in the absence of dexamethasone for HAT resistance, and subsequently tested with or without hormone; clones isolated from these populations were similarly assayed. TK enzyme assays revealed that the TK specific activity in the patK transformants is unaffected by treatment of the cultures with 1- M dexamethasone for 24 hr, whereas the enzyme activity in the paPS1 transformants increases 3- to 20-fold with hormone treatment (2,23). Likewise, blot hybridization of RNA fractionated in formaldehyde agarose gels demonstrated that the dexamethasone-treated paPS1 populations and clones accumulate 5- to 50-fold more 1.3-kb tk mRNA than either their untreated counterparts, or the patK control transformants (2,23).

The finding that the hormone-induced tk mRNA found in paPS1 transformants is indistinguishable in size from that produced by the control wild-type gene implies that fusion with a receptor binding fragment confers a receptor-mediated increase in the activity of the bona fide tk promoter, rather than simply the adjoining of an additional promoter region or the adventitous creation of a promoter in the course of the fusion. The results of two additional experiments are consistent with this idea. First, MTV-specific RNA is not detected in the paPS1 transformants by blot hybridization. Second, S1 nuclease transcript mapping experiments, in which RNA from the tranformants was hybridized to a 1.5-kb DNA fragment spanning the MTV-tk fusion junction and end labeled at a site 54 to 56 bp downstream from the normal tk initiation region, demonstrated that only probe fragments of 54 to 56 nucleotides were protected from S1 digestion. As expected, 3- to 30-fold more probe was protected by RNA from the hormone-treated paPS1 transformants (2).

DISCUSSION

Whether the properties of receptor binding domains correspond fully to all of the characteristics of enhancer elements remains to be determined. Indeed, the results summarized here do not establish rigorously that the receptor binding domain must be in a cis configuration with respect to the regulated gene, but these and other data are consistent with that configuration. In the particular fusion described, MTV sequences bearing a receptor binding domain were situated in the same orientation, but 14 bp further from the tk initiation site than they normally are from the MTV initiation site. Activity of the regulatory region in this altered spatial arrangement is in apparent contrast with the relatively stringent maintenance of spacing between sequence components of functional procaryotic promoters (reviewed in ref. 16). Experiments are underway to define in detail the extent to which the activity of receptor binding domains is affected by orientation and distance from promoters.

In any case, our experiments suggest that a receptor binding domain defined in vitro may be recognized by the hormone-receptor complex in vivo, thereby enhancing tk expression by stimulating the activity of the tk promoter. Thus, as with enhancer elements, this receptor binding fragment is able to affect the activity not only of the promoter next to which

it normally resides, but also of a heterologous promoter. If receptor
binding domains are indeed enhancers, the dependence of their activity
upon the glucocorticoid receptor protein allows the enhancement phenomenon to be investigated unambiguously at the level of transcription,
since prior events such as the entry, stability, potential compartmental-
ization, and integration of DNA could be carried out in the absence of
enhancer action. Moreover, identification and purification of a specific
diffusible factor that regulates the activity of a particular enhancer
would likely contribute toward understanding its biological role and
molecular mechanism.

It is clear from a number of observations that the receptor binding
domain does not itself have promoter activity. The overall size of the
tk transcript is not altered in the paPS1 fusion, hormonal stimulation
results in increased initiation from the normal tk initiation site, and
no new start sites are observed within either the MTV or the tk sequences.
Moreover, when the same MTV fragment is fused to defined tk deletion
mutants in which tk promoter function is diminished or abolished, the
very low yield of TK^+ transformants is not increased by dexamethasone
(2). Thus, we conclude that hormone-responsive enhancement involves two
distinguishable components, a receptor binding domain and an intact
promoter.

This result has interesting general implications for the evolution of
hormone-responsive promoters and regulatory circuits. It has been proposed
that certain conserved signaling molecules such as hormones have acquired
in the course of evolution the capacity to regulate increasingly complex
networks of interacting pathways; in a sense, hormones act as molecular
symbols of the physiological status of these networks (17). We suggest
that a genetic unit of expression might efficiently become regulated by
glucocorticoids as a result of a single transposition event that juxtaposes
a glucocorticoid receptor binding domain nearby. An alternative mode,
in which random simple mutations in a transcriptional regulatory region
eventually yield a promoter that is recognized as well as regulated by
the glucocorticoid receptor, seems relatively unwieldly by comparison.

It is interesting to note that the enhancement phenomenon has not been
observed in vitro. One interpretation of this negative result is that
enhancement operates on particular chromatin and/or DNA configurations.
The expression and regulation of MTV genes has been shown to be subject
to strong chromosomal position effects that apparently reflect differences in proviral chromatin structure at different genomic sites (3);
moreover, hormonal stimulation of transcription may itself involve directed changes in chromatin or template structure. It therefore seems
conceivable that the relationships of genomic structure and expression,
and the rules that govern promoter function might be related to, and
perhaps even revealed by, the mechanism of action of enhancer elements
and glucocorticoid receptor proteins.

ACKNOWLEDGEMENTS

We are greatly indebted to Steve McKnight for generously providing an
extensive series of fully characterized deletion plasmids bearing the HSV
tk gene. In addition, we thank Gordon Hager for XCtk⁻ cells, and colleagues in our laboratory for suggestions on the manuscript, and for con-
structive skepticism. This work was supported by grants from the National
Cancer Institute and the American Cancer Society. KRY is a recipient of
a Camille and Henry Dreyfus Teacher-Scholar Award and held an NIH Research
Career Development Award.

REFERENCES

1. Banerji J, Rusconi S, Schaffner W (1981): Cell 27:299
2. Chandler VL, Maler BA, Yamamoto KR (1983): Cell 33:489
3. Feinstein SC, Ross SR, Yamamoto KR (1982): J Mol Biol 156:549
4. Fujimura FK, Deininger PL, Friedmann T, Linney E (1981): Cell 23: 809
5. Grove JR, Dieckmann BS, Schroer TA, Ringold GM (1980): Cell 21:47
6. Huang AL, Ostrowski MC, Berard D, Hager GL (1981): Cell 27:245
7. Katinka M, Vasseur M, Montreau N, Yaniv M, Blangy D (1981): Nature 290: 720
8. Lee F, Mulligan R, Berg P, Ringold G (1981): Nature 294:228
9. McKnight SL, Gavis ER, Kingsbury R, Axel R (1981): Cell 25:385
10. McKnight SL, Kingsbury R (1982): Science 217:316
11. Olson L, de Villiers J, Banerji J, Schaffner W (1983): Cold Spring Harbor Symp Quant Biol 47: in press
12. Payvar F, Firestone GL, Ross SR, Chandler VL, Wrange O, Carlstedt-Duke J, Gustafsson JA, Yamamoto KR (1982): J Cell Biochem 19:241
13. Payvar F, Wrange O, Carlstedt-Duke J, Okret S, Gustafsson JA, Yamamoto KR (1981): Proc Natl Acad Sci USA 78:6628
14. Ringold GM (1979): Biochim Biophys Acta 560:487
15. Ringold GM, Yamamoto KR, Tomkins GM, Bishop JM, Varmus HE (1975): Cell 6:721
16. Siebenlist U, Simpson RB, Gilbert W (1980): Cell 20:269
17. Tomkins GM (1975): Science 189:760
18. Ucker DS, Firestone GL, Yamamoto KR: (1983) Molec Cell Biol 3:551
19. Ucker DS, Ross SR, Yamamoto KR (1981): Cell 27:257
20. Wasylyk B, Chambon P (1983): Cold Spring Harbor Symp Quant Biol 47: 921
21. Wigler M, Pellicer A, Silverstein S, Axel R, Urlaub G, Chasin L (1979): Proc Natl Acad Sci USA 76:1373
22. Yamamoto KR, Chandler VL, Ross SR, Ucker DS, Ring JC, Feinstein SC (1981): Cold Spring Harbor Symp Quant Biol 45:687
23. Yamamoto KR, Payvar F, Firestone GL, Maler BA, Wrange O, Carlstedt-Duke J, Gustafsson J-A, Chandler VL (1983): Cold Spring Harbor Symp Quant Biol 47:977

Gene Transfer and Cancer, edited by M. L. Pearson and N. L. Sternberg. Raven Press, New York © 1984.

Study of DNA Modification and X Inactivation in the Mouse Using DNA-Mediated Gene Transfer

*R. Michael Liskay, **Verne M. Chapman, **Paul G. Kratzer, and Linda D. Siracusa

*Departments of Therapeutic Radiology and Human Genetics, Yale School of Medicine, New Haven, Connecticut 06510; and **Department of Molecular Biology, Roswell Park Memorial Institute, Buffalo, New York 14263*

ABSTRACT. Early in the development of mammalian females one X chromosome becomes functionally inactive. The initial event is, in general, a random event because in any particular cell either the maternal or paternal X can become inactivated. Once established, however, the pattern is stable through many somatic cell divisions. We have investigated the role of DNA modification in the X chromosome inactivation process utilizing a) DNA transfer of the X chromosome-linked hprt gene, and b) an electrophoretic variant of hprt in the mouse. We have produced female mice heterozygous for both this hprt variant and a reciprocal translocation between the X chromosome and chromosome 16 (TX:16 females). Unlike normal X/X females, TX:16 females are not mosaic for X chromosome-linked expression and express only genes on the translocated X chromosome material. DNA from the brain, liver, and kidney of TX:16 females genetically heterozygous for hprt but expressing only the B form of hprt was used to generate 59 independent hprt transformant cell lines. All but one of these lines expressed the hprtB, indicating that the inactive X hprtA allele is not efficient in hprt gene transfer. Control experiments indicate that when the hprtA allele resides on the active X chromosome it is functional in gene transfer. These results are consistent with the hypothesis that DNA modification plays a role in X chromosome inactivation in adult somatic tissues. We have also examined the gene transfer efficiency of inactive X chromosome from a derivative of trophectoderm, yolk sac endoderm, which undergoes preferential paternal inactivation. Yolk sac endoderm tissue of a heterozygous female fetus expresses only the maternally inherited form of hprt. DNA from yolk sac endoderm was used in hprt gene transfer and surprisingly both paternal allele- and maternal allele-expressing transformants were well represented showing that the inactive X hprt allele from yolk sac endoderm is functional. These findings suggest a difference between inactive X DNA of randomly vs nonrandomly inactivated tissues.

INTRODUCTION

Early in the development of eutherian mammalian females, embryos one X chromosome in each cell becomes genetically inactive. The initial inactivation event is usually random resulting in either a paternal inactive X(X_i) or a maternal X_i in any given embryonic cell. Once the pattern of inactivation is established it is stable and becomes part of each embryonic cell's somatic heredity. Therefore, adult females are mosaic for X chromosome expression in their somatic tissue (for review see 4). Until recently our knowledge of the mechanism(s) responsible for the maintenance of the inactive state was nonexistent. However, recent experiments by ourselves (5) and others (6,8) provide evidence that is consistent with DNA modification (e.g., methylation) playing a crucial role in X chromosome inactivation.

We have analyzed the role of DNA modification in X chromosome inactivation using the technique of DNA-mediated cell transformation (or gene transfer). Our basic rationale assumed that if DNA modification is responsible, wholly or in part, for the inactivity, we might expect that DNA of the X_i to be inefficient in gene transfer of the X chromosome-linked hprt gene. A recently detected electrophoretic variant of hprt in the mouse [from Mus castaneus (1)], and an X chromosome:autosome translocation resulting in nonrandom expression of the X chromosomes have enabled us to determine the relative efficiencies of X_a- and X_i-purified DNAs from adult tissues to elicit transformation for hprt. In brief, our findings indicate that X_i DNA of adult tissues is impressively inefficient in hprt gene transfer.

RESULTS AND DISCUSSION

To exploit the electrophoretic variation for hprt in gene transfer, we needed to obtain tissue material in which all inactive X chromosomes carried the same hprt allele. We crossed males carrying the hprt variant A form with females homozygous for the hprtB allele and heterozygous for a reciprocal X chromosome:autosome translocation between the X chromosome and chromosome 16 (so-called TX:16 females). Such TX:16 females are not mosaic for X chromosome expression and, in fact, express only genes on the translocated X chromosome (1,3,7). There are two types of female progeny, a) chromosomally normal X/X females mosaic for hprt expression (hprtAB), and b) TX:16 females that express only hprtB, or the allele on the translocated X chromosome. Therefore, the X_i chromosomes of such TX:16 females all carry the hprtA allele. If DNA from such TX:16 females is used in hprt gene transfer, the ability of X_i DNA to function will be signaled by the frequency of hprtA-expressing transformants. To serve as a control, DNA from X/X females that are hprtAB was used in parallel experiments. Because these females are mosaic for hprt expression both hprtA and hprtB transformants should be seen with approximately equal frequencies, assuming that when these alleles reside on an X_a chromosome they are both active in gene transfer.

DNA was extracted from the brain, liver, or kidney of adult TX:16 and X/X females heterozygous for hprtAB and was used to transform a Chinese hamster hprt⁻ recipient as previously described (5). Independent transformants were grown and tested for the hprt form being expressed (1,2). Results indicate that of 59 transformants produced from TX:16 DNA only one was hprtA (i.e. or from X_i DNA). In the control experiments DNA from X/X females produced a significantly higher fraction of hprtA transformants (9 of 31) implying that when the hprtA allele is from the

X_a it is efficient in gene transfer. Importantly, it should be mentioned that one of the TX:16 females that was used as a DNA source was able to transmit her hprtA allele to offspring, thus showing that the X_i hprtA allele in our DNA preparations was intact. We conclude from these experiments that the X_i allele of hprt as naked DNA from adult mouse tissues is inefficient in gene transfer. This finding is consistent with the hypothesis that DNA modification plays a crucial role in the maintenance of X chromosome inactivation. We do know at what stage gene transfer with X_i DNA is blocked. One could argue that X_i DNA cannot be extracted efficiently and is lost during purification. We consider this a highly unlikely possibility.

Recently, we have begun to inquire into the state of the X_i from an unusual tissue, yolk sac endoderm. This tissue is derived from the primitive endoderm and is part of the extraembryonic yolk sac membranes. Importantly yolk sac endoderm shows preferential paternal inactivation (9), therefore resulting in expression in that tissue of only the hprt type inherited from the mother.

Using the hprtAB system, we have preliminary results suggesting that X_i DNA of the yolk-sac endoderm of 14-day-old fetuses is functional in gene transfer. This suggests that in terms of DNA modification, X_i DNA of mouse adult tissues (or cell lines) is different from X_i DNA of yolk sac endoderm taken from 14-day-old mouse fetuses. Such a contrasting finding could reflect a difference in the mechanisms involved in random versus nonrandom inactivation, or alternatively could be due to a difference between "young" X_i DNA vs. adult X_i DNA. Regarding the latter possibility, DNA modification might occur in the initial stages but not affect gene transfer. Subsequently, the nature of this modification might change during development (e.g., increase) so that the level of modification affects the ability of the DNA to function in our gene transfer system. Distinguishing between these two possibilities should be possible by examining early (12 to 14 day-old) fetal proper DNA of TX:16 females heterozygous for hprt. Finally, the results presented here speak only to the issue of DNA modification in the maintenance of X inactivation. The nature of the initial event of inactivation need not necessarily involve DNA modification.

REFERENCES

1. Chapman VM, Kratzer PG, Siracusa LD, Quarantillo BA, Evans R, Liskay RM: (in press) Proc Natl Acad Sci USA
2. Chasin LA, Urlaub G (1976): Somatic Cell Genet 2:453
3. Disteche CM, Eicher EM, Latt SA (1981): Exp Cell Res 133:357
4. Gartler SM, Andina RJ (1976): Adv Hum Genet 7:99
5. Liskay RM, Evans RJ (1980): Proc Natl Acad Sci USA 77:4895
6. Mohandas T, Sparkes RS, Shapiro LJ (1981): Science 211:393
7. Takagi N (1980): Chromosoma 81:439
8. Venolia L, Gartler SM, Wassmann EM, Yen P, Mohandes T, Shapiro LJ (1982): Proc Natl Acad Sci USA 79:2352
9. West JD, Frels WI, Chapman VM, Papaioannou VE (1977): Cell 12:873

Gene Transfer and Cancer, edited by M. L. Pearson
and N. L. Sternberg. Raven Press, New York © 1984.

Alternative View of Mammalian Repetitive DNA Sequence Organization

*,†Robert K. Moyzis, *Jacques Bonnet, †Brian D. Crawford,
*Maria Dani, †Paul J. Jackson, *Jung-Rung Wu,
and *Paul O. P. Ts'o

*Division of Biophysics, School of Hygiene and Public Health, The John Hopkins
University, Baltimore, Maryland 21205; and †Genetics Group, Los Alamos Scientific
Laboratory, Los Alamos, New Mexico 87545*

ABSTRACT.   Recently our laboratory presented biochemical and biophysical studies of the arrangement of repetitive DNA sequences in the Syrian hamster genome (42,43).   These experiments suggested that a) traditional methods of measuring repetitive DNA sequence spacing potentially overestimate the amount of spacing distances shorter than 1 kb (kilobase), b) hyperchromicity experiments potentially underestimate the weight average length of repetitive DNA regions, and c) short 0.3-kb S1 nuclease-resistant repetitive DNA duplexes can be produced from the reassociation of either repetitive sequences surrounded by nonrepetitive regions or larger repetitive DNA regions.   An alternative model of mammalian repetitive DNA sequence organization was proposed in which repetitive sequences are either frequently spaced at distances of 7 ± 2 kb or randomly spaced on a number average basis.   The model further proposed that short 0.3-kb repetitive DNA sequences are often found in larger repetitive sequence clusters.   These studies have now been extended to include the rat and human genomes, and similar results have been obtained.   We have constructed libraries of rat, Syrian hamster and human genomic DNA in bacteriophage λ Charon 4A, as well as libraries of human S1 nuclease-resistant reassociated repetitive DNA in plasmid pBR322 and bacteriophage M13mp7. Studies utilizing these libraries have confirmed our previous findings and have, in addition, indicated that the repetitive sequences present in long (> 2 kb) S1 nuclease-resistant structures are widely interspersed in the genome (at least once every 15-20 kb).   This suggests that interspersed repetitive sequences are often longer than 0.3 kb, or that some members of 0.3-kb interspersed repetitive sequences are also found in longer repetitive sequence clusters.   Repetitive sequences highly conserved in Syrian hamster and human DNA (approximately 10% of the total) are included in this interspersed long S1 nuclease-resistant class.

INTRODUCTION

The genomes of most eucaryotic organisms contain DNA sequences present in multiple copies (9).   This repetitive DNA is operationally defined by its ability to reassociate more rapidly than expected for sequences present only once per haploid genome. Although suggestions have been made that repetitive DNA may be involved in the regulation of gene expression, DNA replication, chromosome folding, or DNA transposition (Figure 1), the functional significance of over 99% of the repetitive DNA found in mammalian genomes has remained speculative (7,15,22,44).

A prerequisite to an understanding of the functional importance of repetitive DNA is an accurte description of its organization in the genome. Beginning with the pioneering experiments of Davidson et al. (17) on the Xenopus genome, and Graham et al. (25) on the sea urchin genome, many reports of the pattern of interspersion of repetitive and nonrepetitive DNA sequences have appeared. In general, it has been reported that two contrasting patterns of repetitive DNA sequence interspersion are present in eucaryotic genomes (33). In most organisms examined, an interspersion of short 0.3-kb repetitive DNA sequence alternating with nonrepetitive sequences approximately 1 to 2 kb long has been reported (1,16,24,45,48). This pattern has been referred to as a short-period interspersion or the Xenopus pattern.

In contrast, the genome of Drosophila melanogaster was reported to consist of an interspersion of repetitive and nonrepetitive DNA sequences at least an order of magnitude longer than that found in the short period interspersion pattern (35). Although it initially appeared that this Drosophila or long-period interspersion pattern was exceptional, the list of eucaryotic organisms reported to lack short-period interspersion has continued to grow (3,4,13,14,21,23,28,47).

The relationship, if any, between these two contrasting patterns of DNA sequence organization has remained obscure. Considerable variability has been reported in the measured length of repetitive sequence spacing found in the short-period interspersion pattern (i.e., 0.6 to 2.7 kb; for a recent summary, see ref. 33). In most organisms thought to exhibit a short-period interspersion pattern, nonrepetitive DNA regions longer than 1 to 2 kb are also present. It is important to distinguish the extent to which this reported variability may be attributed to actual differences in repetitive DNA sequence interspersion or to the use of different experimental methods. Recently, we presented a critical reevaluation of the biochemical and biophysical techniques commonly used to determine the organization and length of repetitive and nonrepetitive DNA sequences (42,43). A few key experiments are presented that have led to the proposal of an alternative model of mammalian DNA sequence organization.

RESULTS

A precise evaluation of the pattern of repetitive sequence interspersion in Syrian hamster, rat, and human DNA has been conducted, with the use of the technique pioneered by Davidson et al. (17) as modified by Moyzis et al. (42). In this procedure, trace amounts of radiolabeled DNA of various fragment lengths are incubated with a short driver DNA to a C_0t value (C_0t = product of initial nucleotide concentration in mol/ℓ and time in sec) at which, ideally, only repetitive sequences will have hybridized. If repetitive sequences are interspersed in the genome, the amount of radiolabeled DNA tracer bound to hydroxyapatite should increase with increased tracer fragment length, because of the covalent linkage of repetitive and nonrepetitive sequences. It is possible to construct an expected interspersion curve, given particular assumptions regarding the sequence organization of repetitive and nonrepetitive DNA. For example, Figure 2 presents five hypothetical models of repetitive sequence

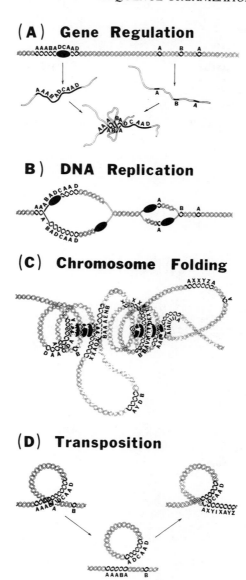

(A) Gene Regulation

B) DNA Replication

(C) Chromosome Folding

(D) Transposition

FIGURE 1. Models of repetitive DNA sequence function. Proposed repetitive DNA sequence functions are diagrammed. Repetitive DNA regions are represented by dark portions of the double helix, nonrepetitive regions are represented by light portions. Different repetitive regions have been assigned arbitrary letters (A, B...Z). The relative average length of repetitive and nonrepetitive regions are drawn approximately to scale; the size of the helix has been greatly exaggerated. Single-strand RNA transcripts of repetitive and nonrepetitive sequences are shown in A and putative DNA binding proteins are represented in A, B, and C by dark oblongs.
    Selected references: A) Gene Regulation: 7, 15, 18, 19, 32, 46, 52. B) DNA replication: 20, 26, 29, 36, 49. C) Chromosome Folding: 11, 31, 37, 53, 56. D) Transposition: 8, 10, 12, 22, 44, 49.

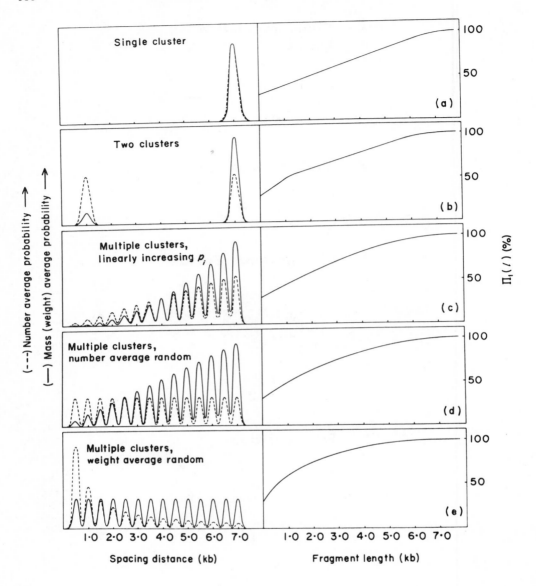

FIGURE 2. Models of repetitive DNA sequence spacing. Various models of repetitive DNA sequence spacing (left) and their computed interspersion curves (right) are depicted. All curves have been computed using the equation:

$$\Pi_1(\ell) = \sum_{s=0}^{\ell - 2h_o} \frac{m_1 + s}{m_1 + ES} f(s) + \sum_{s=1-2h_o+1}^{x} \frac{m_1 - 2h_o + 1 + i}{m_1 + ES} f(s)$$

where $\Pi_1(\ell)$ is the probability of binding to hydroxyapatite for a fragment of length ℓ; m_1 is the length of an ordinary repetitive DNA sequence; h_o is the number of adjacent duplex bases from a repeat necessary for hydroxyapatite binding (assumed to be 50 for all computed models); and s is the length of nonrepetitive DNA regions, assumed to be a discrete random variable with mass function f(s), expected value ES, and standard deviation SS.

Letting k be the number of values of s with positive probability and $p_i = f(s)$, then:

$$\sum_{i=1}^{k} p_i = 1 \quad \text{and} \quad \sum_{i=1}^{k} p_i \, s_i = ES$$

Both the number average probability (p_i; broken line) and the mass average probability (unbroken line) are indicated for each model distribution. The ordinate scale for each model has been drawn arbitrarily to aid visual comparison. All interspersion curves have been computed such that the proportion of repetitive sequences in each model is assumed to be:

$$\Pi_1(h_o) \approx \frac{m_1}{m_1 + ES} = 0.30$$

(Reprinted, with permission from Moyzis et al. (42).

⟵ ──────────────────────────────

spacing with their computed interspersion curves. One can compare various computed curves to experimentally observed data and, if the hypothesized model is not inconsistent with the experimental data, certain parameters can be estimated. Parameters of particular interest are the degree of randomness or order in repetitive sequence spacing, and estimates of the average distance(s) between repetitive regions (42) (Figure 2).

As shown in Figure 3a, when interspersion experiments with Syrian hamster DNA were performed using the protocol originated by Davidson et al. (17), a bend in the curve is apparent at approximately 1 kb. When an alternative protocol was used, however, no indication of a major 1-kb spacing distance was obtained (Figure 3b). This alternative protocol includes a) the use of purified repetitive sequence DNA rather than total DNA as drive, b) correction for the lack of complete binding of short DNA fragments to hydroxyapatite, and c) the redetermining of all tracer DNA fragment lengths after incubation (42).

Similar modified interspersion experiments conducted with rat and human DNA indicate that previous reports (45,48) had overestimated the amount of 1- to 2-kb spacing distances present in these organisms (40,41).

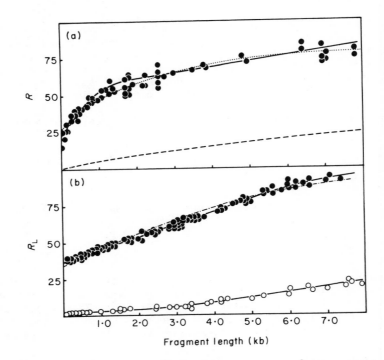

FIGURE 3. Interspersion of repetitive sequences. ^{3}H–Labeled hamster
cell DNA tracers of various average fragment lengths were hybridized to
a 500- to 15,000-fold excess of (a) 0.2 kb total hamster nuclear DNA or
(b) 0.2 kb purified repetitive DNA. The reaction was terminated at a
corrected $C_o t = 50$ and the percentage binding of radiolabeled tracer DNA
to hydroxyapatite was measured (●). Binding of tracer at $C_o t = 5 \times 10^{-6}$
is also plotted (O). Details of the experimental methods are in Moyzis
et al. (42). Reprinted, with permission from Moyzis et al. (42).

Curve fitting, using the equations proposed in Moyzis et al. (42) suggest
that repetitive sequences are either frequently spaced at 7 ± 2 kb or
randomly spaced (on a number average basis) in all three organisms (Figures 2 and 3).

    From these interspersion experiments, the average length of all re-
petitive regions in Syrian hamster DNA can be computed to be approximately
3 to 4 kb (42). This value has been confirmed by hyperchromicity studies
of hydroxyapatite-fractionated reassociated repetitive DNA (43). In
this technique, sheared DNAs of various average fragment lengths are
reassociated to a $C_o t$ value where only repetitive sequences will have
formed successful nucleations whereas nonrepetitive sequences will be
predominantly single stranded. After fractionation on hydroxyapatite to
remove the unreassociated nonrepetitive sequences, the repetitive DNA
duplexes are denatured, and the increase in absorption at 260 nm is
measured spectrophotometrically. Interspersion of repetitive and nonrepetitive regions in the genome will result in a decrease in hyperchromicity due to the presence of nonrepetitive DNA tails attached to
the repetitive DNA duplexes that bind to hydroxyapatite. This experimental approach yielded the first estimate that repetitive sequences
in Xenopus and sea urchin DNA were approximately 0.3 kb long (17,25).

During our investigations (43), we found that the extent of reassociation, as well as the nonrandom elution of hyperpolymers from hydroxyapatite, profoundly effect the observed hyperchromicity. When care is
taken during reassociation and fractionation, little decrease in the hyperchromicity of reassociated hamster repetitive DNA was observed over that
expected for any large, randomly sheared simple sequence DNA (such as
Escherichia coli) reassociated to the same extent.

Although the interspersion and hyperchromicity data indicate that the
average length of mammalian repetitive regions is significantly greater
than 0.3 kb, S1 nuclease digestion of reassociated mammalian DNA yields
substantial amounts of 0.3-kb nuclease-resistant duplexes (42,43). Assuming our interpretations of interspersion and hyperchromicity experiments
is correct, our computations indicate that the mass of 0.3-kb S1 nuclease-
resistant duplex obtained is, in fact, too large to have arisen only from
isolated repetitive regions alternating with nonrepetitive regions. This
suggests that many short repetitive DNA duplexes are formed during reassociation from larger repetitive regions present in the genome. One such
organization is diagrammed in Figure 4, in which short repetitive sequences are arranged in scrambled tandem arrays. After denaturtion and
reassociation, such repetitive sequence blocks would form both long
(> 2 kb) and short (0.3 kb) S1 nuclease-resistant duplex structure (43).

A number of tests of this hypothesis have been conducted. First,
reassociation analysis indicates that extensive sequence homology exists
between long and short nuclease-resistant DNA duplexes in Syrian hamster,
rat, and human reassociated repetitive DNA (41,43).

Second, isolated long S1 nuclease-resistant duplexes from hamster, rat,

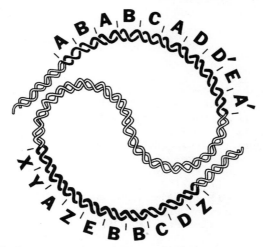

FIGURE 4. A model for repetitive DNA sequence organization. A diagram-
matic representation of a segment of DNA including two blocks of repetitive sequences organized into scrambled tandem clusters. Repetitive DNA
regions are represented by dark portions of the double helix whereas nonrepetitive DNA regions are represented by light portions. The repetitive
DNA sequence blocks are divided into distinct shorter repetitive DNA
regions, designated by letters (A, B...Z). Two inverted repetitive DNA
sequences are designated A' and D'. The average length of these individual
short repetitive DNA sequences (0.3 kb) is not drawn to scale, and would,
in fact, consist of approximately 30 turns of the helix.
(Reprinted with permission, from Moyzis et al. (43).

or recombination errors, or from the "scars" of aborted viral infections. The finding that repetitive sequences may be randomly distributed in mammalian DNA, inferred from interspersion experiments (Figures 2 and 3) (41, 42), is certainly consistent with this idea, as is, perhaps, the scrambled tandem cluster arrangement of short repetitive elements (Figure 4) (5). We have shown previously that repetitive sequences capable of forming well-matched duplexes upon reassociation are also interspersed in the hamster genome, but either at a greater distance, or in only a portion of the genome (42). Under hybridization conditions that allow only 10% of the repetitive sequences to cross hybridize in solution between human and hamster DNA, extensive cross hybridization to most genomic recombinant DNA plaques is observed (Dani & Moyzis, unpublished data). We have recently constructed libraries of human S1 nuclease-resistant repetitive DNA in plasmid pBR322 (6) and bacteriophage M13mp7 (38). Highly conserved repetitive sequences isolated from these libraries may include repetitive sequences whose nucleotide sequence is intimately related to their function.

Another possibility to explain repetitive sequence variability, however, is that the functional significance of many DNA sequences may be only mildly related to their linear nucleotide sequences. The observation that DNA may exist in various three-dimensional structures (2,54,55) suggests that the functional significance of many DNA regions may ultimately depend on these subtle conformational changes, rather than a unique and invarient base sequence. The resolution of these issues awaits further experimentation. Clearly, a crucial goal of future investigations will be the ability to define a functional DNA repetition from the viewpoint of the cell, rather than the investigator. Gene transfer techniques will undoubtedly prove invaluable in such investigations.

REFERENCES

1. Angerer RC, Davidson EH, Britten RJ (1975): Cell 6:29
2. Arnott S, Chandrasekaran R, Birdsall DL, Leslie AGW, Ratliff RL (1980): Nature (London) 293:743
3. Arthur RR, Strauss NA (1978): Canad J Biochem 56:257
4. Beauchamp RS, Pasternak J, Strauss NA (1979): Biochem 18:245
5. Benton WD, Davis RS (1977): Science 196:180
6. Bolivar F, Rodriguez RL, Greene PJ, Betlack MC, Heyneker JL, Boyer HW (1977): Gene 2:95
7. Britten RJ, Davidson EH (1969): Science 165:349
8. Britten RJ, Davidson EH (1971): Quart Rev Biol 46:111
9. Britten RJ, Kohne DE (1968): Science 161:529
10. Calabretta B, Robberson DL, Barrera-Saloana HA, Lambrou TP, Saunders GF (1982): Nature (London) 296:219
11. Chao MV, Gralla J, Martinson HG (1979): Biochem 18:1068
12. Calos MP, Miller JH (1980): Cell 20:579
13. Crain WR, Eden FC, Pearson WR, Davidson EH, Britten RJ (1976a): Chromasomo 56:309
14. Crain WR, Davidson EH, Britten RJ (1976b): Chromosomo 59:1
15. Davidson EH, Britten RJ (1979): Science 204:1052
16. Davidson EH, Galau GA, Angerer RC, Britten RJ (1975): Chromosomo 51:253
17. Davidson EH, Hough BR, Amenson CS, Britten RJ (1973): J Mol Biol 77:1
18. Davidson EH, Klein WH, Britten RJ (1977): Dev Biol 55:69
19. Davidson EH, Posakony JW (1982): Nature (London) 297:633

20. De Pamphilis ML, Wassarman PM (1980): Ann Rev Biochem 49:627
21. Dons JJM, Wessels JGH (1980): Biochim Biophys Acta 607:383
22. Doolittle WF, Sapienza C (1980): Nature (London) 284:601
23. Eden FC, Hendrick JP (1978): Biochem 17:5838
24. Goldberg RB, Crain WR, Ruderman JV, Moore GP, Barnett TR, Higgins RC, Gelfand RA, Galau GA, Britten RJ, Davidson EH (1975): Chromosoma 51:225
25. Graham DE, Neufeld BR, Davidson EH, Britten RJ (1974): Cell 1:127
26. Hand R (1978): Cell 15:317
27. Houck CM, Rinehard FP, Schmid CW (1979): J Mol Biol 132:289
28. Hudspeth MES, Timberlakes WE, Goldberg RB (1977): Proc Natl Acad Sci USA 74:4332
29. Jelinek WR, Toomey TP, Leinwand L, Duncan CH, Biro PA, Coudary PV, Weissman SM, Rubin CM, Houck CM, Deininger PL, Schmid CW (1980): Proc Natl Acad Sci USA 77:1398
30. Klein WH, Thomas TL, Lai G, Scheller RH, Britten RJ, Davidson EH (1978): Cell 14:889
31. Lawson Gm, Knoll BJ, March CJ, Woo SLC, Tsai M-J, O'Malley BW (1982): J Biol Chem 257:1501
32. Lerner MR, Boyle JA, Mount Sm, Wolin SL, Steitz J (1980): Nature (London) 283:220
33. Lewin B (1980): Gene Expression - 2. Eukaryotic Chromosomes, 2nd edition, John Wiley and Sons, New York
34. Maniatis T, Hardison RC, Lacy E, Lauer J, O'Connel C, Quon D, Sim GK, Efstratiadis A (1978): Cell 15:687
35. Manning JE, Schmid CW, Davidson N (1975): Cell 4:141
36. Mattern MR, Painter RB (1977): Biophys J 19:117
37. McGhee JD, Felsenfeld G (1980): Annu Rev Biochem 49:1115
38. Messing J, Crea R, Seeburg PH (1981): Nucl Acids Res 9:309
39. Moore GP, Scheller RJ, Davidson EH, Britten RJ (1978): Cell 15:649
40. Moyzis RK (1978): Ph.D. Dissertation, The Johns Hopkins University
41. Moyzis RK, Crawford BD, Dani M, Jackson PJ, Wu J-R, Ts'o POP (1984) in preparation
42. Moyzis RK, Bonnet J, Li DW, Ts'o POP (1981): J Mol Biol 153:841
43. Moyzis RK, Bonnet J, Li DW, Ts'o POP (1981): J Mol Biol 153:871
44. Orgel LE, Crick FHC (1980): Nature (London) 284:604
45. Pearson WR, Wu J-R, Bonner J (1978): Biochem 17:51
46. Robertson HD, Dickson E (1975): Brookhaven Symp Biol 26:240
47. Schachat F, O'Conner DJ, Epstein HF (1978): Biochim Biophys Acta 520:688
48. Schmid CW, Deininger Pl (1975): Cell 6:345
49. Schmid CW, Jelinek WR (1982): Science 216:1065
50. Smith GP (1976): Science 191:528
51. Tashima M, Calabretta B, Torelli G, Scofield M, Maizel A, Saunders GF (1981): Proc Natl Acad Sci USA 78:1508
52. Wallace B, Kass TL (1974): Genetics 77:541
53. Walker PMB (1971): Prog in Biophys Mol Biol 23:145
54. Wang AH-J, Quigley CJ, Kolpak FJ, Crawford JL, van Boom JH, van der Marel G, Rich A (1979): Nature (London) 282:680
55. Wang AH-J, Quigley GJ, Kolpak FJ, van der Marel G, van Boom JH, Rich A (1981): Science 211:171
56. Weintraub H (1980): Nucleic Acids Res 8:4745

Gene Transfer and Cancer, edited by M. L. Pearson
and N. L. Sternberg. Raven Press, New York © 1984.

Host Specificity of Enhancement of Gene Expression by Activator Elements

*Laimonis Laimins, *George Khoury, **Cornelia Gorman,
**Bruce Howard, and *Peter Gruss

*Laboratory of Molecular Virology and **Laboratory of Molecular Biology,
National Cancer Institute, Bethesda, Maryland 20205*

ABSTRACT. Although the 72-bp tandem repeat sequences of simian virus 40 (SV40) and the 72-bp repeat sequence of Moloney murine sarcoma virus (MoMSV) bear very little sequence homology, both activate gene expression. The degree of activation is host cell dependent. As an indicator of gene activity, we utilized plasmid constructs with an easily quantifiable pro-caryotic gene, chloramphenicol acetyl-transerase (EC 2.3.1.28). These constructs differ only with respect to which 72-bp repeat sequence they contain. Using an in vitro assay for expression the following conclusions were drawn: a) In CV-1 and AGMK cells, the SV40 repeats were seen to activate expression at a rate 5 times that seen with the MoMSV-derived repeats. Both repeat sequences activate expression will above that seen with a control plasmid missing 72-bp repeats. b) In L-cells and NIH/3T3 cells, the MoMSV repeats were seen to activate expression at a rate of 2 times that seen with the SV40 repeats. These results suggest that the MoMSV repeats are more host sensitive than the SV40 repeats. c) Since the sequences responsible for activation of viral gene expression exhibit a host preference, but not an absolute preference, we suggest the presence of a discriminating factor in cells that assists in polymerase binding of transcription itself.

INTRODUCTION

One level at which gene expression is regulated involves the initiation of transcription through the action of RNA polymerases or modifying proteins that bind to specific DNA regulatory sequences. In procaryotic organisms, these sequences are rather well defined and include the 10 to 15 nucleotides of the Pribnow box (22) and adjacent operator sequences located approximately 10 to 20 nucleotides from the 5' end of the gene. In eucaryotes, sequences important for transcriptional control are still being identified and some appear to bear little resemblance to their pro-caryotic counterparts.

Sequence analysis (2,10) of the 5' flanking region of many eucaryotic genes reveals homologous sequences approximately 30 nucleotides upstream from many polymerase II transcribed genes. These sequences, referred to as Goldberg-Hogness or "TATA" boxes, appear to act in setting the 5' ends of transcripts (9). The TATA sequences are not absolutely required for transcription, as shown for example in the case of SV40 in which transcription of early genes is maintained even when the TATA box is deleted (13). These findings suggest that additional sequences are required for accurate transcription of eucaryotic genes.

In SV40 deletion of a set of tandem repeated sequences, located 150 bases upstream from the 5' end of the SV40 early transcript eliminates transcription and destroys the viability of the virus (3,14). Surprisingly, deletion of a single repeat has no obvious effect on transcription. This tandem repeat sequence, referred to as an activator or enhancer, has the ability to enhance the expression of other genes, such as -globin (1), when located 5' to the natural promoter of these genes. In addition, these enhancer sequences have been shown to increase the transformation frequency of the herpes thymidine kinase (tk) gene (5) when associated with these sequences in a cis arrangement. Other studies have suggested that enhancer sequences can function when located 5' or 3' to a gene, in either orientation, and at a distance from the gene (20, M. Fromm, P. Berg, personal communication, L. Laimins, C. Gorman, B. Howard, G. Khoury, P. Gruss, unpublished observations). Enhancer sequences are not restricted to SV40 but are also found in other papovaviruses such as polyoma (6,24) BKV (our unpublished results) and BPV (Bocham, Lusky, personal communications) as well as in retroviruses such as MoMSV (19). The long terminal repeat of retroviruses like MoMSV contain sequences responsible for the initiation of transcription of the integrated provirus (4,15,21). Like SV40, the LTR of MoMSV contains a 72-bp tandem repeat sequence about 150 nucleotides upstream from the putative 5' end of the major transcript. In a recent study, Levinson et al. (19) used this 72-bp tandem repeat from MoMSV, which bears little sequence homology to the SV40 repeat, to replace the SV40 repeat, forming a viable recombinant virus (SVr[MSV]) expressing both early and late genes. However when equal amounts of wild-type SV40 and SVr[MSV] were used to infect CV-1 monkey cells, the wild-type SV40 virus appeared to express T antigen at a rate considerably higher than that of the recombinant virus, SVr[MSV]. Since the only structural difference between the two viruses was in the enhancer sequences, this observation suggested that the variability in expression could be attributed to different strengths of these enhancer sequences in monkey cells. Since MoMSV is a mouse virus, it seemed possible that the MSV enhancer sequences might function better in their natural host than in a heterologous system.

We have investigated the host specificity of the 72-bp tandem repeats from SV40 and MoMSV in monkey and mouse cells. Initially, we compared the production of T antigen in cells infected with either SV40 or SVr[MSV]. Since SVr[MSV] does not generate detectable plaques, the titers of SVr[MSV] and SV40 were measured indirectly by determining the total amount of viral DNA in the viral stock. This method, however, cannot access differences in the amounts of defective virus in the stocks. Equal amounts of each virus were used to infect either confluent CV-1 cells or MEFC mouse cells. To eliminate any advantage wild-type SV40 might have over SVr[MSV] due to enhanced DNA replication, hydroxyurea, an inhibitor of DNA replication, was added to the infected CV-1 cells. Since neither virus replicates in MEFC cells, no inhibitor was added to these cultures. Cells were labeled at 24 hr postinfection, T antigen was immunoprecipitated and analyzed by gel electrophoresis. Five times more T antigen was produced in SV40-infected CV-1 cells than in SVr[MSV]-infected CV-1 cells. In contrast, approximately equal amounts of T antigen were expressed after infection of MEFC mouse cells by either virus, although the level of T antigen produced in these cells was low. Although this

finding suggested a host preference for activator sequences, the difficulty of quantitating T antigen expression required a more accurate assay
system before a definitive conclusion could be made.

RESULTS AND DISCUSSION

Gorman et al. (11) recently developed a quantitative assay for gene
expression in eucaryotes using the synthesis of the procaryotic enzyme,
chloramphenicol acetyltransferase (CAT) as an indicator. A sensitive
assay has been developed for CAT that has no known eucaryotic counterpart.
Expression of CAT in eucaryotic cells is thus dependent upon joining
eucaryotic regulatory sequences to the cat gene. A plasmid, pSV2cat (see
Figure 1) was constructed in which the cat gene replaces the SV40 T antigen coding region. This plasmid was used to examine activation of expression by the SV40 tandem repeats. A corresponding plasmid (pSrM2cat)
was constructed consisting of the MoMSV repeats coupled to the SV40 21-bp
repeats, the SV40 TATA box, and cat gene. As a control, a plasmid,
pA10cat$_2$ carrying only the 21-bp repeats of SV40 and the SV40 TATA box,
without enhancer sequences, was also constructed.

These three plasmids were individually transfected onto either CV-1
cells or mouse L cells by the Ca^{2+}-phosphate precipitation method (12).
At 48 hr posttransfection, cells were harvested, and cell lysates were
prepared. In the presence of acetyl-CoA, chloramphemicol acetyltransferase acetylates chloramphenicol. The acetylated forms of ^{14}C chloramphenicol are easily separated from the nonacetylated substrate form by
thin layer chromatography, which allows for easy analysis and quantitation of enzyme activity. Incubation of cell lysates of transfected cells
with acetyl-CoA and ^{14}C-chloramphenicol to determine the relative amounts
of CAT activity provide an indication of gene expression.

In CV-1 cells the SV40 repeats were found to enhace cat to levels of
expression 5 times those seen with the MoMSV repeats (see Figure 1). Both
activating sequences however enhanced expression well above levels observed with the plasmid pA$_{10}$cat$_2$ lacking either activator. In L cells,
however, the MoMSV repeats activated expression at a rate approximately
twice that of the SV40 repeats, again well above the level seen in the
control plasmid, pA$_{10}$cat$_2$ (22). Similar results were obtained with mouse
NIH/3T3 and African green monkey kidney cells. These results suggest
that some enhancers act in a host-specific manner.

Host specificity for enhancer sequences has also been suggested by
the isolation of polyoma virus mutants that grow on otherwise restrictive
lines of undifferentiated mouse teratocarcinoma cells (9,16,17,23). One
feature of many of these mutants is the acquisition of a second repeated
set of nucleotides, often analogous in size and position, but not in
sequence to the SV40 tandem repeats.

In our study, the MoMSV tandem repeats were found to exhibit a higher
degree of host specificity than the SV40 tandem repeats in the activation
of gene expression. Although the level of activation is highly dependent
on the host cells, the MoMSV enhancers induce a significant level of expression in CV-1 cells, well above the level seen with no enhancer present (pA$_{10}$cat$_2$). The activation of the SV40 tandem repeats is not as host
sensitive as enhancement of expression, it is only slightly less efficient
in mouse cells than in the natural host monkey cells. These results suggest that discriminatory factors exist in each cell that act through the
enhancers to assist in transcription. It has been suggested that these
discriminatory factors may bear a resemblance to the   factors that confer sequence specificity on transcription by bacterial RNA polymerase (12).

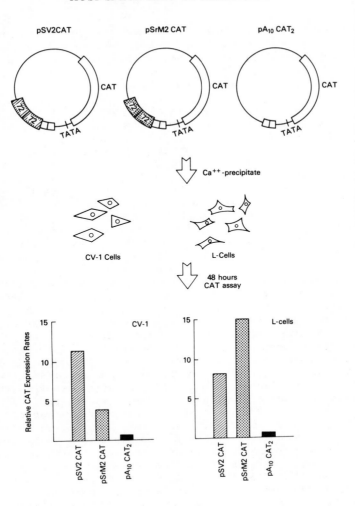

FIGURE 1. Host specificity of activation of gene expression by the 72-bp
tandem repeats from SV40 and MoMSV. Plasmids were constructed in which
the cat gene coding for chloramphenicol actyletranstase was inserted
 into the T antigen-coding sequence of a plasmid carrying the SV40 erly
transcription unit (pSV2cat). The plasmid pSrM2cat carrying the early
transcription unit of SVr^{MSV} consisting of the 72-bp repeats of the LTR
of MoMSV coupled to the SV40 21-bp repeats and TATA box was constructed
in a similar manner. ▨ SV40 72-bp repeats, ▧ MoMSV 72-bp repeats;
 ☐   21-bp repeats). The plasmid pA$_{10}$ was the enhancer deletion control plasmid. The plasmids were transfected onto either L cells or CV-1
cells by the Ca^{2+} phosphate precipitation method. Cell lyates were prepared 24 hr after transfection and analyzed for CAT activity. The relative rates of cat gene expression, indicative of activator strength, are
shown in the associated graphs. In monkey cells, the SV40 repeats activated expression at a rate 5 times that seen with the MoMSV repeats. In
mouse cells, the MoMSV repeats activate expression at a rate approximately
twice that seen with the SV40 repeats.

Several models have been postulated for the mechanism of action of enhancers. These models include sites for topoisomerase activity, sequences for the transport and binding to the transcriptional areas on the nuclear matrix, and sites for polymerase binding. In some respects the third model is most consistent with the data on distance and orientation of the enhancers with respect to promoter sequences of associated genes. Preliminary data have suggested that enhancers, although functional in both orientations, have a preferred sense orientation for transcription (L. Laimins, G. Khoury, C. Gorman, B. Howard, P. Gruss, unpublished results). One might expect both topoisomerase recognition sequences and sequences required for binding to the nuclear matrix to be independent of orientation, and perhaps even independent of position.

In the polymerase binding or entry site model, a polymerase-cofactor-complex would first bind to the recognition site of an activator-enhancer. Upon binding, the complex would slide along the DNA backbone, scanning for appropriate promoter sequences. These sequences might include, in the case of SV40, the 21-bp repeats in conjunction with the TATA box (7). This model would allow the activator-enhancer to be physically well separated from the static promoter.

The existence of viral enhancers has suggested the possibility that similar sequences could be associated with endogenous cellular genes. No cellular enhancers have been found, but such sequences probably do exist. It is possible that these cellular activators, though similar in function, do not activate gene expression to the levels seen with viral enhancers. Viruses must compete with cellular genes for polymerase activity and so may have evolved very efficient mechanisms for inducing high levels of transcription.

In this study we have examined the host specificity of the activation of transcription by enhancer sequences from SV40 and MoMSV. The MoMSV enhancer sequences were found to act in a very host-specific manner; in contrast the SV40 enhancer sequences, at least in the cells examined, were not found to be as host specific. Host specificity is thus an attribute of at least some enhancer sequences, suggesting that these sequences may play a role in determining the host range of eucaryotic viruses.

REFERENCES

1. Bannerji J, Rusconi S, Schaffner W (1981): Cell 27:299
2. Benoist C, Chambon P (1980): Proc Natl Acad Sci USA 77:3865
3. Benout C, Chambon P (1981): Nature 290:304
4. Blair DG, Oskarsson M, Wood TG, McClements WL, Vande Woude GF (1981): Science 212:914
5. Capecchi MR (1980): Cell 22:479
6. deVilliers J, Schaffner W (1981): Nucleic Acids Res 9:6251
7. Efstradiadis A, Pasakony J, Maniatis T, Juan R, O'Connell C et al: (1980): Cell 21:653
8. Fujimara FK, Deininger PL, L Friedmann T, Linney E (1981): Cell 23:809
9. Ghosh PK, Lebowitz P, Frisque RJ, Gluzman Y (1981): Proc Natl Acad Sci USA 78:100
10. Gluzman Y, Sambrook J, Frisque RJ (1980) Proc Natl Acad Sci USA 77:3898
11. Gorman C, Howard B (1982): Mol Cell Biol 2:1044
12. Graham F, Vander Eb A (1973): Virology 52:456
13. Grosschedl R, Birnesteil ML (1980): Proc Natl Acad Sci USA 77:1432

14. Gruss P, Dhar R, Khoury G (1981): Proc Natl Acad Sci USA 78:943
15. Huang AL, Ostrowski MC, Berard D, Hager GL (1981): Cell 27:245
16. Katinka M, Yaniv M, Vasseur M, Blangy D (1980): Cell 20:393
17. Katinka M, Vasseur M, Montreau N, Yaniv M, Blangy D (1981): Nature 290:720.
18. Laimins L, Khoury G, Gorman C, Howard B, Gruss P (1982): Proc Natl Acad Sci USA 79:6453
19. Levinson B, Khoury G, Vande Woude G, Gruss P (1982): Nature 295:568

20. Moreau P, Hen R, Everett R, Gaub MP, Chambon P (1981): Nucleic Acids Res 9:6251
21. Payne GS, Bishop JM, Varmus HE (1982): Nature 295:209
22. Pribnow D (1982): Proc Natl Acad Sci USA 72:784
23. Sekikawa K, Levine AJ (1980): Proc Natl Acad Sci USA 77:6556
24. Tyndall C, LaMantia G, Tacker CM, Favaloro J, Kamen R (1981): Nucleic Acids Res 9:6231

Gene Transfer and Cancer, edited by M. L. Pearson and N. L. Sternberg. Raven Press, New York © 1984.

Use of Gene Transfer to Study the Properties of Long Terminal Repeats of Retroviral DNA

Sheau-Mei Cheng and Nat Sternberg

Cancer Biology Program, National Cancer Institutes, Frederick Cancer Research Facility, Frederick, Maryland 21701

ABSTRACT. Lambda and pBR327 vectors containing the long terminal repeat (LTR) of Moloney murine leukemia virus (M-MuLV) and the herpes simplex virus thymidine kinase (tk) gene were constructed and then used in gene transfer experiments with a mouse cell line that is deficient in tk activity (LMtk⁻) to assess the effect of the LTR on the gene transfer process. Our results indicate that, in the absence of homologous carrier DNA, the LTR increases the number of tk⁺ transformants by a factor of 20- to 100-fold. Transient expression experiments indicate that the levels of TK mRNA and enzymatic activity are stimulated 3- to 10-fold by the presence of the LTR. The enhancement of tk gene transfer cannot be attributed to the promoter activity of the LTR, nor does it appear attributable to recombination events associated with the LTR. Rather, we propose that the 73-base-pair "enhancer" sequence of the M-MuLV LTR increases the efficiency of tk gene transfer by stimulating tk gene expression. This proposal is supported by the observation that a deletion of the enhancer sequence eliminates the stimulation of gene transfer.

INTRODUCTION

The technique of DNA and/or phage-mediated gene transfer presently represents one of the best methods available for manipulating specific genes and for studying their expression and recombination in somatic cells. In this report we describe experiments that use that technique to study the properties of the LTR of retroviruses. The repeat contains several interesting features that could be important in regulating gene expression and gene rearrangement: a) it resembles procaryotic transposable elements (2,4,6) and thus may play an important role in gene rearrangement; b) it contains a promoter from which adjacent genes can be transcribed; and c) it contains enhancer sequences that have the ability to stimulate transcription from nearby promoters located either on the 3' or 5' side of the enhancer (2,4,5).

To study the properties of LTR elements, vectors were constructed containing the M-MuLV LTR and the HSV tk gene and these were then used to transform LMtk⁻ cells to tk⁺. We observed that the presence of an LTR increases the efficiency of tk transformation 20- to 100-fold, probably by stimulating tk gene expression.

RESULTS

The vectors used to study the properties of the LTR are shown in
Figure 1. The first two vectors, designated λLTR-tk2 and λLTR-tk2a,
were constructed by cleaving a circular molecule of M-MuLV DNA containing
two tandemly repeated copies of the LTR at an XhoI site and then cloning
that DNA into the single XhoI site of phage λgtWES·λB DNA (8). A portion of the M-MuLV DNA was then replaced by the 3.4-kb HSV tk BamHI fragment. The two constructions differ in the orientation of the tk fragment.
In both cases the tk gene is located on the 5' side of the LTR promoter.
A third vector, λ-LTR-tk1, is derived from λ-LTR-tk2 and contains a
single LTR. Using either calcium phosphate-mediated DNA transfer (9) or
polyethylene glycol-mediated phage transfer (10), DNA from the three λ
hybrids were transferred into LMtk⁻ cells in the absence of carrier DNA
and tk⁺ transformants selected in HAT (hypoxanthine, aminopterin, thymidine) medium. As a control we used a vector, designated λ-tk, containing the 3.4-kb BamHI HSV tk fragment cloned into the BamHI site of λDam
DNA (3) (Figure 1). The efficiency of tk gene transfer with the three
LTR vectors is about the same and is 50-100 times higher than with λ-tk
(Table 1).

Several of the tk⁺ transformants were isolated, and their DNA were
analyzed after BamHI digestion by Southern transfer and hybridization.
The analysis showed that the LTR tk transformants differ from the tk
transformants in two important respects: First, the former invariably
retain the 3.4-kb BamHI tk fragment and the DNA within 9-kb XhoI M-MuLV
tk fragment, whereas the latter frequently show rearrangements of the
3.4-kb BamHI tk fragment; second, the copy number of the former is usually
low (1-3 copies per diploid genome), whereas the copy number of the
latter is usually high (>5 copies per diploid genome).

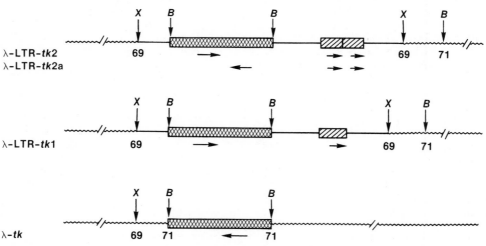

FIGURE 1. λ-tk vectors. The M-MuLV-LTR-tk XhoI fragment (9 kb) of
λ-LTR-tk1, λLTR-tk2 and λLTR-tk2a is cloned at the XhoI site of λgtWES.λB
(λ map coordinate 69). The 3.4-kb BamHI tk fragment of λ-tk is cloned
at the BamHI site of the λDam vector (λ map coordinate 71) (3). Arrow,
direction of tk transcription. ▨, LTR. ▨, 3.4-kb HSV-tk fragment
(〰) = λ sequences. (——) = M-MuLV sequences. B = BamHI, X = XhoI.

TABLE 1. tk Gene Transfer Efficiency with Various λ-tk and pBR327-tk hybrids[a]

Source of tk	Relative transformation efficiency
λtk	1[b]
λLTR-tk1	71
λLTR-tk2	109
λLTR-tk2a	63
pBR327-tk	1[c]
pBR327-LTR-tk	23
pBR327-ΔLTR-tk	3

[a] Experiments with λ vectors were performed using both phage- and DNA-mediated gene transfer. All of the experiments were performed without carrier DNA and at a concentration of vector DNA that gives a linear response. Each result is the average of four determinations with variations of + 20%.
[b] 10 HAT^R colony/μg λ-tk DNA/10^6 recipient cells.
[c] 17 HAT^R colonies/μg pBR327-tk DNA/10^6 recipient cells.

In order to localize that portion of the LTR responsible for the stimulation of gene transfer, the XhoI M-MuLV tk fragment of λLTR-tk1 was cloned at the SalI site of plasmid pBR327 (Figure 2). The resulting plasmid DNA is called pBR327-LTR-tk. A 700-bp deletion of this plasmid was constructed by removing an XbaI-HpaI fragment that contains a portion of the LTR and a portion of the M-MuLV DNA. We call this DNA pBR327-ΔLTR-tk. It is missing the 73-bp tandemly repeated sequence of the LTR that constitutes the enhancer sequence, as well as one end of the LTR, but retains the LTR promoter and the other end of the LTR. pBR327-tk is plasmid pBR327 with the 3.4-kb BamHI tk fragment cloned at the BamHI site of pBR327 (Figure 2). pBR327-LTR-tk transforms LMtk$^-$ cells to tk$^+$ 10 to 20 times more efficiently than does either pBR327-ΔLTR-tk or pBR327-tk (Table 1).

The three plasmids containing tk were used in transient expression experiments to measure the levels of Tk enzyme and Tk mRNA two days after the addition of calcium phosphate-precipitated DNA to LMtk$^-$ cells. The results indicate that an intact LTR stimulates both Tk enzyme and mRNA levels by a factor of 3- to 10-fold over that observed in the absence of that sequence.

DISCUSSION

We have analyzed the effect of LTR on the ability of the HSV tk gene to transform LMtk$^-$ cells to tk$^+$. The following conclusions can be drawn: First, the presence of an intact LTR on the same DNA molecule as that containing the tk gene stimulates the efficiency of gene transfer by 20- to 100-fold; second, the LTR works at a distance of 1.5 kb and can be located either on the 3' or 5' side of the tk gene; third, the stimulatory effect is more pronounced in the absence of carrier DNA. Only a 2- to 5-fold effect is seen in the presence of carrier (data not shown); fourth,

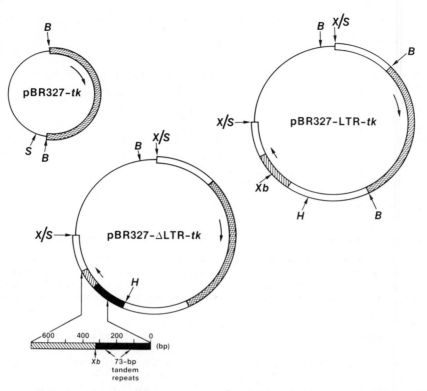

FIGURE 2. pBR327-tk vectors. Arrow, direction of tk transcription.
(━━━━━━), pBR327. ▢ , M-MuLV sequences. ▨ , LTR.
▧ , 3.4-kb HSV-tk fragment. ▰ , deletion. B = BamHI,
H = HpaI, S = SalI, Xb = XbaI, X = XhoI.

transformants obtained in the presence of the LTR usually have a lower tk
copy number and have undergone fewer DNA rearrangements than those obtained
without the LTR; fifth, a deletion of the LTR enhancer sequence and one
end of the LTR eliminates the stimulation; and sixth, the level of both
Tk mRNA and enzyme activity is stimulated 3- to 10-fold by the LTR in
transient expression experiments.

With these facts we can begin to address the questions of how LTR act
to increase the efficiency of gene transfer. In the introduction we proposed three alternative models for LTR action: promoter-initiated transcription, recombination, and promoter enhancement. Since we can observe
stimulation when the tk gene is situated on the 5' side of the LTR promoter
in either orientation, the promoter initiation model is ruled out. Stimulation of recombination by LTR sequences is a possibility because a limiting event in the transformation process is likely to be the integration
of vector DNA into the cell chromosome. Our data at least allow us to
rule out the possibility that such integration occurs at the termini of
the LTR since, in all of the transformants analyzed, the junctions between
LTR and flanking vector DNA were intact after DNA integration. A similar
conclusion has been reached by Copeland, et al. (1). However, we cannot
rule out the possibility that the LTR promotes integration by stimulating
recombination elsewhere in the vector DNA in a manner similar to the
action of chi sites in procaryotes (7). The third possibility, promoter

enhancement, is supported by the observation that a deletion of the LTR enhancer sequence eliminates the stimulation. If we further assume that transformation with tk always requires the juxtaposition of a cellular enhancer and tk, much of our data can be explained. Thus, in the absence of an LTR, transformation with tk is highly dependent upon carrier because the tk gene must become associated with cellular enhancer sequences in order to become efficiently expressed. This also explains the frequent rearrangement of sequences flanking tk and the higher tk copy number of transformants. In contrast, if the added tk DNA already contains an enhancer sequence, the efficiency of transformation is less carrier dependent, and transformants have fewer DNA rearrangements and a lower tk copy number.

ACKNOWLEDGEMENTS

We thank Dr. C. Wei for gifts of λ–LTR–tk2 and λ–LTR–tk2a. Research sponsored by the National Cancer Institute, DHHS, under contract No. NO-CO1-75380 with Litton Bionetics, Inc. The contents of this publication do not necessarily reflect the views or policies of the Department of Health and Human Services, nor does mention of trade names, commercial products, or organizations imply endorsement by the U.S. Government.

REFERENCES

1. Copeland N, Jenkins N, Cooper G (1981): Cell 23:51
2. Dhar R, McClements WL, Enquist LW, Vande Woude GF (1980): Proc Natl Acad Sci USA 77:3937
3. Enquist LW, Sternberg NS (1979): Methods Enzymol 68:281
4. Levinson B, Khoury G, Vande Woude G, Gruss P (1982): Nature 295:568
5. Moreau P. Hen R, Wasylyk B, Everett R, Gaub MP, Chambon P (1981): Nucleic Acids Res 9:6047
6. Shoemaker C, Goff S, Gilboa E, Paskind M, Mitra SW, Baltimore D (1980): Cold Spring Harbor Symp Quant Biol 45:711
7. Stahl F (1979): Annu Rev Genet 13:7
8. Tiemeier D, Enquist L, Leder P (1976): Nature 263:526
9. Wigler M, Silverstein S, Lee L-S, Pellicer A, Cheng Y-C, Axel R (1977): Cell 11:223
10. Yamamoto KR, Chandler VL, Ross SR, Veker PS, Ring, JC, Feinstein, SC (1980): Cold Spring Harbor Symp Quant Biol 45:687

Gene Transfer and Cancer, edited by M. L. Pearson
and N. L. Sternberg. Raven Press, New York © 1984.

Molecular Cloning and Expression of a Gene that Encodes a Novel Transplantation-Related Antigen

Michel Kress, David Cosman, Ernest Jay, George Khoury, and Gilbert Jay

Laboratory of Molecular Virology, National Cancer Institute, National Institutes of Health, Bethesda, Maryland 20205

ABSTRACT. We have recently identified a novel class of H-2-related cDNA clones from a library derived from mouse liver mRNA (4). Sequence analysis of these clones reveals a gene with extensive homology to the H-2K and H-2D antigens except for the transmembrane region. In this region, nucleotide substitutions and a short deletion result in the replacement of hydrophobic residues with charged and polar amino acids. In addition a translational termination codon has been introduced near the end of this structurally important region of the molecule. This H-2-related gene can be distinguished from H-2 genes on the basis of its unique 3' noncoding sequence. Unlike the H-2K and H-2D products, the expression of this gene is tissue specific; the liver is the only tissue where its mRNA is detected. Although lymphoid tissues do not normally express this gene, they are activated in leukemic mice. All mouse strains tested express this gene in their liver, but the level of expression varied significantly and may correlate with specific immunological disorders. The product of this gene may serve as a tolerogenic form of the H-2 antigen, and perturbations in its level of expression may affect immune functions in general.

INTRODUCTION

The first indication that graft rejection is under genetic control came from studies reported about 45 years ago involving skin grafts in mice (6). Subsequent studies have mapped the responsible genetic loci to the major histocompatibility complex (MHC) on chromosome 17 of the mouse and on chromosome 6 of humans (8).

Three different genetic loci coding for the classical transplantation antigens in mice (H-2K, H-2D and H-2L) and in humans (HLA-A, HLA-B and HLA-C) have been identified. The products of these loci, the class I antigens, are highly homologous as revealed by amino acid sequence analysis (12,13). Recent molecular cloning of H-2 sequences has identified other regions both from within the MHC (like the Qa2,3 and Tla loci) as well as outside the MHC (but yet to be mapped) that can code for related molecules (9,15,16).

These class I antigens are unique in several ways (8). Apart from being expressed on the surface of all cells in the body, they are also highly polymorphic with at least 56 alleles at the H-2K locus and 45 alleles at the H-2D locus. In addition, more than 90% of mice are heterozygous at these class I loci. Since they are encoded by a family of genes exhibiting extensive genetic polymorphism and heterozygosity, it is not surprising that the variability in the combination of class I antigens among individuals in the population is extraordinary.

Although it has been generally recognized that the risk of graft rejection can be somewhat reduced if there is a good tissue match between the donor and the recipient, the likelihood of finding a compatible donor is poor. The usual method of overall suppression of the recipient's immune system to prevent rejection of the graft is unsatisfactory because it markedly increases the individual's susceptibility to infections and cancer. The future of organ transplantation will depend upon our ability to provoke in that recipient a specific tolerance to incompatible donor antigens while at the same time preserving his/her immunological defenses (11).

One area of clinical research that has attracted much attention and has proven encouraging is the incorporation of blood transfusion for the potential recipient before the transplant, a procedure which has significantly improved the survival rates of individuals receiving kidney grafts (10). One possible explanation for this apparent success is the induction of tolerance in the recipient as a result of the transfusions. However, until we can identify the component(s) in the blood that can render the recipient tolerant to the donor tissue, this clinical observation remains an art.

We describe here the identification and expression of an H-2 related gene which is expected to encode a secretory form of the transplantation antigens. The prospect of this circulating antigen playing a role in inducing H-2 tolerance is conceptually challenging and merits consideration.

RESULTS

The class I antigens are classical cell-surface glycoproteins composed of a single polypeptide chain about 346 amino acids long, noncovalently associated with a molecule of β2-microglobulin. Biochemical analyses have demonstrated that the N terminal ~280 amino acids are external to the plasma membrane and contain the alloantigenic determinants (12,13). This extracellular portion of the molecule is followed by a stretch of about 25 hydrophobic residues that penetrate the lipid bilayer of the plasma membrane and an adjoining 4 to 5 basic amino acids that serve to anchor it to the membrane. The remaining C terminal 30 to 40 residues are intracellular and presumably function to transmit external signals to the inside of the cell.

Analysis of H-2 cDNA clones has allowed us to define a novel class of H-2 molecules whose nucleotide sequence is closely related to those of the classical H-2 antigens except for the transmembrane domain (4). Within this region of the molecule, extensive nucleotide substitutions and a short deletion result not only in the replacement of hydrophobic residues with charged and polar amino acids, but also in the introduction of a translational termination codon toward the end of this structurally important region of the molecule (Figure 1). Such a messenger RNA would encode a shortened polypeptide containing the biologically active portion of the H-2 antigen located N terminal to the transmembrane

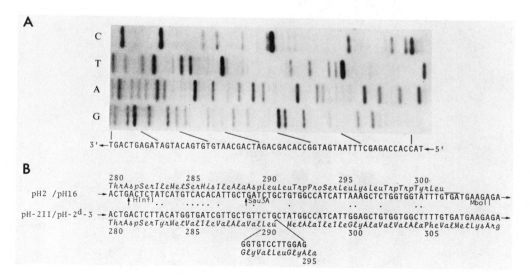

FIGURE 1. Comparison of the amino acid sequence around the transmembrane region of the classical H-2 antigen with the predicted amino acid sequence of the corresponding region from the nonclassical molecule (clone pH2). <u>Panel A</u>: Autoradiogram of a sequencing gel showing the nucleotide sequence of the antisense strand of pH2 DNA around amino acid 280-300. <u>Panel B</u>: Comparison of the pH2 sequence with the corresponding sequence from two previous isolates, pH-2II (15) and pH-2^d-3 (16). The sequences are aligned for maximum homology showing the 13-bp deletion of pH2 relative to pH-2II and pH-2^d-3. All differences in nucleotide sequences are indicated by dots. The numbers correspond to the amino acid sequence of H-2K^b (3).

region but lacking the intracellular domain. Because of the nonconservative replacement of hydrophobic residues in the transmembrane region (Ser285, His286, Asp289, Pro293, Ser294, Lys296), the predicted product would not be expected to insert into the plasma membrane but most likely would be secreted.

Further studies on this novel class of H-2-related molecules are feasible because of our observation that the 3' noncoding region of their RNA transcripts are distinguishable from those that encode the classical H-2 antigens. In order to compare the expression of this unique class of RNA molecules with those encoding the classical H-2 antigens, the following cDNA probes were used: a) probe <u>A</u>, a common 250-bp fragment from the coding region that spans amino acids 151 to 236. This probe includes the coding sequence that is suspected to be highly conserved among all class I (H-2) antigens and is responsible for the binding of β2-microglobulin; b) probe <u>B</u>, a unique 185-bp noncoding fragment derived from clone pH8, a representative of the class of cDNA clones that codes for an H-2 antigen with a classical transmembrane domain composed of entirely hydrophobic residues; c) probe <u>C</u>, a unique 170 bp noncoding fragment derived from clone pH2. This clone is a representative of the class of cDNA clones that codes for the H-2-related

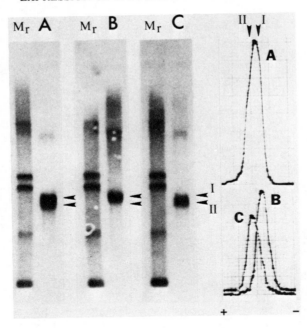

FIGURE 2.   Detection of different classes of H-2-related RNA.   Total polyadenylated RNA from SWR/J mouse liver was fractionated by electrophoresis in a formaldehyde-containing agarose gel, transferred to a nitrocellulose membrane, and hybridized with either probe A, B or C. Autoradiograms of the blots after hybridization are shown on the left, and densitometric scans of the autoradiograms are shown on the right. The scans of B and C are superimposed to demonstrate the different mobilities of the two hybridizing components, designated I and II, respectively.   Molecular weight markers (M_r) were ^{32}P-labeled DNA fragments of 4400, 2300, 1950, 1100 and 600 bp.

molecule with a nonclassical transmembrane region where extensive nonconservative substitutions of hydrophobic residues have been detected and which lacks the cytoplasmic domain.

These cDNA probes were hybridized to Northern blots of total poly(A)$^+$ RNA obtained from livers of SWR/J mice (Figure 2).   Probe A, which is expected to detect transcripts for all class I (H-2)-related antigens, hybridized to a heterogeneous population of RNA molecules with a size range of about 1700 to 1800 bases (Figure 2A).   The heterogeneity in this RNA population is further confirmed by densitometric scanning of the autoradiogram (Figure 2, right), which indicated a main peak (component I) which a distinct shoulder on the leading edge (component II). A minor component about 4000 bases probably represents the unspliced nuclear RNA precursors.

Probe B, derived from the 3' noncoding region of a classical H-2 molecule, hybridizes to a more discrete RNA component about 1800 bases long (Figure 2B), which by denistometric scanning overlaps the major RNA species (component I) detected with probe A.   Considering the known specific activities of the two DNA probes and their differences in size, it can be estimated that 30 to 40% of all the H-2 transcripts detected with probe A are also detected with probe B.

In contrast, probe C, derived from the 3' noncoding region of the nonclassical H-2 molecule, is found to hybridize almost exclusively to the faster-migrating RNA species (component II) that is about 1700 bases long (Figure 2C). A conservative estimate indicates that this DNA probe detects between 20 to 30% of all H-2 transcripts identified by the coding probe. This suggests that the class of cDNA clones represented by pH2 is derived from a pool of stable mRNA that represents a significant fraction of all class I-related transcripts present in liver RNA.

The unusually high level of accumulation of the nonclassical H-2 transcripts in the liver prompted us to analyze other tissues for its expression. Total RNA extracted from kidney, brain, testis, thymus, and spleen was compared to that obtained from liver. With probe A, a component of similar size (about 1800 bases) is detected in all of the tissues (Table I). Analysis with probe C, the noncoding probe specific for the class of H-2 molecules with a nonclassical transmembrane region, produced significantly different results. Hybridization with this probe detected an RNA species present only in liver; none was found in RNA from kidney, brain, testis, thymus or spleen.

The above experiments were carried out with RNA and cDNA probes derived from SWR/J (H-2^q) mice. To access the generality of these observations, we examined the livers of other strains of mice for the expression of this novel class of H-2 related RNA. The additional mouse strains tested include: C57BL/10 (H-2^b), BALB/c (H-2^d), RF (H-2^k), NZB (H-2^d), C3H (H-2^k), and AKR (H-2^k). In each case, there was hybridization of both the coding probe, probe A, and the nonclassical/non-

TABLE 1. The expression of histocompatibility-related RNAs in different tissues of the SWR/J mouse[a]

	DNA Probes		
RNA	A Coding ($\alpha\alpha$ 151–236)	B Noncoding (classical)	C Noncoding (nonclassical)
Liver	++++	++++	+++
Kidney	+++	+++	−
Brain	++	++	−
Testis	++	++	−
Thymus	++	++	−
Spleen	++	++	−

[a] Total RNA extracted from different tissues of SWR/J mice was electrophoresed, blotted and hybridized to ^{32}P-labeled cDNA probes. The relative amount of DNA in each of the tissues was determined from autoradiograms of the blots after hybridization.

TABLE 2. The expression of histocompatibility-related RNAs in the liver of various strains of mice[a]

RNA	DNA Probes	
	A Coding ($\alpha\alpha$ 151-236)	C Noncoding (nonclassical)
SWR/J	+++	+++
C57BL/10	+++	+++
BALB/c	+++	+++
RF	+++	+++
NZB	+	+
C3H	+++	+++
AKR	++++	++++

[a] Total liver RNA was electrophoresed, blotted and hybridized to ^{32}P-labeled cDNA probes. The relative amounts of RNA were determined from the autoradiograms of the blots after hybridization.

coding probe, probe C, to an RNA species of the expected size, demonstrating that the expression of this novel H-2-related molecule is not unique to SWR/J mice (Table 2).

DISCUSSION

Analysis of cDNA clones has allowed us to identify a novel class of H-2 related genes that could encode a shortened polypeptide (4,5). This protein would contain the entire biologically active portion of the H-2 antigen, located N terminal to the transmembrane region, but probably would not be able to insert into the plasma membrane or to interact with cytoplasmic components of the cell. Such a molecule seems likely to be secreted.

Our estimate shows that this novel class of RNA comprises about one-fourth of all class I (H-2) transcripts present in the liver, a substantial proportion in view of the fact that the class I antigens are encoded by a family of genes (16). This analysis, however, does not indicate whether the RNA is composed of a single molecular species or represents a population of related molecules encoded by a family of genes.

Of particular interest is the apparent tissue-specific expression of this novel class of H-2 related RNA. The liver is the only tissue where significant quantities are detected. In contrast, the H-2K and H-2D products are expressed on virtually all cells in the body. Other membrane-associated class I antigens, such as Qa2,3 and T1a, do show a more restricted tissue distribution, but one that is very different from that of the novel RNA described here.

Is there any evidence in support of the secretion of H-2 antigens by the liver? It has been observed in different animal systems that orthotopic transplants of liver are not rejected even when the MHC barrier is crossed (3,7). Instead of sensitizing the recipient, these enduring liver grafts actually induce a state of donor-specific unresponsiveness (immunological tolerance), to the extent that subsequent grafts of other organs become accepted permanently. Because liver allograft protection from rejection is specific only for tissues from the same donor, transplantation antigens are presumably involved (3). Furthermore, liver grafts transplanted into previously sensitized animals not only failed to reject, but converted the state of heightened reactivity to donor grafts (characteristic of immune recipients) into one of nonreactivity characteristic of tolerant animals (7). Since there is no evidence of cell-mediated suppression, this state of unresponsiveness is presumably associated with the presence of specific blocking materials in the circulation (2). We would like to suggest that the expression of the non-classical form of the H-2 gene in the liver is responsible for this phenomenon. Such an altered form of the H-2 antigen would fulfill the expected requirements of having H-2 reactivity and being selectively secreted by the liver into the circulation.

Recent studies suggest that the risk of graft rejection can be significantly reduced if blood transfusions are given to the recipient before the actual transplant (10). It is tempting to speculate that a circulating form of the transplantation antigen may be responsible for inducing tolerance in this case.

What is the physiological role of such a secreted H-2 molecule? Since H-2 is a self antigen, present on the surface of all cells in the body, the immune system must be rendered tolerant to it. It is possible that immunocompetent cells with H-2 reactivity are regulated by some form of suppression in the adult (active tolerance), instead of the complete deletion of H-2-specific immunoreactive cells during prenatal and/ or neonatal life (passive tolerance). A molecule with H-2 specificity that is constantly secreted into the circulation may well act as a blocking factor to suppress H-2 recognition.

It will be important in the future to confirm the presence of secretory H-2 molecules, to determine if they are polymorphic, and to define the molecular mechanism for their constitutive expression in the liver and apparent repression in other tissues. If the product of these H-2-related genes can act to induce tolerance to self and/or foreign H-2 antigens, the prospect for inducing their expression will have profound implications in the field of transplantation immunology.

ACKNOWLEDGEMENTS

This work was supported in part by grants (to E.J.) from the National Cancer Institute of Canada and the Natural Science and Engineering Research Council of Canada.

REFERENCES

1. Bregegere F, Abastado JP, Kvist S, Rask L, Lalanne JL, Garoff H, Cami B, Wiman K, Larhammar D, Peterson PA, Gachelin G, Kourilsky P, Dobberstein B (1981): Nature 292:78
2. Calne RY, Davis DR, Hadjijannakis E, Sells RA, White D, Herbertson BM, Festenstein H (1970): Nature 227:903

3. Calne RY, Sells RA, Pena JR, Davis DR, Millard PR, Herbertson BM, Binns RM, Davis DAL (1969): Nature 223:472
4. Cosman D, Khoury G, Jay G (1982): Nature 295:73
5. Cosman D, Kress M, Khoury G, Jay G (1982): Proc Natl Acad Sci USA 79:4947
6. Gorer PA (1937): J Pathol Bacteriol 44:691
7. Kamada N, Davis H ff S, Roser B (1981): Nature 292:840
8. Klein J (1979): Science 203:516
9. Margulies HD, Evans GA, Flaherty L, Seidman JG (1982): Nature 295:168
10. Marx JL (1980): Science 209:673
11. Maugh TH (1980): Science 210:44
12. Nathenson SG, Uehara H, Ewenstein B, Kindt TJ, Coligan JE (1981): Annu Rev Biochem 50:1025
13. Ploegh HL, Orr HT, Strominger JL (1981): Cell 23:289
14. Steinmetz M, Frelinger JG, Fisher D, Hunkapiller T, Pereira D, Weissman SM, Uehara H, Nathenson S, Hood L (1981): Cell 24:125
15. Steinmetz M, Moore KW, Frelinger JG, Sher BT, Shen FW, Boyse EA, Hood L (1981): Cell 25:683
16. Steinmetz M, Winoto A, Minard K, Hood L (1982): Cell 28:489

TABLE 1. Molecular Phenotypes of Adh⁻ Mutant Flies

Mutants	Phenotypes			Analyses	
	CRM[a]	RNA[b]	Genomic DNA[c]	DNA Structure[d]	Functional Promoter[e]
Adh^fn4	−	reduced amount of larger size RNA	deletion at N terminus	17 bp deleted from 65-bp IVS at 3' splice site	+
Adh^fn6	−	reduced amount of larger size RNA	deletion at N terminus	6 bp deleted from 65-bp IVS at 5' splice site	+
Adh^fn24	−	reduced amount of wild-type size RNA	deletion at N terminus	11 bp deleted from coding region; ↠ frame shift at amino acid 63; ↠ early termination[f] at codon 196	+
Adh^fn23	+	normal amount of shorter DNA	deletion at C terminus	34 bp deleted from coding region; ↠ frame shift at amino acid 242; ↠ new termination[f] at codon 247	+

[a] CRM (cross-reacting material) was detected by goat anti-ADH-antibody.
[b] RNA was analyzed by Northern blot hybridization and quantitative solution hybridization.
[c] Genomic DNA was analyzed by Southern blot hybridization.
[d] DNA sequence analysis was according to Maxam and Gilbert (4).
[e] Promoter activity was assayed by transcription in vitro using HeLa cell nuclear extracts (8).
[f] The wild-type monomeric ADH protein has 255 amino acids.

five nucleotides 5' of both RNA start sites, we find the TATA boxes, which we have described earlier in this report. The larval transcript start site and its promoter are thus located within the 654-bp IVS of the adult transcript. Both transcripts share part of the 5' transcribed, untranslated sequence, the same protein-coding sequence, and the same 3' transcribed, untranslated region. The existence of the two-promoter arrangement of this single-copy gene, which is developmentally-regulated, raises the possibility that stage-specific and/or tissue-specific expression in eucaryotes can be regulated by selection of promoters and transcription initiation sites.

ACKNOWLEDGEMENTS

I am grateful to Bill Sofer for introducing me to the Drosophila alcohol dehydrogenase gene enzyme-system and for the mutant flies used in
this study. Bill Sofer and Allen Place's ongoing collaboration with me
is greatly appreciated. Thanks are due to Mark Pearson for his enthusiasm and continuous support, morally and scientifically, of this work.
Jim Dray has been providing excellent technical assistance. This research was sponsored by the National Cancer Institute, DHHS, under Contract No. NO1-CO-75380 with Litton Bionetics, Inc. The contents of this
publication do not necessarily reflect the views or policies of the Department of Health and Human Services, nor does mention of trade names,
commercial products, or organizations imply endorsement by the U.S. Government.

REFERENCES

1. Benyajati C, Place AR, Powers DA, Sofer W (1981): Proc Natl Acad
   Sci USA 78:2717
2. Darnell Jr JE (1982): Nature 297:365
3. Fitzgerald M, Shenk T (1981): Cell 24:251
4. Maxam SM, Gilbert W (1980): Methods Enzymol 65:499
5. Mount SM (1982): Nucleic Acids Res 10:459
6. O'Donnell J, Mandell HC, Krauss M, Sofer W (1977): Genetics 86:553
7. Schwartz M, Sofer W (1976): Genetics 83:125
8. Weil PA, Luse DS, Segall J, Roeder RG (1979): Cell 18:469

Gene Transfer and Cancer, edited by M. L. Pearson and N. L. Sternberg. Raven Press, New York © 1984.

Amplification and Regulated Expression of a Modular Dihydrofolate Reductase cDNA Gene

[1]Randal J. Kaufman and Phillip A. Sharp

Department of Biology, Center for Cancer Research, Massachusetts Institute of Technology, Cambridge, Massachusetts 02139

ABSTRACT. A dihydrofolate reductase (DHFR) modular gene has been constructed in pBR322 from a DHFR cDNA and the adenovirus 2 major late promoter. DNA-mediated transfer of this gene, in the absence of carrier DNA, transforms Chinese hamster ovary (CHO) DHFR-deficient cells to the DHFR[+] phenotype at a low efficiency. With the addition of the entire or even portions of the SV40 genome, the transformation efficiency is increased. SV40 DNA containing sequences for a polyadenylation signal and sequences for the transcription enhancer (72-bp repeat) enhance the efficiency. Transformants arising from transfection with the modular gene linked to SV40 DNA contain one to five copies of the transfected DNA integrated into the host genome and, upon growh in increasing concentrations of methotrexate, give rise to lines containing several hundred copies of the transfected DNA. The mRNA encoding DHFR in these amplified transformants comes from transcription initiation at the adenovirus major late promoter. The adenovirus first late leader is properly spliced to a 3' splice site cloned into the modular gene. The mRNA is not efficiently polyadenylated at sequences in the 3' end of the DHFR cDNA, but rather uses polyadenylation signals downstream from the DHFR cDNA either in SV40 DNA or cellular DNA sequences. Since DHFR synthesis is regulated with cell growth (i.e., its synthesis is specifically repressed as cells are arrested in stationary phase of growth), independent amplified transformants were tested for growth phase regulation. Several clones do exhibit growth-dependent DHFR synthesis, and further analysis indicated the 3' end of the cDNA gene is responsible for the growth-dependent change in DHFR mRNA levels.

INTRODUCTION

The analysis of DNA transcription and its regulation has been facilitated by the ability to isolate specific genes, modify them in vitro, and reintroduce them into cells in order to study the effects of specific DNA sequence alterations on the expression and the regulated expression of the gene in question. We as well as others (7,8,11,17) have utilized DHFR cDNA clone and added segments of DNA encoding specific functions to produce an active modular gene capable of efficient DHFR

---

[1]Present address: Genetics Institute, Boston, MA 02115.

expression. There are several advantages in utilizing DHFR to construct
chimeric genes in order to study gene expression and its regulation.
First, a CHO cell line deficient in DHFR provides a sensitive assay for
minimal DHFR expression from modular DHFR recombinants (4). Efficiency
of transformation of DHFR cells to the DHFR[+] phenotype after DNA transfection can be quantitated for different modular DHFR cDNA genes in
order to define DNA sequences necessary for efficient expression. Second, growth in increasing concentrations of methotrexate (MTX) selects
for cells containing amplified DHFR genes (1). Thus, it is possible to
amplify sequences cotransfected with DHFR in order to study gene dosage
effects of particular genes on cell metabolism as well as to isolate
cell lines which overproduce proteins that are difficult to obtain by
other means. In addition, the amplification of the sequences introduced
facilitates the analysis of signals utilized for mRNA production and
the analysis of regulatory events. Third, the level of cellular DHFR
synthesis may be easily monitored by enzyme activity, immunoprecipitation
of DHFR by monospecific antisera, or inhibition of cell growth by MTX,
or by fluorescence intensity after saturation with a fluorescent derivative of MTX (6). Thus, regulated expression imparted by the introduction
of specific DNA segments may be studied by monitoring DHFR expression.

RESULTS

Construction of a Modular DHFR cDNA Gene

The murine DHFR cDNA [pDHFR26 from Chang et al. (3)] contains intact
the coding region for DHFR and several polyadenylation signals in its
3' end. When this cDNA was transfected into CHO DHFR[-] cells, no DHFR[+]
transformants were observed (Figure 1). Subsequently, proper segments
encoding transcription initiation, RNA splicing, and polyadenylation were
added to convert the cDNA into an active gene. pAdD26-1 (Figure 1, no. 2)
is a plasmid that contains a 900-bp segment from the adenovirus 2 major
late promoter (Ad2 MLP) containing the first leader and 5' splice site
of the adenovirus tripartite leader fused to the 5' end of a 100-bp segment encoding a 3' splice site isolated from a variable region immunoglobulin gene (see 7 for details). This has been positioned upstream
from the DHFR cDNA. Transcription initiation at the Ad2 MLP should generate an mRNA with the adenovirus late leader spliced to the 3' splice
site and contain a poly A tract at sequences in the 3' end of the DHFR
cDNA. The first AUG on this mRNA is that for DHFR translation. However,
this recombinant is very inefficient in transforming DHFR[-] cells to the
DHFR[+] phenotype. Since a number of reports have implicated the 72-bp
repeat of SV40 in enhancing the expression of DNA in a cis manner (15,5),
a full genome of SV40 was inserted by fusion of its EcoRI site in the late
region to the EcoRI site in pBR322 of pAdD26-1. The resulting plasmids
pASD11 and pASD12 contain the SV40 genome in either orientation and have
higher biological activity in transforming DHFR[-] cells to the DHFR[+] phenotype (Figure 1, nos. 3 and 4).

Amplification of the Transforming DNA

Clones transformed to the DHFR[+] phenotype by pASD11 or pASD12 contain
one to five copies of the transforming DNA integrated into the CHO genome.
Three clones (1B, 1C, and 1D) transformed by pASD11 and one clone (2B)
transformed by pASD12 were subjected to growth in increasing concentrations
of MTX. At 1 μM MTX resistance, the transforming DNA had been amplified

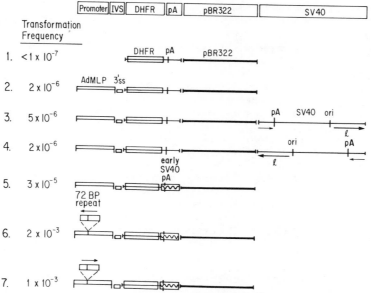

FIGURE 1. DHFR⁻ to DHFR⁺ transformation frequency from various cDNA genes. Calcium phosphate-mediated transfection of plasmid DNA (1 μg/10⁶ cells) in the absence of carrier DNA into CHO DHFR-deficient cells has been described (7). Transformation frequencies are determined from the number of DHFR⁺ transformants arising per number of cells plated into selective media. Recombinants indicated are 1) pDHFR26 (3), 2) pAdD26-1 (7), 3) pASD11, 4) pASD12 which contain the entire SV40 genome in either orientation cloned into the recombinant by their EcoRI sites (in the late region of SV40 and in pBR322 of pAdD26-1) (7), 5) pAdD26SV(A) which contains an early SV40 polyadenylation site (8), and 6) pCVSVE, and 7) pCVSVL which contain the 72-bp repeat in either orientation (8). The arrows depict the late transcription unit of SV40 in no. 3 and no. 4 and the direction of the SV40 late promoter in no. 6 and no. 7. Also shown is the inefficient polyadenylation site in the 3' end of the DHFR cDNA and the location of polyadenylation sites supplied by SV40 sequences (pA).

several hundredfold (7). However, clones 1C and 2B had deleted pBR322 sequences from the transforming DNA during the transfection and amplification process, and clone 2B had dramatically rearranged its DNA upon amplification.

Since the early region of SV40 was present intact on the original plasmid, it was possible to determine whether any SV40 early proteins were expressed after amplification of the transforming DNA. Indeed, clone 2B produced both large and small T antigen of SV40 and clone 1B produced only small t antigen of SV40. When clone 1B cells were selected for resistance to 50 μM MTX, a small t-antigen-related polypeptide accounted for more than 10% of the total protein synthesis (8). This directly demonstrates the coexpression and overproduction of a gene product after coamplification (see 11 for similar results of coexpression after amplification).

Signals Utilized in DHFR mRNA Production

The amplification of the transforming DNA facilitated the analysis of the DHFR mRNA produced in transformed clones 1B, 1C, 1D, and 2B (see Figure 2 for summary). Primer extension and sequencing of the extended products indicated that all transformants utilize the AD2 MLP for transcription initiation and that the adenovirus late leader is correctly spliced to the 3' splice site introduced from an immunoglobulin gene to remove a hybrid intron of 200 bases.

Analysis of the 3' end of the mRNA by S1 nuclease mapping indicated inefficient polyadenylation in the 3' end of the DHFR cDNA in all transformants (8). The mouse endogenous DHFR gene contains multiple polyadenylation signals in its 3' end, thus generating heterogeneity in the size of DHFR-specific mRNAs. Mouse cells produce four DHFR mRNA species of 750, 1000, 1200, and 1600 bases in length (16). The cDNA utilized to construct the modular DHFR cDNA genes described here contains the polyadenylation signals for the 3 shorter of these mRNAs but not the signal specifying the 1600-base polyadenylation site. Surprisingly, these signals for polyadenylation are not used efficiently in the amplified transformants 1B, 1C, 1D, and 2B. Instead, most DHFR mRNA in these transformants is polyadenylated at signals downstream from the signals specifying poly-

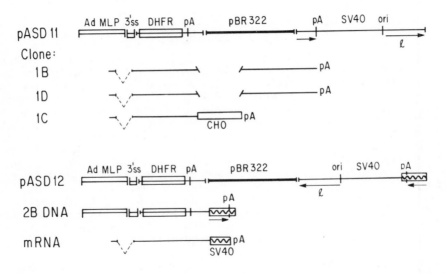

FIGURE 2. Major DHFR mRNA in amplified lines. Clones isolated by transformation with pASD11 (1B, 1C, 1D) and pASD12 (2B) are indicated. pASD11 DNA is shown with the major mRNA species from 1B and 1D below. The adenovirus major late leader is properly spliced to the 3' splice site. An additional segment of RNA (approximately 1 kb) is removed presumably by splicing of sequences in pBR322. The mRNA is polyadenylated at the late polyadenylation signal. Clone 1C is identical to 1B and 1D at the 5' end, but its 3' end is derived from cellular DNA sequences that are joined to plasmid DNA sequences (open box). pASD12 is depicted with the DNA in transformant 2B indicating a rearrangement of DNA sequences so that the SV40 late transcription unit and polyadenylation signal are positioned 3' to the dhfr segment. The 5' end of DHFR mRNA produced in 2B is identical to that produced in clones 1B, 1D, and 1C; however, the sequences 3' of the DHFR portion differ. The mRNA from 2B cells does not contain pBR322 sequences but is polyadenylated at the SV40 late polyadenylation signal. The arrows depict the SV40 late transcription unit.

adenylation in the 3' end of the DHFR cDNA. Clones 1B and 1D produce very similar DHFR mRNAs that contain pBR322 sequences and are polyadenylated at the SV40 late polyadenylation signal. Clone 1C has integrated into cellular DNA to produce a DHFR mRNA that contains CHO-derived sequences in its 3' end. Polyadenylation of this mRNA occurs in CHO sequences downstream from the plasmid integration site in the CHO genome. Clone 2B, derived from transformation by pASD12 (which contains SV40 in the opposite orientation compared to pASD11), has become dramatically rearranged upon MTX selection. The rearrangement of the plasmid DNA in transformant 2B has involved the inversion of sequences containing the SV40 late polyadenylation signal and their insertion downstream from the DHFR coding region. DHFR mRNA in this line also utilizes the SV40 late polyadenylation signal for polyadenylation; however, it lacks the pBR322 sequences present in the 3' end of DHFR mRNA in transformants 1B and 1D. In conclusion, all transformants have identical 5' ends, which contain the Ad2 major late leader spliced to the 3' splice site, and differ in their 3' ends. Three transformants have derived polyadenylation signals from the SV40 late region and another transformant utilizes a cellular polyadenylation signal approximately 2-kb downstream from the point of plasmid integration into the genome.

Optimization of DHFR Expression from the Modular DHFR cDNA Gene

The analysis of the DHFR mRNA in these four transformants indicated that one way SV40 DNA might increase the efficiency of DHFR expression is by providing more efficient polyadenylation signals. This has been directly tested by introducing an SV40 early polyadenylation signal into the 3' end of the DHFR cDNA in pAdD26-1. Figure 1 indicates that this recombinant (no. 5) is capable of transforming DHFR$^-$ cells to the DHFR$^+$ phenotype 10-fold more efficiently than similar plasmids containing the entire SV40 genome (compare either recombinant 3 or 4 to recombinant 5 in Figure 1). Since the DHFR modular gene transforms CHO DHFR-cells, we were also able to test the effect of addition of the 72-bp repeat on the transformation frequency. The 72-bp repeat has been introduced into the modular cDNA gene in either orientation 250 bp upstream from the Ad2 MLP. The introduction of this segment further increased transformation frequency 50- to 100-fold (Figure 1, nos. 6 and 7). Thus, one in a thousand cells subjected to selection after DNA transfection of this latter plasmid become transformed to the DHFR$^+$ phenotype.

Growth-Dependent Protein Synthesis Requires Signals in the 3' End of the Gene

The synthesis of DHFR is dependent on the growth state of the cell. Like other enzymes important in DNA symthesis, it is synthesized in logarithmically growing cells and specifically repressed in quiescent stationary-phase cells (9,19). This growth dependence can be explained by the specific synthesis of DHFR in the S phase of the cell cycle (13) since logarithmically growing cells have a larger percentage of the cells in S phase than do quiescent stationary-phase cells. Several transformants containing amplified DHFR modular cDNA genes also exhibit growth-dependent synthesis. Figure 3 shows results from [^{35}S]methionine pulse-labeled extracts prepared from early-logarithmic-phase or stationary-phase cells from transformants 1B, 1D, 2B resistant to 1 μM MTX. Transformants 1B, 1D, and 2B all specifically repress (approximately 10-fold) DHFR synthesis in stationary-phase cells as compared to early-logarithmic-phase cells.

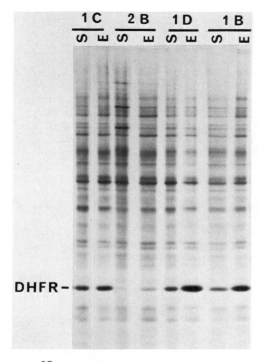

FIGURE 3. Analysis of [^{35}S]methionine pulse-labeled proteins from growing
and resting amplified transformants. Duplicate confluent plates of transformants 1B, 1C, 1D, and 2B resistant to 50 μM MTX were either subcultured (1:6) into fresh media (E) or left untreated (S), and 24 hr later
incubated with [^{35}S]methionine for 1 hr. Cells were washed and extracts
were prepared by sonication and centrifugation at 100,000 x g. Equal
numbers of incorporated counts were electrophoresed on a 15% SDS-poly-
acrylamide gel, and the gel was prepared for autoradiography.

Transformant 1C shows a negligible effect. All transformants have identical DHFR mRNA at their 5' end. All transformants that exhibit the growth-
dependent DHFR synthesis utilize the SV40 late polyadenylation signal for
DHFR mRNA production. Transformant 1C shows very little response and
utilizes a different signal for polyadenylation. Thus, there is an association between the ability to exhibit growth-dependent synthesis and
specific sequences in the 3' end of the gene.
    Whether the growth-dependent synthesis is a translational effect or
a result of differences in DHFR mRNA levels was examined by S1 nuclease
mapping in DNA probe excess (2). A 3'-end-labeled DNA probe was prepared
from a DHFR cDNA plasmid that contains the entire 3' sequence of DHFR
encompassing the four polyadenylation sites at 750, 1000, 1200, and 1600
bases (Figure 4). When this probe is hybridized to 3T3-R500 mouse MTX-
resistant cell DNA (a cell line containing amplified endogenous DHFR genes),
4 DNA fragments (corresponding to the four polyadenylation signals) should
be protected after S1 nuclease digestion. After electrophoresis of the
S1-nuclease-digested hybrids on denaturing agarose gels, there appear
four protected fragments (Figure 4, fragments 1 through 4) generated by
hybridization to RNA from logarithmically growing 3T3-R500 cells. The
band intensity is proportional to the quantity of each specific mRNA. RNA

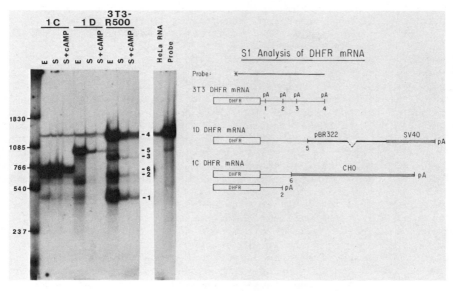

FIGURE 4. S1 analysis of DHFR mRNA. Total cytoplasmic RNAs from 50 μM
MTX-resistant 1C and 1D transformants and from murine 3T3-R500 MTX resistant cells were prepared from confluent stationary-phase cells (S),
from stationary-phase cells that were treated for 24 hr with 1 mM dibutyryl
cyclic AMP and 1 mM theophylline (S+ cAMP), and from confluent cells that
had been subcultured 1:6 into fresh medium for 24 hr (E). A DNA probe
uniquely labeled at its 3' end was prepared by flushing a TagI site in
the DHFR coding region of pDHFR12 (3) using Klenow fragment of polymerase
1 and [^{32}P]deoxytriphosphates. pDHFR12 contains sequences for the four
major polyadenylation sites in the 3' end of the DHFR gene. The labeled
DNA was digested with PstI, and the specific DHFR end-labeled fragment
was isolated from an agarose gel. Equal amounts of total RNA were hybridized to an excess of end-labeled DNA probe, and the hybrids digested
with S1 nuclease and electrophoresed on a denaturing glyoxal agarose gel.
Results show amounts of 3' protected fragments from each cell line under
different growth conditions. Also shown are results from hybridization
to HeLa RNA which contains no homologous DHFR sequences (HeLa) and another
lane containig 1/10 the amount of undigested probe DNA used in these experiments (Probe). Molecular weight markers are indicated at the left.
The diagram on the right shows the homology of the probe to the various
mRNA species. The DHFR coding regions (box) are identical in all mRNA
species. 3T3-R500 DHFR mRNA contains 4 major species (denoted 1 through
4) by differences in polyadenylation which protect four different-sized
probe DNAs from S1 nuclease digestion (bands labeled 1 through 4). 1D
DHFR mRNA produces a major species that represents the position at which
the 3' sequences from DHFR diverge and enter pBR322 in recombinant pASD11
(band number 5). 1C DHFR mRNA diverges at the position (band number 6)
where the plasmid DNA has integrated into the CHO genome. It also produces a slightly smaller protected fragment derived from hybridization to
an mRNA produced by polyadenylation at site 2 in the 3' end of the DHFR
cDNA. This fragment comigrates with the respective fragment protected
after hybridization of the probe to murine 3T3-R500 RNA.

from stationary-phase cells also generates these four bands but in 10- to 20-fold less abundance. Thus, the four DHFR mRNAs are all reduced in level as the cell progresses from the growing to resting state. In addition, stationary-phase cells that are treated for 24 hr with 1 mM dibutyryl cAMP and 1 mM theophylline show a further reduction in the level of all DHFR mRNAs. cAMP inhibits many cellular functions that are correlated with serum stimulation of cell growth (10). When the DNA probe hybridized to RNA isolated from the MTX-resistant transformant 1D, a predominant band (Figure 4) is protected which corresponds to the point of divergence of the RNA from the DNA. This point represents the fusion between the cDNA and pBR322 sequences in the modular gene. The reduction in the quantity of this protected fragment in progression from early-growth-phase cells to stationary-phase cells and further to staionary-phase cells with dibutyryl cAMP and theophylline is like that observed for the 3T3-R500 DHFR mRNAs. Thus, the specific change in DHFR protein synthesis is due to a change in the DHFR mRNA level.

Hybridization of the probe to MTX-resistant transformant 1C RNA generates a doublet after S1 nuclease digestion and gel electrophoresis. The upper band (Figure 4, band 6) corresponds to the breakpoint where the DHFR mRNA procedes into genomic CHO sequences at the point of plasmid DNA integration. The level of this S1-nuclease-protected fragment changes only several-fold as cells progress from the growing (early-logarithmic-phase cells) to the resting (stationary-phase cells or stationary-phase cells with dibutyryl cAMP and theophylline) state. In transformant 1C, a second protected fragment (Figure 4, band 2) is generated by hybridization to an mRNA which is polyadenylated at the 2nd polyadenylation site (corresponding to the 1000-base DHFR mRNA) in the DHFR cDNA. This band is repressed as cells progress from the growing to the resting state. Thus, clone 1C produces two different-sized DHFR mRNAs that differ in the polyadenylation signal utilized. The mRNA produced by polyadenylation in the DHFR cDNA is specifically repressed in quiescent cells, whereas the mRNA produced by polyadenylation at a cellular site into which the plasmid DNA integrated shows only minor quantitative differences when growing cells are compared to resting cells.

DISCUSSION

A DHFR cDNA clone has been converted into an active gene by addition of the adenovirus major late promoter for transcription initiation and a 3' splice site from an immunoglobulin gene in order to create a hybrid intron that can be excised. This clone has been tested for biological activity by testing its efficiency in transforming CHO DHFR⁻ cells to the DHFR⁺ phenotype. Recombinants constructed subsequently contain either the entire or only specific portions of the SV40 genome and transform DHFR⁻ cells to the DHFR⁺ phenotype more efficiently. Analysis of the DHFR mRNA in four independent MTX-resistant transformants has indicated that the adenovirus major late promoter is utilized for transcription initiation and that a hybrid intron consisting of a 5' splice site from the adenovirus first late leader and a 3' splice site from an immunoglobulin gene is properly excised. However, polyadenylation signals in the 3' end of the DHFR cDNA are not efficiently utilized. Three transformants utilize the SV40 late polyadenylation signal for polyadenylation, and the fourth utilizes a cellular polyadenylation signal downstram from the point of plasmid integration (see ref. 8 for details). Thus one function SV40 provides to increase transformation efficiency is an efficient polyadenylation signal. This has been directly demonstrated by showing that the addition of the early polyadenylation site of SV40 into the 3' end of the DHFR gene cDNA (without any other SV40 sequences) can transform DHFR⁻ cells to the DHFR⁺ phenotype 15-fold more efficiently. Another function SV40 may provide to increase transformation efficiency is the enhancement of transcription through its enhancer or 72-bp repeat. This has been demonstrated by finding a 50- to 100-fold increase in transformation efficiency after the insertion in either orientation of a segment of SV40 DNA which contains the 72-bp repeat.

The DHFR gene is normally subject to growth-dependent regulation. Actively growing cells produce DHFR mRNA and in stationary-phase cells dhfr mRNA synthesis is specifically repressed. It was surprising to find that DHFR synthesis was similarly regulated in cells expressing modular DHFR cDNA genes. Cell cycle regulation of DHFR synthesis was correlated with the presence of sequences in the 3' end of the gene. Only the mRNAs which are polyadenylated at DHFR polyadenylation signals or the late SV40 polyadenylation signal show growth-dependent mRNA accumulation. A transformant that contains a DHFR cDNA gene that utilizes a cellular DNA site for polyadenylation shows constitutive DHFR synthesis. These results indicate that the growth state of the cell can have profound effects on altering the steady-state levels of mRNAs and that this change in steady-state mRNA level is dependent upon sequences in the 3' end of the gene, possibly the polyadenylation signal. It is generally assumed that large increases in protein synthesis and mRNA levels in differentiation and in response to hormonal stimuli result from increases in the transcription rate by protein-DNA interactions at the 5' end of specific genes. This is based on the study of gene expression of specialized products of highly differentiated cells. In contrast, our studies on growth-dependent protein synthesis predict that posttranscription events may be important in controlling RNA levels by altering mRNA stability. These findings are consistent with those of Leys and Kellems (12) who have demonstrated the rate of DHFR mRNA synthesis is not altered in growing versus resting cells, but rather the DHFR mRNA is preferentially stabilized in growing cells.

Several transformants that we have characterized utilize the SV40 late polyadenylation signal for DHFR mRNA synthesis and show growth-dependent DHFR mRNA accumulation. The SV40 late polyadenylation signal may have evolved to preferentially generate mRNAs in growing (S phase of the cell cycle) cells. Early SV40 infection produces large and small tumor antigens which stimulate cells to enter the S phase of the cell cycle to allow replication of SV40 DNA (18). At this time accumulation to late SV40 mRNA begins. An important signal for synthesis of this late mRNA may be the preferential stabilization of late mRNA due to sequences in the 3' end of the late transcript.

ACKNOWLEDGEMENTS

R.J.K. is a Helen Hay Whitney Postdoctoral Fellow. This work was supported by grants NSF PCM78-23230 and NIH CA26717 to PAS and partially by NIH Center for Cancer Biology at MIT grant CA14051.

REFERENCES

1. Alt FW, Kellems RM, Bertino JR, Schimke RT (1978): J Biol Chem 253: 1357
2. Berk AJ, Sharp PA (1977): Cell 12:721
3. Chang ACY, Nunberg JH, Kaufman RJ, Erlich HA, Schimke RT, Cohen SN (1978): Nature 275:617

4. Chasin LA, Urlaub G (1980): Proc Natl Acad Sci USA 77:3216
5. Fromm M, Berg P (1983): J Mol Appl Gen 2:127
6. Kaufman RJ, Bertino JR, Schimke RT (1978): J Biol Chem 253:5852
7. Kaufman RJ, Sharp PA (1982a): J Mol Biol 159:601
8. Kaufman RJ, Sharp PA (1982b): Mol Cell Biol 2:1304
9. Kellems RE, Morhenn VB, Pfendt EA, Alt FW, Schimke RT (1979): J Biol
    Chem 254:309
10. Kram R, Mamont P, Tomkins GM (1973): Proc Natl Acad Sci USA 70:1432
11. Lee F, Mulligan R, Berg P, Ringold G (1981): Nature 294:228
12. Leys EJ, Kellems RE (1981): Mol Cell Biol 1:961
13. Mariani BD, Slate DL, Schimke RT (1981): Proc Natl Acad Sci USA 78:
    4985
14. Ringold G, Dieckmann B, Lee F (1981): J Mol Appl Gen 1:165
15. Schaffner W (1980): Proc Natl Acad Sci USA 77:2163
16. Setzer DR, McGrogan M, Nunberg JA, Schimke RT (1980): Cell 22:361
17. Subramani S, Mulligan R, Berg P (1981): Mol Cell Biol 1:854
18. Tooze J, ed. (1981): DNA Tumor Viruses, Molecular Biology of Tumor
    Viruses (2nd edition), Cold Spring Harbor, NY: Cold Spring Harbor
    Laboratory
19. Wiedemann LM, Johnson LF (1979): Proc Natl Acad Sci USA 76:2818

Gene Transfer and Cancer, edited by M. L. Pearson and N. L. Sternberg. Raven Press, New York © 1984.

Mouse *dhfr* Minigenes: Transfer, Expression, and Amplification

Gray F. Crouse, Robert N. McEwan, and Mark L. Pearson

Cancer Biology Program, National Cancer Institute, Frederick Cancer Research Facility, Frederick, Maryland 21701

ABSTRACT. We have studied the expression of the mouse dihydrofolate reductase gene (dhfr), which is normally 31 kb long, by constructing a series of dhfr minigenes using recombinant DNA methods in conjunction with standard phage crosses. These minigenes have 1500 bp of 5' flanking region; however, as many as five intervening sequences were deleted specifically, producing genes as small as 2.9 kb. Plasmids containing the engineered dhfr minigenes rescued CHO Dhfr⁻ cells with transfection frequencies of more than 10^{-4}. Detectable levels of DHFR were produced in all selected clones, but the levels were generally much lower than in the parent CHO cells. Clones differing in gene copy number by as much as a hundred-fold produced comparable levels of DHFR, indicating that the levels are unrelated to the copy number of these initial clones. Cells with increased gene copy number and levels of DHFR were subsequently selected by growth in increasing amounts of methotrexate. One cell line has over 2,000 copies of the dhfr minigene arranged in a tandem array. Other cell lines contain an amplified and rearranged minigene. These results indicate that the expression of transfected genes can depend on other factors, in addition to gene structure and copy number.

INTRODUCTION

The dihydrofolate reductase gene (dhfr) codes for an enzyme that is necessary for the biosynthesis of nucleotides and some amino acids in all eucaryotic cells. Thus, unlike most eucaryotic genes studied to date, it is not the product of a differentiated cell type; it is a "housekeeping" enzyme that is found in all cells. An additional feature of interest is that cells selected for resistance to increasing concentrations of methotrexate (MTX), a specific inhibitor of DHFR, most frequently acquire resistance by amplification of the dhfr gene (1).

We wanted to study the regulation of expression of the cloned gene by DNA transformation methods in order to study its transcription and to determine whether the transfected DNA could be amplified as a result of selection with MTX. The difficulty with this approach is that even though DHFR has only 186 amino acids, the dhfr gene is 31 kb in size (3). Although a gene of this size could be carried in cosmid vectors, any subsequent manipulation of the gene structure in vitro could be very difficult because of its size. Therefore, we decided to construct dhfr

minigenes that would have all the necessary 5' flanking regulatory sequences, coding sequences, and 3' sequences, but would lack most of the
intervening sequences in the dhfr gene.

RESULTS

Construction of Minigenes

The method we developed to construct the minigenes is shown in Figure
1. λrva and λrvb are λ phages developed by Carroll et al. (2) in
order to study genetic recombination. They are designed such that recombination between selectable phage markers conferring the Spi and Imm
phenotypes must occur in homologous DNA sequences inserted at the unique
HindIII site. Therefore, a genomic DNA fragment containing the 5' flanking regions and the first two coding sequences of the dhfr gene was
cloned into λrva, and a dhfr cDNA containing the entire coding sequence
and 3' untranslated region was cloned into λrvb. Selection for phage
recombinants in a λ,P2 double lysogen yielded the two types of recombinant molecules shown at the bottom of Figure 1. Both types have 5' genomic flanking sequences, coding sequences, and the 3' end of the cDNA,
which in this case is a complete copy of the 3' end of the 1600-bp mRNA
including some of the polyA tail. The only difference between the two
molecules is the presence of intervening sequence I in pdhfr3.2 and its
absence in pdhfr2.9.

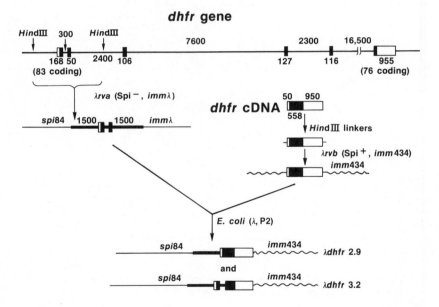

FIGURE 1. Construction of dhfr minigenes. The top line illustrates the
mouse dhfr gene drawn to scale (with the exception of the 16.5-kb intervening sequence). The boxes represent the sequences found in the mRNA
as determined from dhfr cDNA clones. The filled-in boxes represent
coding sequences and the open boxes represent the 5' and 3' untranslated
regions. Underneath each box is the number of nucleotides as determined
by DNA sequencing of the region (3).

This approach can be used to generate dhfr minigenes with any desired combination of intervening sequences and does not depend on conveniently located restriction sites for the piecing together of desired parts of genes. It should permit the generation of hybrid genes from various members of multigene families so that genes with novel properties can be created.

Transfer and Expression of the dhfr Minigenes

In order to see whether these minigenes were functional, the dhfr HindIII fragments from the recombined λ phage were cloned into pBR327. The dhfr plasmids pdhfr3.2 and pdhfr2.9 were then transferred into dhfr⁻ CHO recipient cells (6) by calcium phosphate coprecipitation with or without carrier mouse DNA. The transfectants were then selected in medium lacking hypoxanthine, thymidine, and glycine so that any survivors would be required to have a functioning dhfr gene. Both plasmids, with or without carrier, gave rise to Dhfr$^+$ colonies at frequencies of $> 10^{-4}$ transformants/cell. The number of minigene copies and the level of DHFR protein were measured in various clones and are shown in Table 1.

As can be seen, there is a wide variation in the amount of DHFR produced in independent transfectant clones. This level appears to be unrelated to the number of minigene copies present in the cell. Possible explanations for this finding include the following: 1) not all copies may be expressed; 2) not all copies may have an intact structure; and 3) chromosomal location could greatly affect levels of expression. There appears to be a tendency for greater levels of DHFR to be found in cells transfected in the presence of carrier DNA compared to cells transfected in the absence of carrier, although this may be due to the generally higher copy numbers found in the transfectants obtained with carrier DNA.

There does appear to be a difference in the structure of the minigenes in clones obtained with or without carrier (results not shown). In eight of nine clones obtained with carrier DNA, a restriction enzyme digest of the DNA gave dhfr and plasmid bands of the expected size, as well as bands of other sizes in some cases. Most clones appeared to have multiple copies of the expected size. However, in clones obtained without carrier DNA, there were very few copies of the minigene; furthermore, four of six clones had no bands of the expected size and the other two had only one band of the expected size and additional bands of different size. Apparently, in the presence of carrier DNA, multiple copies of the minigene arranged in tandem arrays are likely to be formed. In contrast, in the absence of carrier, even when a large amount of plasmid is used (20 µg/10^6 cells), only a few copies of the minigene are stably integrated, and these are extensively rearranged.

Minigene Amplification

Several transfected clones were subjected to selection in increasing concentrations of MTX. Resistance to MTX was correlated with an increased level of DHFR and an increased dhfr minigene copy number. Some representative data are shown in Table 2. In all three cases shown, high levels of amplification were obtained. Although the gene copy number continues to increase in the later steps of selection in 29CF4 and 32CF4, the measured level of DHFR does not proportionately increase. We do not know whether this result is caused by problems in the DHFR assay or whether it reflects changes in the cell. The structures of the am-

TABLE 1. dhfr minigene copy number and DHFR enzyme
levels in various pdhfr-transfected clones[a]

Clone	dhfr copy no.	DHFR assay ^{3}H-MTX binding (mouse liver = 1 U/mg)
pdhfr3.2 DNA		
32S1	5–10	0.16 ± 0.02(5)
32S2	450	1.2 ± 0.3(5)
32S3	< 5	1.1 ± 0.2(5)
32S6	10–20	0.26 ± 0.03(6)
32CF1	< 5	0.13 ± 0.03(14)
32CF4	< 5	0.26 ± 0.06(11)
pdhfr2.9 DNA		
29S3	< 5	0.29 ± 0.06(9)
29S4	300	0.14 ± 0.01(4)
29CF1	< 5	0.08 ± 0.02(6)
29CF4	< 5	0.12 ± 0.03(7)
K1 (parent)		1.7 ± 0.26(8)
DUK XB11		< 0.01

[a]The clones with a CF in their disignation were obtained by calcium
phosphate transfection with 20 µg of plasmid DNA per 100-mm dish
(10^6 cells) without carrier DNA; all other clones were obtained with
0.3 µg of plasmid DNA and 20 µg mouse DNA carrier per dish. The
copy number/genome was determined by a DNA dot blot hybridization (5)
using pdhfr3.2 as a standard. The standard for the MTX binding (4)
was an extract from mouse liver; 1 mg of this extract bound 35,000
cpm of ^{3}H-MTX. The numbers in parentheses represent the number of
determinations. K1 is the parent CHO cell line from which the dhfr⁻
line DUKXB11 was derived.

plified genes were examined by restriction digestion and Southern hybridization, with the results shown in Figure 2. 32S3M.1a was derived from
a clone obtained with carrier DNA; the minigene in this transfectant is
contained in amplified head-to-tail tandem arrays. The digestion results
indicate that each array has only a few copies of the minigene and that
the minigenes are broken at random locations in the joints with genomic
DNA. There is apparently only one structure of the minigene in the amplified unit of 32CF4M.3 and 29CF4M.3, transfectants obtained with
pdhfr3.2 and pdhfr2.9, respectively, and no carrier DNA. Both have
undergone substantial rearrangement (29CF4M.3 has even lost all plasmid
sequences). In addition, flanking genomic DNA has been amplified. This
result suggests that the dhfr minigenes can be used to amplify linked
sequences, as demonstrated with the genomic dhfr gene by Wigler et al.

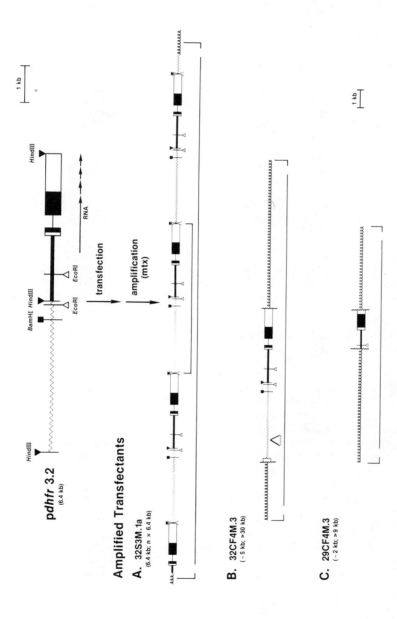

FIGURE 2. Proposed structures for the amplified dhfr minigenes. At the top of the figure is shown pdhfr3.2 with the location of some restriction enzyme sites. The structure of the minigenes in 32S3M.1a(A), 32CF4M.3(B and 29CF4M.3(C) are shown at half the scale for pdhfr3.2. Estimates of the sizes of the amplified minigenes (6.4 kb in A, ~ 5 kb in B, and ~ 2 kb in C), and a minimum size for the amplified region are also shown. The curly line represents genomic sequences not part of the minigene.

TABLE 2. <u>dhfr</u> minigene copy number and DHFR protein in amplified
clones selected for MTX resistance[a]

Clone	Selected in MTX (μM)	<u>dhfr</u> copy no.	DHFR assay ^{3}H-MTX binding (mouse liver = 1 U/mg)
32S3 (parent)	–	< 5	1.1 ± 0.18(6)
M1.a	0.1	2200	14 ± 2.7(10)
32CF4 (parent)	–	< 5	0.26 ± 0.06(11)
M.01	0.01	35	6.3 ± 0.4(5)
M.05	0.05	120	9.8 ± 0.7(5)
M.1	0.1	170	35 ± 4.9(5)
M.3	0.3	340	30 ± 1.0(3)
29CF4 (parent)	–	< 5	0.12 ± 0.03(7)
M.01	0.01	30	1.9 ± 0.2(3)
M.05	0.05	90	6.3 ± 1.6(6)
M.1	0.1	200	4.7 ± 0.4(4)
M.3	0.3	370	3.8 ± 0.3(3)

[a]Clones selected stepwise for resistance to the MTX concentration shown
were assayed for copy number and DHFR as in Table 1. For the 29CF4 and
32CF4 clones, populations of cells were subjected to selection in increasing concentrations of MTX, and cells at each stage of the selection
were analyzed.

(7), and thereby obtain increased levels of expression from cotransferred
genes.

CONCLUSIONS

We have been able to engineer substantially shortened <u>dhfr</u> genes
which are still functional in animal cells. The methods used for the
minigene construction should be applicable to a wide variety of genes.
The <u>dhfr</u> minigenes can be amplified to high copy number and enzyme
levels by selection with MTX; the <u>dhfr</u> amplification is accompanied by
amplification of the flanking sequences.

ACKNOWLEDGEMENTS

Research sponsored by the National Cancer Institute, DHHS, under
Contract No. NO1-CO-75380 with Litton Bionetics, Inc. The contents of
this publication do not necessarily reflect the view or policies of the
Department of Health and Human Services, nor does mention of trade names,
commercial products, or organizations imply endorsement by the U.S. Government.

REFERENCES

1. Alt FW, Kellems RE, Bertino JR, Schimke RT (1978): J Biol Chem 253:
    1357

2. Carroll D, Ajioka RS, Georgopoulos C (1980): Gene 10:261
3. Crouse GF, Simonsen CC, McEwan RN, Schimke RT (1982): J Biol Chem 257:7887
4. Haber DA, Beverley SM, Kiely ML, Schimke RT (1981): J Biol Chem 256:9501
5. Kafatos FC, Jones CW, Efstratiadis A (1979): Nucleic Acids Res 7:1541
6. Urlaub G, Chasin LA (1980): Proc Natl Acad Sci USA 77:4216
7. Wigler M, Perucho M, Kurtz D, Dana S, Pellicer A, Axel R, Silverstein S (1980): Proc Natl Acad Sci USA 77:3567

Subject Index

A

abl gene, 180
Acute transforming virus(es)
  from chemically transformed cells, 170–171,220–225
  gene analogs of, in human tumors, 197–203
  interspecies transmission of, 164–166
  phosphotyrosine levels in, 173–175
  as replication defective, 169,171
  as retroviruses, 163–165,169–177,207
  type C RNA helper viruses and, 163,169–175,179,197
Adenosine phosphoribosyl transferase *(aprt)* gene, 271
Adenoviruses
  in cell transformation, 237–246,351
  as gene vectors, 81,135–140
  in transcription promotion, 135–140,352–354
Alcohol dehydrogenase *(adh)* gene
  cloned mutant strains of, 346–349
  promoter regions of, 345–349
  transcription of, 345–346
α-Amanitin resistance
  creatine kinase activity and, 75–78
  DNA-mediated gene transfer of, 67–71,73–79
  myogenesis defect development and, 73–79
  RNA polymerase II effect in, 67–71,73–79
  stability of, 74–75
  temperature sensitivity of, 67–71
Amplicons (HSV derived); *see also* Defective viral genomes
  characterized, 105
  designation system for, 108
  DNA introduction and transfer via, 105–113
  replicative functions of, 107–109
  sequence arrangements in, 106
Antibiotic resistance markers, 15–18
Antigens
  class I, 337–338
  generic loci for MHC, 337
  transplant tolerance and, 343
Asparagine synthetase gene
  albizziin (Alb) in drug resistant mutant selection for, 59–65
  β-aspartyl-hydroxamate in drug resistant mutant selection for, 59–65
  gene amplification in mutant selection for, 59–65
Avian leukosis virus (ALV), neoplastic induction mechanism of, 207–215

Avian sarcoma virus (AVS)
  Fujinal strain, 179,180
  long-term repeat sequence of, 153
  PRC-II strain, 179
  in transformed mouse cell phenotype analysis, 227–234
5-Azacytidine, in gene expression activation, 265–271,273–275,278,291
5-Azacytosine, 273,276

B

B-cell lymphoma
  avian leukosis virus induced, 207–210
  promoter insertion in, 212
B-lymphocyte neoplasms, 219,222,225
Baboon enodgenous virus, transcription control element in, 153
Bacteriophage lambda, 90
bas gene, 197,214
BK virus, enhancer sequence in, 326
Blebs, in genetic transformation competence, 9–12
Bovine papilloma virus (BPV)
  characteristics of, 126
  as cloning vector, 81–88,126,297
  human papilloma virus sequence compared with, 130,131
  transcriptional enhancer sequences in, 326
  transformation efficiency of, 81–83
Burkitt's lymphoma, chromosomal abnormalities in, 202–203,215

C

Cell transformation; *see also* Gene tranfer; Malignant transformation; Oncogenesis
  amplicons in, 105–113
  antibiotic resistance transfer via, 15–18,53–56
  cellular vs. viral genes in, 219–220
  chemical carcinogens in, 169–177,219–225
  defective viral genomes in, 105–113,207
  dihydrofolate reductase *(dhfr)* gene in, 351–359
  early transcription region in, 135–140
  efficiency of DNA fragment insertions in increasing, 31–35,48–50,81,86,89,193–194,297
  glucocorticoid hormone effects on, 297–301,303–308
  high-molecular-weight DNA in efficiency of, 220,222

Cell transformation *(contd.)*
   homologous recombination in, 43–44,47–51
   human *beta*-globulin DNA in, 81,86
   human chromosomes in, 214
   in human malignancies, 198,202–203,212–
      215
   indirect activation of, by lymphoid leukosis
      viruses, 220
   integration in, 135
   large tumor antigen encoding in, 41–43
   long-term repeats in, 219–225,297–301,
      331–335
   methylation and, 274
   neoplastic gene identification in, 111–113,
      208,220,219–225
   plasmid digestion in, 32–33
   procaryotic sequences in, 81
   restriction endonucleases in, 32–35,220–221
   retroviruses in, *see* Retroviruses
   simian virus-40 in, 31–35,47,125–131,227–
      234
   specificity of gene activation in, 220–221
   tandem repeat sequences in, 37–44
   thymidine kinase *(tk)* gene in, *see*
      Thymidine kinase *(tk)* gene
   tumor antigens in, 38,41–43,115–116
Chemical carcinogens
   activated transforming genes and, 169–177,
      219–225
   DNA methylation and, 274,277–278
   enzymatic DNA modification by, 273–278
   phenotype expression analysis via, 227–234
   tumor-inducing virus derivation via, 169–
      171
Chicken syncytial virus (CSV), 163–165
Chloramphenicol acetyltransferase *(cat)* gene,
   325,327
Chloramphenicol resistance marker, 16
Chromatin, DNase sensitivity and, 255,
   289,292
Chromosome folding, 317
Chromosome mapping, of human oncogenes,
   197–203
Chromosome transfer/translocation
   in Chinese hamster cells, 21–28
   in *emt* gene expression, 268–269
   in gene mapping, 27–28
   by Ig genes, 202–203,215
   microcell hybridization in, 21–22,268
   in monochromosomal marker detection, 21–
      28
   in oncogene activation, 198
CI-3 virus, 170–171,176
Class I antigens
   amino acid structure of, 337,338
   characteristics of, 337–338
   membrane specificity among, 337,342–343
   single vs. multiple RNA coding of, 342
Colchicine resistance
   chemotherapy and, 53,56
   DNA-mediated gene transfer of, 53,54,55
   glycoprotein expression and, 53,55–56
   multiple drug resistance and, 53–56
Condyloma acuminata, 126
Creatine kinase activity, 73–78
Cytosine, 273–278

D
Defective viral genomes (Herpes simplex
      derived)
   amplicons for amplifying and cloning in,
      105–113; *see also* Amplicons
   chimeric DNA sequences cloned into, 106–
      109
   cis replication function sequences required
      in, 106–109
   deletion of chimeric sequences from
      transfected, 109–111
   eucaryotic DNA insertions into, 109–112
   viral gene expresion by, 111–113
Dihydrofolate reductase *(dhfr)* gene
   amplification and regulation of, 351–359
   in CHO cell transformation, 351–359
   coding sequences of, 352–353,358,362–366
   copy DNA cloning for, 362
   DHFR enzyme coded by, 351,361
   expression efficiency of, 355
   methotrexate amplification of, 361,363–
      364,366
   minigene construction for, 361,366
   in modular gene construction, 351–359
   size of, as complication, 361
Dimethylsulfoxide (DMSO), 23,54
DNA
   chromosomal site integration of, 290,293
   gene transfer mediation by, *see* Gene
      transfer
   repetitive sequence organization in, *see*
      DNA sequence organization
   transforming potential of high molecular
      weight, 219–225,290
   transcriptional onset sequences, *see* Early
      transcriptional promoter sequences;
      Transcriptional enhancer elements;
      Transcriptional promoter
DNA-adenine methylase activity
   in *Mu mom* gene modification, 281–286
   site specificity of, 284
DNA methylation, *see* Methylation
DNA-protein interactions, 237–238,274–276
DNA sequence organization
   in defective genomes (HSV), 105–113
   Drosophila type, 316
   eucaryotic, 81,111–113,315–322
   functional repetition models for, 317
   in gene expression, 237–238,249–250,252–
      257,262,291,293,316,334–335
   heterologous, 90,95

length of sequences in, 315–322; *see also*
    Long-term repeats
mapping of, *see* Gene mapping
multiple copies in, 315–316
nonrepetitive sequences in, 315,316,320,321
repetitive, in mammals, 315–322
short period interspersions in, 316,321–322
variability in, as experimental artifact,
    316,319–321,322
Xenopus pattern of, 316
DNA uptake
    active transport and, 290
    in bacterial gene transformation, 1–6,9–12
    cell-surface vesicles in, 10–12
    flanking nucleotide effects on, 1–6
    foreign gene expression and, 290
    recognition site determination in, 1–6
DNase I, 255,299
Drug resistance
    in asparagine synthetase gene transfer, 63–
        65
    in cloned-mutant cell selection, 60–61
    colchicine resistant mutants as, 53–56
    DNA-mediated transfer of, 53–56
    gene amplification and, 60
    glycoprotein expression and, 53–56
    membrane permeability and, 53–56
Duck infectious anemia virus (DIAV), 163

E

Early transcriptional promoter sequences; *see
    also* Transcriptional enhancer elements
    in polyoma tranformed cells, 116
    in polyoma virus DNA, 115–122
    tumor-antigen binding relative to, 115,
        116,119
Early transcriptional region
    in human adenovirus 5 DNA, 135–140
    localization of, 135–136
    mutant-induced defective transformant types
        of, 135–140
    polypeptide coding by, 136
Emetine, sensitivity to, as gene marker, 265–
    266
Emetine responsive *(emt)* genes
    chromosone transfer in expression of, 268–
        269
    inactivation and reactivation of, 265–271
Endogenous virus-1 (EV-1), 152,153
Enhancer sequences, *see* Transcriptional
    enhancer elements
Envelope *(env)* gene, 165
Epidermodysplasia verruciformis, 126

F

Feline leukemia virus (FeLV), 179
Feline sarcoma virus (FeSV), 179–186
fes gene, sequential analysis and comparison
    of, 179–186

fps gene, sequential analysis and comparison
    of, 179–186
Friend spleen focus-forming virus (SFFV)
    long-term repeat of, 144,145,152
    malignancy of, 90
    sequential structure of, 91,148
    as *tk* gene transfer vector, 89–96

G

gag gene, 165,171
Gene amplification; *see also* Gene expression
    in asparagine synthetase gene cloning, 60
    dihydrofolate reductase cDNA and, 351–353
    drug resistance and, 60–62
    homogeneously staining region in, 59,60
    membrane glycoprotein expression and, 53–56
    tk gene reverse hypermethylation and, 255
Gene expression
    activation of, as host dependent, 325–329
    by cellular oncogenes, 208; *see also*
        Oncogenes
    chloramphenicol acetyltransferase as
        indicator of, 327
    chromatin structure and, 250,255,259,289–
        294
    in defective genome repeat units, 111
    dihydrofolate reductase cDNA and, 352
    DNA methylation and, 237–246,250–256,
        259–264,273–274,291–292
    DNA sequencing organization in, 237–238,
        249–250,252–257,262,291,293,
        316–317,334–335
    glucocorticoid hormones and, 297–301
    heterozygosity and detection of, 265
    inactivation and reactivation of, 255–256,
        265–271
    integration sites and, 293
    quantitative assay for, 327
    repetitive DNA sequence activation of, 325
    by retroviruses, 157,214,257
    RNA polymerase activity and, 67,73–79,
        325,327
    segregation mechanisms in *emt*, 267–268
    by *tk* genes, 256–257,289–294
    transcription enhancer effects on, 121–
        122,303–308,331–335
    transcriptional level modulation of, 289–294
    variability of, and gene regulation,
        237,249,259
Gene mapping; *see also* DNA sequence
    organization
    of *adh* gene in *Drosophila*, 345–349
    chromosome transfer in, 27–28
    of *Haemophilus* recognition sites, 1–6,9
    of Herpes simplex virus-*tk* gene, 47–51, 97–
        102,256–257,289–291
    of human papilloma virus, 125–131
    of long-term repeat sequences, *see* Long-
        term repeats

Gene mapping *(contd.)*
  of major histocompatability complex
    (MHC), 337
  of mouse mammary tumor virus sequences,
    297–301,304–306
  microcell hybridization in, 21–22,27–28
  polyoma virus early promoter sequences,
    116–119,121
  of retroviruses, 143–147
  sequential loss of selectable markers in, 27–
    28
Gene transfer
  of *alpha*-amanitin resistance, 67–71,73–79
  cell surface blebs in competence for, 9–12
  of drug resistance capability, 53–56
  chromosome mediated, 21–28; *see also*
    Chromosome transfer/translocation
  competence for, in *Haemophilus*
    transformation, 1–6,9–12,15–18
  via defective genomes/amplicons, 105–113
  direct vs. indirect methods, 1–2,289–290
  DNA-calcium phosphate precipitation in,
    31,63,67,289,290,332
  DNA uptake and incorporation in, 1–6,9,
    12,22,63–65,67–71,293
  drug resistance in, 15–18,53–56,59–65
  gene amplification in, 60,62–63
  gene expression and, 237,249,289,351
  of glycoprotein expression, 53–56
  homologous DNA recombination in, 15–
    18,37,43–44,47–51
  interspecies retroviral, 164–165
  long-term repeats in efficiency of, 152–
    153,208–210,287–301,331–335
  microcell hybridization in, 21–28,268
  from normal vs. malignant cells, 219–220
  phenotypic instability and, 74–75
  plasmid-chromosomal, 15–18,37–44,47–
    51,97,163–166
  polyethylene glycol-mediated phage method
    in, 332
  RNA polymerase activity in, 67–71,73–79,
    115,329,335
  selectable marker transfer by, 22
  specific transforming gene activation in,
    220–221
  tandemly arranged plasmid sequences in,
    37–44
  temperature sensitivity transmission in, 67–
    71
  transcriptional enhancement in, 331–335
  tumor antigen in, 38,40–42
Gibbon ape leukemia viruses (GALVs), 143–
  145
gin gene, 281
α-Globin DNA, 97,101–102,251
β-Globin DNA
  DNase I hypersensitive, 154
  duplication of, 154

  in transforming efficiency, 81,86
Glucocorticoid hormones
  in DNA transcription enhancement, 303–
    308
  in gene expresion regulation, 297–301
Glycoprotein expression
  in defective genome repeat units, 111
  DNA-mediated gene transfer of, 53–56
  mammary tumor virus genes and, 221,303–
    308
  multidrug resistance and, 53–56
gpt gene, 31–35
Guanine residue, carcinogens and, 274

H
H-2 antigen
  genetic loci coding for, 337
  H-2 related, cloned, nonclassical gene
    compared with, 338–340,342–343
  nucleotide structure of, 338–339
  physiological role of, 343
H-2-related gene
  classical type H-2 antigen compared with,
    338–340,342–343
  immune function aspects inticated for,
    337,343
  liver tissue specificity of, 337,342,343
  nucleotide sequence characteristics of, 337–
    339
  transmembrane domain distinctiveness of,
    338–339
Harvey murine sarcoma virus (HaMuSV)
  90,165,189–194,297–301
Helper virus DNA, in replication-defective
  gene generation, 105–113; *see also* Type
  C viruses
Herpes simplex virus-thymidine kinase (HSV-
  tk) gene, *see* Thymidine kinase *(tk)* gene
Heterologous sequences, 90,95
Homogeneously staining region, gene
  amplification and, 60,62
Homologous recombination
  in eucaryotic somatic cells, 47
  in polyoma viral DNA transfected
    mammlian cells, 43–44
  in thymidine kinase gene defective cell
    reconstruction, 47–51
Human chorionic gonadotropin subunit alpha,
  111
Human chromosomes
  cell transformation by, 214
  translocations of, in human malignancies,
    202–203
  tumor virus transforming gene location in,
    197–203
Human lung carcinoma DNA, 179–186
Human papilloma virus (HPV)
  in cell cultures, 125
  cloning of, 125–126

genetic mapping of, 126–131
origin site determination for, 131
wart types produced by variants of, 126
Hypermethylation, in *tk* gene inactivation,
249–257,262,293; *see also* Methylation
Hypoxanthine quanine phosphoribosyl
transferase *(hprt)* gene, 21–28,311–313

I

Immunoglobulin (Ig) genes
chromosomal location and translocation,
202–203,215
lymphoid neoplasms and abnormal, 215
Immunological tolerance, 342
Infected cell polypeptide (ICP), 111
Integration, in cell transformation, 135
Isozyme expression, 26–27

J

Juvenile laryngeal papillomatosis, 126

K

Kirsten sarcoma virus, 165,189–194

L

Large T-antigen, 41–43,115–116,122; *see also*
Tumor antigen
Leukemia viruses, *see specific types*
Long-term repeats (LTR)
DNase hypersensitivity in, 154,155
duplication function of, 153,154
gene-transfer efficiency of, 331–335
glucocorticoid regulation of transcription in,
300–301
hairpin sequences in, 148–152
in mammalian DNA, 143–155,315–322
in mouse mammary-tumor virus, 297–301
oncogenes in relation to viral, 212
in retroviruses, 143–155,325–329; *see also*
specific types
sequences of murine and gibbon retrovirus
compared, 143–155
tandem repeat sequences and, *see* Tandem
repeat sequences
tk gene transfer efficiency and, 331–335
transcription initiation function of, 148,
152,154–155,208–210,297–301,326,
331–335
vector construction for study of, 332–333
Lymphocytes
gene regulation in, 249,255–257
methylation of, 255–257
Lymphoid leukosis viruses (LLV), 220

M

Macaque viruses, 164
Major histocompatability complex (HMC),
337–338
Malignant transformation

in vitro, *see* Cell transformation
in vivo, *see* Oncogenesis; Tumorigenicity
Mammary tumor(s)
glycoprotein antigen in, 221
transforming gene activation in, 220–221
Mammary tumor virus genes, 303–308
Metallothionein gene, 259,273
Methylation
cell transformation and, 274
chemical carcinogens and, 274,277–278
gene activity modulation by, 237–246,249–
256,259–264,265–271,273–278,281–
286
heritability of, 256,274,278
inhibition of, 259,277–278
in lymphocytes, 255–257
maintenance of, 273–278
site specificity of, 238–241,276–277,284
tissue specificity of, 274
X chromosome inactivation by, 311–313
5-Methylcytosine, 244,274,275,278
Methyltransferase
in adenovirus infected human cells, 244–
246
inhibition of, 276–278
preparation and extraction of, 274–276
Microcell(s)
characteristics of, 22
cytological analysis of hybrid, 24–28
preparation of, 23–24
Microcell fusion/hybridization
chromosome transfer by, 21–28
gene mapping and, 21–22,27–28
gene transfer in, 21–28,268
micronucleation in, 23–24
selectable marker transfer in, 22,268
Moloney murine leukemia virus (MoMuLV),
143,171
infectivity change in, with methylation, 160
long-term repeat characteristics of,
144,153,331–335
Moloney murine sarcoma virus (MoMuSV),
143,325
in human chromosome mapping, 200–203
long-term repeat characteristics of,
144,148,152–153
mom gene, 281–286
mos gene, 197,202–203
Mouse mammary tumor virus–long term
repeat (MMTV-LTR)
in cell-transforming gene activation, 219–
225,297–301
in glucocorticoid regulated transcription,
297–301
hypomethylation and expression by, 273
sequencing of, 153,297–301
mtx gene, 266
Murine leukemia virus(es) (MuLV); *see also*
specific types

Murine leukemia virus(es) (MuLV) *(contd.)*
  infectivity of DNA transfected via embryo
    culture, 157–161,220
  long-term repeat characteristics of, 144,
    149–152,153
Murine sarcoma virus(es) (MuSV); *see also*
    specific types
  Abelson strain, 180
  as acute transforming viruses, 169–177
  isolation of, 169
  oncogenic characteristics, of 3611 strain,
    169,172,175
  replication defectiveness, of 3611 strain,
    169,171
myb gene, 197
myc gene, 165,197
  avian leukosis virus induction of, 207–215
  malignant transformation induction by, 207–
    215
  promoter insertion activation of, 212
Myoblasts, 75–77
Myogenesis, defective via drug resistant-RNA
    polymerase mutation, 73–79

N
Novobiocin resistance marker, plasmid transfer
    of, 16–18
Nuclease-resistant complex, in cell surface
    vesicle binding, 12

O
Oncogenes; *see also specific genes*
  in B-lymphocyte neoplasms, 222–225
  as cellular, 208
  chemical carcinogens and, 170,220–221
  chromosomal mapping of, 197–203
  detection of transmissable, 219–225
  differential expression of, 208
  indirect activation of, 220
  malignancy potential of cellular, 208
  methylation of, 237–246,259–264,274
  potentialities of human *ras* genes as, 189–
    194
  promoter insertion enhancement of, 207–
    215
  sequential differential activation of cellular,
    219–221
  in T-lymphocyte neoplasms, 219,222–225
Oncogenesis; *see also* Cell transformation;
    Tumorigenicity
  chromosomal location and translocation of
    oncogenes in, 197–203
  DNA methylation and, 274
  gene amplification and, 212,215
  inappropriate cell differentiation and, 274
  interspecies DNA mediated gene transfer
    and, 164–165
  promoter insertion enhancement of,
    198,207–215

viral oncogenes in induction of, 38,90,164–
    166,173,198,207–208,214,220

P
Papilloma viruses
  bovine, *see* Bovine papilloma virus
  characteristics of, 125–126
  classification of, 125
  human, *see* Human papilloma virus
  propagation of, 125
Papovaviruses, 125,326
Phosphoserine, 173
Phosphothreonine, 173
Phosphotyrosine, 173–175,208
pol gene, 165
Polyadenylation signals, 148,152,351–359
Polyoma virus
  characteristics of, 37–38,125
  deletion mutations in mapping, 116–119
  early transcription promoter in, 115–122
  homologous recombination after mammalian
    transfection with, 37,43–44
  lytic sequences in infection by, 115–116
  non-replicating cell transformation by, 116
  replication vs. transforming effects of
    recombinant, 38–42
  tumor antigen encoding and binding by,
    38,40,43,115–116,120–121
  tumorigenicity of, 38
Promoter, *see* Transcriptional promoter
Promoter activation hypothesis, 212
Protein kinase activity, tyrosine specific
  in acutely transformed virus gene
    sequences, 173–175
  oncogenic sequences in human encoding of,
    179–186
  in retrovirus transformed cells, 173
  virus polyprotein gene products and,
    179,208
Proviruses
  characterized, 143
  DNA sequences of retroviral integrated,
    143–155
  transcription promoter insertion and, 208–
    210,212

R
ras gene, 189–194,214,297
Rasheed rat sarcoma virus, 165
Rauscher murine leukemia virus (RMuLV),
    long-term repeat of, 143,144
Recognition sequences, in DNA
    transformation, 1–6
rel gene, 163,165
Repetitive DNA sequences; *see also* DNA
    sequence organization; Long-term
    repeats; Tandem repeat sequences
  characteristics of, 315–316
  in gene expression, 325

models of, illustrated, 317
traditional measurement of, queried, 315–322
Restriction endonuclease(s)
  B- and T-lymphocyte responses to, 222–225
  in cell transformation frequency, 32–35
  cloning from human normal DNA, 189
  in polyoma mapping, 118
  in retrovirus long-term repeat sites, 153
  transforming gene differentiation by, 220–221,225
Reticuloendotheliosis virus (REV)
  avian affinities of, 163–164
  core DNA sequence and mammalian affinities of, 163–164
  horizontal (interspecies) transmission of, and oncogenesis, 163–166
  strain A, as helper viral DNA, 98,100
Retroviruses; see also specific types
  as acute transforming viruses, 163–165,169–177,197,207
  DNAse hypersensitivity site in, 154,155
  duplication in long-term repeats of, 153,154
  expression diversity of endogenous, 157
  as gene vectors, 81,89,90,97–102,157–161
  hairpin inversion sequences in, 148–155
  methylation and gene inactivation in, 256
  neoplastic transformation by, 90,164–166, 173,207,214,220
  protein kinase activity and, 173
  proviruses in, 143–145,152
  replication defective, 169,171
  RNA genome in, 143–144
  transcription initiation by, see Long-term repeats; Transcriptional promoter
Reverse transcriptase gene, 165
RNA polymerase activity
  α-amanitin resistance mutation and, 67–71
  DNA mediated gene transfer and, 67–71, 73–79,115,329,335
  gene expression and, 67,73–79,325,327
  myogenic defects and, 73–79
  in polyoma early region transcription, 115
  second site suppressor effects of, 67
  temperature-sensitive effects of, 67–71
ros gene, 180
Rous associated virus-2, 152,153
Rous sarcoma virus, 208

S
Sarcoma virus(es)
  avian, see Avian sarcoma virus
  feline (FeSV), 179–186
  Harvey, 90,165
  Kirsten, 165
  Rasheed rat, 165
  simian, 197
  wooly monkey, 165
Shuttle vectors, 125,126

Simian virus-40 (SV-40)
  classification of, 125
  in DNA methylation and gene inactivation, 241
  as gene vector, 31–35,47,81,82,125–131, 227–234,351–352,355
  host specificity in tandem repeat activity of, 325–329
  long-term repeat in viability of, 154
  tandem repeat sequences in, 325–329
  transcription enhancement sequences in, 122,154,212,351
sis gene, 197,199–200
Spleen necrosis virus (SNV)
  avian, 90,163
  long-term repeat sequence of, 153
  as tk gene cloning vector, 97–102
src gene, 208

T
T-antigen, see Tumor antigen
T-lymphocyte neoplasms, 219,222–225
Tandem repeat sequences
  in cell transformation, 41–43
  host specificity of, 326–327
  in recombinant plasmid molecules, 15–18,37–44
  in simian virus-40, 325–329
  in transcriptional enhancement, 326
TATA box sites, 122,148,152,325
Temperature sensitive mutations, 67–71,207
Terminal inversion sequences, 152
Thymidine kinase (tk) gene (HSV)
  cellular enhancer sequences in expression of, 326,331–335
  in Chinese hamster ovary transformation, 31–35
  cluster arrangements of, 251–252,255
  DNase I sensitivity of, 292
  expression variability and integration site for, 256–257
  glucocorticoid regulation of transcription and, 303–308
  homologous recombination of, in mouse L cells, 47–51
  in lambda phage vector construction, 47–51,332–333
  hypermethylation vs. methylation of, 253–254
  hypermethylation in transformed cells, 249–257,262,293
  inactivation of, by methylation, 237–246, 249–257,259–264,293
  in long-term repeat effects on gene transfer, 331–334
  transfer of, via viral vectors, 41–51,85–96, 97–98,289–294,332–333
Topoisomerase activity site, 329

Transcriptional enhancer elements; *see also*
    Early transcriptional promoter sequences;
    Early transcriptional region;
    Transcriptional promoter
  in BK virus, 326
  in BP virus, 326
  characteristics of, 115–122,303–304,326,
    329
  gene expression responses to, 121,122,331–
    335
  glucocorticoid hormone effects on, 297–
    301,303–308
  glucocorticoid receptor binding and, 307–
    308
  in papovaviruses, 326
  polymerase binding site and, 329
  in retrovirus long-term repeats, 326,331–
    335
  in simian virus-40, 212,325–326,351–352
  tandem repeat sequences as, 326
  transcriptional promoters compared with,
    212–213,297,298,303–304,329
Transcriptional promoter; *see also*
    Transcriptional enhancer elements
  of adenoviruses, 351–352
  in B-cell lymphomas, insertion of, 212
  in cellular oncogene enhancement, 198,207–
    215
  in *Drosophila adh* gene, 345–349
  methylation of, 241–242
  in polyoma virus, 115–122
  in polyoma transformed cells, 116
  in retrovirus long-term repeats, 148,152–
    155,334
Transformed phenotype, genetic analysis of,
    227–234
Transgenome, 21–23
Tumor antigen (T-antigen)
  binding sites of, in polyoma virus, 120–122
  duplication of, in SV-40 long-term repeats,
    154
  early promoter and, in polyoma virus DNA,
    115–122
  enhancer sequences and expression of, 326–
    327
  in gene transcription inhibition, in polyoma,
    116
  in polyoma viral DNA replication, 40–43,
    115–116,122

Tumor viruses; *see also specific types*
  acute transforming, in human tumors, 197–
    203
  transformation integration in mammalian
    cells vs., 135
Tumorigenicity; *see also* Cell transformation;
    Oncogenesis
  glycoprotein antigen and, 221
  human papilloma viruses and, 126
  polyoma virus and, in rodent cells, 38
  transforming gene activation and, 220–221
Type C virus
  acute transforming viruses and, 169–175,
    179,197
  cellular oncogenes and, 179,197
  in chimeric defective gene activation, 106–
    111

U
Uptake sites, in *Haemophilus* transformation,
    1–6; *see also* DNA uptake

V
Vesicles, cell surface, in DNA interactions,
    10–12
Viral DNA; *see also* DNA sequence
    organization; Long-term repeats; *specific
    viruses*
  in defective genomes, 111–113
  early transcription region in, 135–140
  in gene expression activation, 255–257,265–
    271,289–294,325
  methylation in activation of, 242–244,
    259,273
  replication of, 38,40

W
Warts
  development of, 125
  human papilloma virus types and, 125–126;
    see also Human papilloma virus (HPV)
  varieties of, 126
Woolly monkey sarcoma virus, 165

X
X chromosome, methylation and inactivation
    of, 256,311–313
XGPRT (xanthine guanine phosphoribosyl
    transferase), 28

THE LIBRARY
UNIVERSITY OF CALIFORNIA
San Francisco
666-2334

THIS BOOK IS DUE ON THE LAST DATE STAMPER BELOW
Books not returned on time are subject to fines according to the Library
Lending Code. A renewal may be made on certain materials. For details
consult Lending Code.

14 DAY JAN 3 1 1985 RETURNED JAN 3 1 1985	14 DAY APR 1 2 1985 RETURNED APR 1 2 1985	
14 DAY FEB 2 2 1985 RETURNED MAR - 1 1985	14 DAY OCT 2 2 1986 RETURNED OCT 2 2 1986	
14 DAY MAR 2 1 1985 RETURNED MAR 2 2 1985		

Series 4128